Living with Cancer:
A Journey

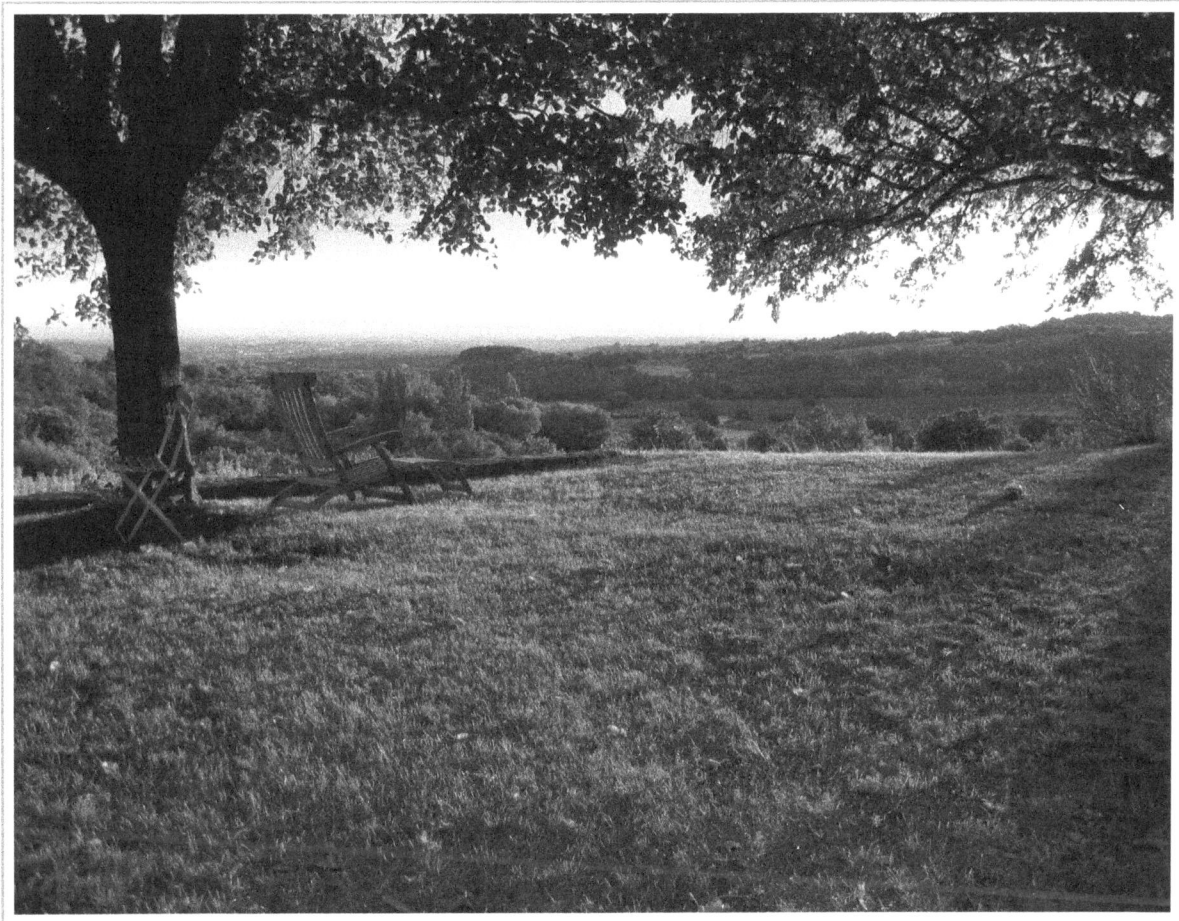

Andrew Griffith

Published by Anar Press

Library and Archives Canada Cataloguing in Publication (for electronic editions)

Griffith, Andrew

Living with cancer [electronic resource] : a journey / Andrew Griffith.

Electronic monograph.
ISBN 978-0-9880640-3-4

1. Griffith, Andrew--Health. 2. Cancer--Patients--Canada--Biography.
I. Title.

RC265.6.G75A3 2012   362.196'9940092   C2012-906187-5

Dedication

To Nazanine, Alex and Roxanne, who supported and continue to support me throughout this journey, and who make life worth living.

To other family and friends who also supported and continue to support me.

Lastly, to my medical team at the Ottawa Hospital - General Campus, Blood and Marrow Transplant Clinic, who epitomized both professionalism and grace, and showed patience with my many questions and concerns.

50 percent of author proceeds will go to The Ottawa Hospital Foundation as a small gesture of thanks.

TABLE OF CONTENTS

The Home Stretch

Preface

Ring the bells that still can ring

Forget your perfect offering

There is a crack, a crack in everything

That's how the light gets in.

Leonard Cohen, from *Anthem*

This book came about as a sharing and coping mechanism following my diagnosis with mantle cell lymphoma (MCL) in June 2009, and my subsequent treatment (intense chemotherapy and an autologous stem cell transplant (SCT), remission, relapse and finally, an allogeneic stem cell transplant in August 2011.

Sharing helped, as I realized more and more that while the lymphoma was 'mine,' my being sick affected family, friends and colleagues. It was not just about me as an individual, but rather about the group of people close to me. Given my need for their support, my mind turned to what kind of support they in turn needed from me. All felt concerned, some felt awkward; some had experience with cancer, some did not.

To encourage their support, I started with a personal journal and weekly updates to friends and colleagues. This progressed to a weekly blog, and then to a more fulsome site with reflection pieces and commentary on health-related issues. As my comfort level with sharing increased, and successive rounds of treatment prompted further reflection, the nature and tone of my posts deepened.

I also shared some of my experience and 'lessons' through other websites, primarily Cancerwise and KevinMD.

As my blog developed, the idea of putting the key elements together in book form – the treatment and recovery 'journey,' the reflection pieces – came to mind. This book about my journey to the edge of death and back (to be melodramatic about it) is the result.

I hope that sharing my journey will help others, whatever their connection to cancer, reflect on how to provide support to those who need it, including their families. I also hope that my journey provides you with an enhanced appreciation of the fragility of life, and the need to live life fully, with compassion, empathy and purpose.

Andrew, August 2012

For updates, check my blog: My Lymphoma Journey or Twitter @LymphomaJourney

Introduction

This book can be read at different levels, depending on whether you have cancer, someone close to you has cancer, you have an interest in the 'what if' scenario (should you be so unlucky), or you are a healthcare professional interested in a patient's experience and reflections on a cancer journey.

My assumption, first in my blog and now here, is that most readers will likely have personal or professional experience with cancer, specifically blood cancers. At the same time, we are not just defined by our 'cancer identity.' We are alive, and have our own histories, beliefs, interests and pastimes. I have shared many of my own interests, primarily by recording the books I read and films I watched. This was partly to ensure that cancer did not 'metastasize my mind,' to use Mark Dery's memorable phrase, and partly to reinforce the need to remain as active and engaged as possible in broader life.

Cancer, like all serious diseases, starts with suffering. Cancer is not a 'blessing,' and it is, to turn around Robert Buckman's book title, a 'sentence, not a word'. For those of us with cancer, we suffer emotionally as we wait for the diagnosis. We suffer physically through the 'torture' of treatment. We continue to suffer emotionally from a worry in the back of our minds that never quite goes away.

One of the underlying themes throughout this book is the role that we all can play in easing suffering, whether that of the person with cancer or that of those close to him or her. Beyond these individual connections to cancer, there is also our communal responsibility to address the widespread nature of cancer in today's world.

Throughout our individual and collective journeys, we seek meaning, and seek to create meaning. As Stanley Kubrick said:

> *The most terrifying fact about the universe is not that it is hostile but that it is*
> *indifferent; but if we can come to terms with this indifference and accept the challenges of*
> *life within the boundaries of death — however mutable man may be able to make them*
> *— our existence as a species can have genuine meaning and fulfillment. However vast*
> *the darkness, we must supply our own light.*

Cancer, in its darkness, provides the impetus to create our own light; to help ourselves and others hopefully get through it all, with our humanity enhanced and a renewed sense of purpose.

Throughout this book, I touch on the following elements of my journey:

- Physical and medical – what my treatment was and what is was doing to me;

- Psychological and emotional – an aspect that became more intense over time;

- Relationships – and how the important ones developed and strengthened.

For readers wondering whether they might prefer to 'dip into' different sections or do a more thorough reading, the following may help.

While a diagnosis of cancer starts off all the 'what if' scenarios and worries, once the diagnosis is known and treatment starts, one quickly focusses on the practical. Chapter 1 (Practical Tips) and Chapter 2 (Navigating Healthcare) aim to help people with cancer and their caregivers with some of the practical issues and questions that they may face. Chapter 3 (Support: A Compact) provides a broader picture of how people with cancer, and those close to them, can support each other through treatment and the journey.

Chapter 4 (The Journey Begins) and Chapter 5 (Transplant and Beyond) provide a week-by-week account of my initial treatment of high dose chemotherapy, and then an autologous stem cell transplant (which used my own cells). This section may be more pertinent to those undergoing comparable chemotherapy and transplant regimes, although my thoughts on the books I read and films I saw may be of interest to all.

Chapters 6 through 8 share my reflections during this period of time, refined through my subsequent experience with relapse and the allogeneic stem cell transplant. Specifically, I focus on how I was pulled, emotionally, in opposing directions (Dualities); some musings on the role played by Faith for someone secular like me; and some general Lessons on what this 'learning experience' means to me.

I then turn to what, in retrospect, was likely my darkest period – when my lymphoma relapsed – and the questioning and decision-making process about whether or not to proceed with an allogeneic stem cell transplant (SCT). My thoughts on being 'between a rock and a harder place' can be found in Chapter 9 (Relapse).

Chapters 10 through 14 (Transplant, Graft vs Host Disease, Recovery, Getting On, The Home Stretch) cover in depth my experience with the allogeneic stem cell transplant, the difficult early months and the slow recovery. Again, this section may be of most pertinent to those undergoing similar transplants (and their caregivers), though as with my initial treatment, some of my readings and viewings may be of interest to all.

I then turn back to reflecting further on what this all means to me and others on similar journeys in Chapter 15 (What We Call Ourselves) and Chapter 16 (Letting Go and Accepting). These focus on the themes of what we (as people living with cancer) call ourselves, and the question of how one knows when to 'fight,' and when to let go and accept one's fate. I then share some general closing thoughts in Chapter 17 (Living with Cancer).

While my focus is on my experience, my reflections, and how I have developed throughout my treatment, my hope is that by sharing these thoughts I will help others with similar 'journeys,' who can then, in their own way and their own circles, share their worries, fears, and hopes. Cancer can bring us together, and I think that all of us, with or without cancer, should take advantage of this opportunity to support each other and, in so doing, affirm the importance of life and living.

Note: This print edition includes all the hyperlinks from the original electronic edition which are not, of course, active in a print edition. These can either be searched directly on Google or through my blog, My Lymphoma Journey.

Chapter 1:

Practical Tips

While we worry about the bigger picture, we need to focus on the here and now of preparing for treatment: finding and understanding information, letting people know about our diagnosis, and organizing our medical file.

GETTING AND LIVING THROUGH CANCER

Over the past few years, I have done more than my share of navigating through the emotional and practical aspects of my treatment for mantle cell lymphoma, while in the back of my mind, the broader questions — Why me? How long will I live? — remain.

Some tips

Once I got over the initial anger and depression that followed my diagnosis (and my relapse), I found these practical tips and approaches helpful:

Be thankful for what you have

I am unlucky. I have an aggressive form of lymphoma that can be treated, not cured. However, though I am unlucky with cancer, I am lucky in the strong emotional and practical support of my wife, family and friends.

I also have a good benefits plan from work, so I have no financial worries. Furthermore, whenever I go to the hospital, I am reminded that there are people worse off than me.

Take it one step at a time

I could not process all the information and the whole treatment plan at the same time. I could not worry about whether the allogeneic SCT would work and whether I would get Graft versus Host Disease (GvHD) at the same time. The best advice I got from the medical team was to take it step by step.

Worry about the current stage, not the future. Dividing treatment into 'chewable chunks' allowed me to celebrate each milestone, like getting through each round of chemo and getting past the first month, and then first 100 days, post-transplant.

Don't get spooked by the stats

In my case, the stats are awful (overall, 50% to 60% mortality within one year of the allo SCT). But these are averages, and I am an individual.

I took the stats seriously. With the help of my medical team, however, I also placed the stats in the context of my age, general health and previous treatment, all of which improved my odds. Some doctors were better than others in walking me through this.

Research, but do not over-research

At the beginning, I spent far too much time trolling the web for medical information and patient experiences. After a while, I found my balance between enough information to be knowledgeable but not so much to become obsessive and worry even more.

I also found that a lot of information was dated, and it was better to focus on getting more recent information from my medical team.

Own your file

It was my life at stake, and I needed to manage my information and interactions with my medical team. I started a binder, organized by topic, and then switched to an iPad to take notes for my appointments.

I always came prepared with questions for my doctors and, because of my previous notes, was able to challenge them when treatment directions changed. My medical team knew me as an empowered and prepared patient, and it strengthened both our relationship and my understanding of the 'why' behind treatment decisions.

Of course, these practical suggestions need to be complemented by deeper reflection on what you want your life to be, during treatment and post-treatment. None of these tips make the journey easy or diminish the fact that cancer is a hard road to travel, but they all helped make it more manageable for my family and I.

FINDING GOOD INFORMATION

When I got a phone call with the diagnosis of mantle cell lymphoma, my instinct was to Google. Today, three years later, I have learned about what to look for, what to avoid, and how to manage my natural desire to know as much as possible.

Google – but wisely

Google (and Wikipedia) are a reflex. Do not fight it. However, when looking at suggested links, go for more reliable sources. These include any national cancer societies (e.g., American Cancer Society, Canadian Cancer Society) or health agency (e.g., National Cancer Institute), major cancer centre (e.g., MD Anderson and others), and any specific cancer organization (in my case, the Leukemia and Lymphoma Society, and LLS Canada).

Be forewarned that for more aggressive cancers, this will be frightening reading.

Ask your medical team

I did not do this at first, but soon learned the error of my ways. When I saw my first hematologist (specialist who treats blood cancer), he warned me that web information was out of date and breezily (almost too much so!), reassured me that better treatments were available. I did not press him, however, on which site he would recommend. Later, when a family member was undergoing what thankfully proved to be a false cancer scare, I did ask for recommendations–and was referred to the kind of sites I have suggested in the previous paragraph.

Complementary and alternative medicine (CAM) – there are no miracles

Invariably, you will find sites that promise alternative cancer treatments. Do not get sucked into what are false hopes at best and money grabs at worst. Respectful Insolence is a good 'debunking' site.

While I believe in complementary approaches to conventional treatments, these are the tried and true advice for everyone: avoid tobacco, eat well (e.g., reducing meat consumption; other nutrition advice here), and exercise.

Prayer, meditation, walking, and being with family and friends are also sound elements of a holistic approach.

Explore – within limits – community forums

There is a risk of losing yourself in these forums. However, they are incredibly powerful in that they connect you with people who have gone through the same treatment.

While I started late – because in some cases, it was depressing – I now ask forum members about side effects that I am not sure about, and give back to people who are at earlier stages by sharing my experience. Start with a forum that deals with your type of cancer first, as it is likely to include the largest number of people in your situation (for Canadians: the US forums are larger than those in Canada, so I tend to go with the former).

Some private cancer forums are also emerging, which can have good logging tools. However, on privacy grounds, I am more comfortable with charitable organizations.

Get efficient with Google Reader

I started off by checking individual sites, fora and blogs, which is inefficient. Use Google Reader (part of your Google account) and set up search terms to capture news stories, blogs and forum updates automatically. You can then scan them quickly and read those of interest.

Lastly, a note of humility. No matter how much you read and how informed you are, you will never have the knowledge and experience of your medical team. Your objectives might be to:

- understand your cancer and treatment better;

- be prepared to ask good questions;

- develop a comfort level in assessing different treatment options; and,

- be able to 'challenge' your medical team if appropriate (e.g., in my case, whether I needed to have more or fewer scans, a colonoscopy, etc. – small stuff in the big scheme of things, but it nevertheless made my journey more bearable).

LETTING PEOPLE KNOW

One of the hardest parts of a cancer diagnosis is telling others: family, friends and colleagues. I preferred a more open approach for a number of reasons:

- keeping everything inside was harder, and talking and writing were a form of release;

- people close to you need to know, to help them support you;

- letting people know avoids awkward questions, and is an invitation for support; and,

- I had previous experience with others who did not share, and their decision made it harder on me and others.

Looking back over the past three years, I can identify a number of steps that helped me talk to people.

Identify your circles

Who needs to know, after close family and friends? Do you have natural support groups (religious or other organizations)? What about colleagues at work – how wide should the net be?

Write out your script and be direct

I think better when I write things out. At work, in particular, a script helped me say what I wanted to and ensure that I did not forget anything important.

Apart from when you are dealing with small children, be direct and honest, and let people know how serious your cancer is. Most people respond better to openness, although it does take them time to get over the initial shock.

Practice on those closest (but it doesn't get easier)

When I was diagnosed, I first told my wife, then our kids, close family and friends, and finally, work colleagues. While my script became more 'automatic,' I was always uneasy when I spoke.

Each group is different and has its own challenges (my kids were the hardest to tell). I found that I just had to plough on, despite the difficulties. Telling people in person (or over the phone) rather than by e-mail was more effective and human.

Set up family 'conferences' as needed

While I never felt the need to do these weekly or monthly, I have held family meetings at various key moments. The hardest was just before my allogeneic SCT, when I had to remind my kids of the poor odds, but that I chose to take the risk to be with them longer (my script helped), and that I needed and counted on their support.

I had an easier meeting with my family after the 100-day mark, but even then I had to temper good news with ongoing longer-term uncertainty.

Tell your colleagues in an orderly manner

I managed a group of 100 people. I had to let them, my boss, and other colleagues know about the duration of my absence.

I informed my boss first, followed by my staff (my immediate staff, then my management team, and then at an all-staff meeting), and lastly other colleagues. I made sure that most people knew within the same week to ensure that office chatter was based on shared information.

Ongoing communications

I started a series of weekly e-mail updates to my colleagues (I generally kept in touch with family and friends by phone or with individual e-mails) to respond to their natural concerns. I then moved to a blog of weekly updates, this time with a broader audience of family and friends as well as colleagues.

After my relapse, I expanded the blog to include articles of interest to me. Through the blog, everyone was kept informed about the health-related questions without having to ask, so we were able to focus our e-mails, telephone calls, and walks on non-cancer, living-our-lives chats.

While each of us has our own comfort level (and initially I was more private myself), sharing reduces rumours and speculation, invites people to support you, and is one of the few areas under your control in the cancer-treatment journey.

The above steps helped me be more open about my journey, come to terms with what I was going through, and become closer to the people supporting me.

ORGANIZING YOUR MEDICAL FILE

Most of us find it challenging to make sense of the wave of information that hits us when we enter our cancer journey. The medical world is foreign territory, with its own language, culture and routines. It takes time to absorb and understand.

We are not oncologists or hematologists. However, we can learn to improve our discussions with our medical team.

Build your knowledge

By the time you start your treatment, you probably will have searched the web and read brochures on your cancer. Ask your medical team about which sites have reliable and up-to-date information to avoid old and possibly discouraging information on treatment outcomes.

While blogs and support fora help give a real-world view of the range of experiences, you are an individual, and too much thinking about what happens to others (good or bad) only increases worry. Moderation!

To save time, set up Google Reader for news sites, blogs and fora, and use the search function (general terms like 'cancer' or 'lymphoma') to narrow down articles of interest.

Keep a notepad

At each appointment, take notes. Even without chemo brain, the information you will be presented with is hard to master. Bring someone to your appointments, either as a listener or a scribe – or use a tape recorder if your doctors agree to it.

My wife played the listener role in my treatment, and that helped ensure that we both heard and understood the consequences the same way.

Start a binder

As you go through treatment, you will accumulate more and more paper. I started a binder, which I organized into these categories: contact info (first page!), treatment plan, test results, background information, and drug information.

The purpose of a binder is to have all the reference material in one place, to consult when necessary and to bring to hospital and clinic visits.

Be prepared

Prepare a list of questions for the medical team before your clinic check-ups (I found it harder during the daily hospital routine). My doctors are busy people. However, they always took the time to answer my questions. Had I not been prepared, appointments would have been limited to a brief summary of my condition.

Since treatment varies depending on the doctor, having detailed notes and questions helps track any changes. Given my clinic has a group practice, where a team of hematologists and doctors treat me, my experience with teams at work, helped me work with them. I questioned my team about changes (scan or not to scan, when to stop immunosuppressants). My intent was not to challenge their judgement, but to ensure that I understood their rationale for the change.

While every patient gets good care, an empowered patient becomes a partner in treatment. My medical team appreciated my proactivity, and it may have resulted in better care.

Go electronic

I started with a paper system. For my second round of treatment, I switched to an iPad (initially just a new toy). I made most frequent use of the following apps (equivalent options available for Android):

- Evernote for clinic notes and questions, as it kept everything easy to find;
- Numbers to track my blood counts;
- Withings to track my blood pressure and weight; and,
- Documents to Go for Word files such as my journal.

These were very effective for keeping me on top of my medical file along with my medical team – they became used to me being prepared!

Organization is one of the few areas of cancer treatment over which one has some control, and it strengthen one's the partnership with the medical team. It may not change the outcome, but it can increase your confidence in the treatment that you pursue.

Chapter 2:

Navigating Healthcare

We need to become experts on how the healthcare system works, how to influence and work better with our medical team, how to prepare for our hospital stay – and our return home – and how to help our recovery.

Overview – Navigating the Healthcare System

The healthcare system is a large, complex bureaucracy, with its own culture and way of doing things. Understanding how it works, and specifically how your medical team and the system work for you, makes things a lot easier. When undergoing treatment for any serious and/or chronic disease, you will likely have a complex, interdisciplinary team comprised of a variety of people, not just one doctor. This is a highly trained, talented and caring group who provide the best care possible while juggling a heavy caseload, and a number of these tips make it easier for them as well.

Since I work for the Canadian government, I had an advantage. I could recognize bureaucratic structures, approval levels and procedures, and develop strategies that helped move things along. The following points helped me help the system.

Second opinion

After one meets with a specialist, who recommends a treatment, the process kicks into high gear. As the specialists all work on a team basis, there is an element of consensus and second opinions built into the process. However, for peace of mind, I consulted with doctors in other jurisdictions to see if the proposed treatment made sense from their point of view. These consultations confirmed that I was getting the current 'state of the art' treatment, and put my mind – and the minds of my family members – at ease.

After my relapse, when I was faced with the higher stakes of an allogeneic SCT, we sought a formal second opinion from Toronto's Princess Margaret Hospital. This was very helpful in confirming the options and identifying some issues with the proposed approach here in Ottawa, which we were then able to raise with my medical team. We also checked on the European approach through the father of one of my son's friends, who again confirmed the general approach but gave some suggestions. These were both crisper than the staging and phasing of information in Ottawa and thus were particularly helpful in assessing options.

Own your file (own yourself)

This may sound trite, but you are the only person who will worry and think about you all the time. Doctors and nurses are juggling many patients, and while they have access to your file, keeping your own parallel file to keep track is indispensable. I started a binder containing all the key documents to keep track of my treatment schedule, medication information, test results, contact numbers, important reference material, and so on. I always brought the binder to the hospital and to appointments so that, for example, whenever I was asked what medication I was taking, I could just pass on the list from the pharmacy.

The healthcare system is overwhelmingly paper-based (we need eHealth!), and I was asked the same standard questions time and time again. Having my reference binder ensured that I was prepared and had everything the medical staff needed (and allowed me to give them paper to copy, rather than have to fill out information again). For example, the patient history form, required at each hospital stay, was easily taken care of: I simply kept a copy in my binder and gave it to the nurses to be photocopied for their records. I transferred most of my important health records to my iPad to avoid carrying the binder, which further simplified things. This was particularly helpful during my second opinion consultation, when I could call up relevant information as needed.

For more details on what worked for me, see the <u>Organizing your Medical File</u> section.

Prepare for clinic (and other) visits

I prepared questions before any appointments or treatments. These were sometimes as simple as asking when to take Neulasta, to make sure that I could order it during weekdays when the hospital pharmacy was open; other times, I had broader questions about how I was doing. For example, I took advantage of the doctor's presence during one treatment to walk me through my mid-point CT scan. During my treatment for relapse, my questions became sharper, my feedback more direct (e.g., providing details of issues to the team quality manager), and my requests and suggestions more pointed (e.g., requesting Neulasta after my fourth round of 'salvage' chemo to reduce my low immunity risk period, reconciling conflicting opinions on whether a CT scan was necessary). At the same time, I ensured that I was respectful of the team treating me.

It is not only important to know your file and quantitative indicators like blood counts. Qualitative 'how do I feel' aspects of treatment also make a difference. My favourite indicator was the 'crumminess' scale, according to which I tracked how I was feeling overall (a 1 being mild chemo taste and 10 being constant vomiting), which could then be supplemented by specifics as required.

Have a partner

There is an incredible amount of information to absorb, and the specialists in particular are time-stretched. Having a second pair of ears at appointments is critical to understanding and recalling all the key points. In addition, when things get rough with side effects (I had to go to emergency because of some of these), a partner is critical for communicating with the hematologist on call and other doctors. On a number of occasions I was not fully coherent, and was unable to articulate what I was undergoing. My wife played this key role in my case, which also ensured that we were on the same page in all aspects of my treatment.

Monitor your care

My daily journal helped me remember reactions to medication and flag those reactions when going in for a repeat cycle. Where there was confusion – such as one week where it was not clear whether I had one appointment or two – I could seek clarity or, as happened in more than one case, benefit from a mix-up in communications that resulted in a second meeting with a doctor during the same week, helping my case move forward more quickly.

As I became familiar with the hospital and treatment routines, I started to understand the standard procedures and could ask appropriate questions when something was not right. Some basic curiosity helped here.

Given my low immunity, I was particularly concerned about minimizing the risk of infections, so if the nurse was not following what I thought was the standard procedure, I would ask, in a non-accusatory manner, about why they were doing it a certain way when I had noticed others doing it a different way. Most times the answer satisfied me (there is a range of acceptable procedures). Only once was I dissatisfied with the precautions taken. In that case, I mentioned my concerns to the head nurse, to make sure that the nurses would be reminded about the procedure. Another example is that I learned how the intravenous worked, so that I could notify the nurse if there seemed to be a problem.

After the introduction of a patient quality manager to the lymphoma and leukemia unit, I was able to point out issues that I noticed to someone who had overall responsibility for implementing a more patient-centered approach. The patient quality manager had the right approach and welcomed feedback, and I found her a useful channel when things were not going as they should.

Know the gatekeepers

All systems have gatekeepers. In healthcare, the doctors play this key role. When I was given an initial consultation date of July 23rd, I asked the scheduling person how I could move it to a sooner date. Her advice? Speak to my referring doctor, as he could contact the specialists and move it up. I did as she suggested, and my appointment was moved up to July 3rd.

The paramount role of doctors was driven home to me when I was discussing a discharge date. The doctor wanted me to go home, but I was not sure. One of the senior nurses was sympathetic and said that she would check with the doctor to see if there was any flexibility. She tried – but he maintained that I was fit to go home, so home I went.

During my relapse, I experimented further with how to get needed information or action between doctors, senior nurses and the assistants. No one formula worked (people are people, after all) but a mix of coming to clinic appointments well armed with questions, engaging with the quality manager, sending e-mails and making phone calls to the senior nurse and assistant, and escalating when things were not being dealt with as quickly as they should be seemed to help. Being forceful and in charge, but maintaining good relations with the team, seemed to be the best approach.

Leverage the team

While the specialists are the top of the pyramid, your time with them is limited compared to that spent with other members of the team. Taking advantage of the knowledge and experience of everyone you work with provides more information and guidance in terms of what you are going through.

The clinical doctors and interns are particularly helpful, as they typically have more time to spend with patients. The interns are more thorough in their physical exams, but can be frustrating since they cannot answer questions directly, almost playing 'telephone' with the doctors. At one point, this was so frustrating that I complained, as it meant I could not engage in discussion – playing 'telephone' – rather than discussing directly with the hematologist my relapse, proposed treatment and implications.

The nurses, particularly the more experienced nurses, are invaluable for practical advice and are always willing to share it. There are other resources, such as social workers, that can help with some of the psychological or other issues facing you and your family. Social workers were particularly helpful in doing a 'check-in' with my kids to make sure that my wife and I had been providing them with the information they needed, and that they understood it fully.

There are also a range of service providers in the broader community that can help further, often with a more holistic perspective than the medical team. I did avail myself of the Canadian Cancer Society peer support program, and spoke to a number of people that had either the same mantle cell lymphoma and treatment as me, or comparable cancers. Through my blog and other online fora, I also had a number of good exchanges with people who had undergone, or who were undergoing, similar journeys.

These were particularly helpful for putting my mind at ease, and it was good to see the common elements that we had faced or were facing. Given my own strong family and friend support network, I did not explore outside sources of support further, but for others this option could be particularly helpful.

Intervention techniques

Given the number and different personalities of people on the medical team, I needed to figure out what intervention style worked best for each role and for each personality. For the past several years at work, I have been using the 3A system: alignment (telling people what to do), appropriation (asking people for input and direction on what to do), and *appui*, or support (providing encouragement and praise to generate a positive attitude).

Ironically enough, the specialists responded best to alignment, as they were practicing alignment with me on the content of my treatment plan. I found this out the hard way. On the number of occasions when I developed complications and had to contact the hematologist on call, one hematologist in particular always had a preference for me to wait and stay home, suggesting that the problem was a 'normal' side effect. In the end, it was not normal. To counter this problem, our modus operandi after the third such discussion became to tell him that I was coming to Emergency and that he should let the staff there know. It worked.

In contrast, the nurses were much more open to appropriation, and appreciated being asked for advice on ways to make the treatment easier. I could ask them questions like, 'What do I need to do to make this easier or more successful?' Most doctors did not respond as well to this approach.

Of course, *appui* is always appreciated by all, and the more I recognized their efforts on my behalf, the more the members of my medical team responded with humanity and made my hospital stays more bearable. Given the range of people looking after you and how busy they all are, small things like expressing thanks or interest in them as people not only makes the experience richer for you, but fulfills the medical team's human need for recognition and acknowledgement.

Another point I want to emphasize is the importance of repetition. I was dealing with a number of different specialists, doctors, nurses, and so on. One of the hematologists gave me the sage advice that if something was important to me, I had to tell every one of them. For example, it was really important for me to be able to drop my son off for his first year at university. I told all the specialists about my desire to do so, as well as the clinical doctor and the nurses. The specialists initially reacted with uncertainty about whether my request could be accommodated, but when the whole medical team met to review my file, they decided to adjust my treatment to suit a life priority.

After relapse, and a few occasions where things seemed to be falling through the cracks, I found that more alignment seemed more effective than the softer techniques. I did try to maintain a balanced tone and approach to reinforce the partnership between myself and the medical team. In Toronto, the intern examining me complimented me on my knowledge and questions, which I found a useful confirmation that I was on the right track in respectfully pressing my concerns.

WORKING WITH YOUR MEDICAL TEAM

Part of the challenge of having cancer is learning how to work with your medical team: doctors, nurses, pharmacists, dietitians, occupational therapists and physiotherapists, and social workers. Figuring out who does what, how the hierarchies are structured, and how best to intervene in decisions is part and parcel of being an informed and empowered patient (one who views treatment and recovery as shared objectives and responsibilities).

A number of people and organizations provide advice on how best to work with your doctor. One of the better documents is by Massachusetts Health Quality Partners and Consumer Reports (here). A number of others worth noting include Pauline Chen's Afraid to Speak Up at the Doctor's Office, Tamara McClintock Greenberg's The New Rules of Modern Medicine, Mary Elizabeth Williams' Listen up, Doctors: Here's How to Talk to your Patients, Marie Meservy's How to Win Friends and Influence Doctors, and Martine Ehrenclou's Tips to Maximize the Relationship with your Doctor.

While there are common threads to all of these (courtesy, respect, preparation, honesty, teamwork), most advice has been written from either the perspective of the patient or that of the doctor, rather than from a shared perspective. With this in mind, I came up with the following list of shared responsibilities.

Be courteous and respectful

We are human. We respond to how we are treated by others, whether consciously or not.

For patients and their caregivers, this means treating everyone in the medical team (and the people who clean the hospital) politely and with respect. In other words, be nice. Saying 'thank you' goes a long way.

If there is an issue – and there will be some – raise it calmly and phrase it in terms of quality control. Use your people skills to get the point across in a clear but non-antagonistic manner. Of course, some occasions may call for a more forceful style, but start off softly and only escalate if necessary.

As patients, we are stressed, sometimes discouraged and even depressed, so we will occasionally overstep the mark. Medical teams understand that and generally handle it professionally and with understanding.

However – again, we are all human – if this is ongoing behavior, it will strain relations and may prevent care from being delivered with the most warmth and empathy.

Medical teams benefit from the experience of dealing with many patients facing the same kind of existential questions, worries and fears. As patients, we expect to be treated as people, not 'a collection of faulty body parts', as Mary Elizabeth Williams so forcefully says.

If, on the other hand, you are a member of a medical team, please strive for the following:

- Empathy and understanding: Do not use the cold style of the oncologist in Hollywood films like 50/50, but instead recognize our vulnerability as you help us through treatment decisions and the treatment itself.

- Eye contact: Do not hide behind the computer when talking to us. We know you need some time to input notes and read us our scan or lab results, but make sure the important messages are delivered directly, not as mumbling from behind a screen.

- Plain language: Use as simple language as possible, and help us through the learning curve as we begin to understand our new vocabulary. 'Cheat sheets,' information booklets and website recommendations can help here.

- Time management: As patients, we should value your time. Similarly, while the juggling act between seeing every patient and providing the time each needs is hard, try not to give the impression that you are rushed, that we are only a number, and that you want to leave as soon as possible. If it really is a crazy day, as is often the case, just let us know. One time, I had a presentation to show my hematologist, which he had asked me to complete as 'homework' (or therapy!). He did not miss a beat – he stepped out of the room, told the next patient that he would be a bit delayed, and then came back in.

Be open and honest

A medical team can only help patients if we are open and honest about our condition, side effects, fears, psychological state, other care we are receiving, what is important to us, and so on.

There is no shame in raising these kinds of issues, and many cancer centers have a range of staff with different expertise to help us.

My family and I chose to have a few joint sessions with the social worker/counsellor to help us work through things together. This was helpful because we were able to start having more open discussions about what I was going through and how it was affecting those around me.

To the medical team: we expect you to be honest with us. Tell us whether things are going well or not. I only had one experience with a hematologist sugar-coating prospects at my initial diagnosis. Otherwise, my medical team has given me dispassionate advice and information, delivered with the requisite empathy and understanding.

Be present, informed and prepared

We surrender much of our life and control to our medical team. They have the expertise and experience that we lack, and we are very much on a learning curve throughout treatment. One of the few areas that we exercise control over is how informed and prepared we are for our discussions with them.

Patients spend too much time on the web trying to become instant experts on their particular cancers and treatment options. We need to recognize our limitations, ask the medical team for sites they recommend (more tips on this here), read the material they give us, and focus on knowing enough to be able to ask good questions and understand the information that the team provides. Generally, the team as a whole will supply the breadth of information required.

Come to appointments with a list of written questions (I keep a running tally). Order them in priority, in case time appears to be running out. When I say I have some questions, my hematologist often tells me, 'Only three!'

While in practice he and his colleagues are more flexible, it is a useful reminder that their time is precious. As patients, we need to focus, take notes and come with another pair of ears for important discussions.

Alternatively, as one of my doctors suggested, come with a tape recorder, as some of us find it hard to listen intently and take notes at the same time – and friends or caregivers may not always be more reliable in their note-taking. But ask your doctor first if he or she is comfortable being taped!

To the medical team: questions are part of the deal in caring for us. Please be patient with us as we may need more time to process our new reality than you would like. Orient us to the websites or other sources of information that could help us and help you.

Also, ask your patients to summarize what you have told them, to ensure that you know whether they have understood correctly (patients can also initiate this 'replay' technique).

Work together as a team

Patients and medical teams are in it together, with the shared objective of as successful a treatment as possible. Being courteous and respectful, informed and prepared, and open and honest is part of this teamwork approach.

Patients can do even more than this and should follow the recommendations of their medical team. Find ways to exercise and be active, commensurate with your condition, and remain engaged in the outside world.

Do not let cancer 'metastasize your life,' to use Mark Dery's wonderful phrase. If you have issues like despondency or depression, seek help, whether from a faith leader, counselor, or trusted family member or friend. Take ownership of what you can, rather than merely submit to treatment. Be as active and engaged as possible; it is your health, after all.

Medical teams can help by encouraging us. My medical team encouraged physical activity and gave me guidelines on how much to push myself. They were less active on other aspects of my well-being, leaving me to take the initiative to see a counselor.

I have been lucky in terms of my medical team, with whom I developed a good and close relationship during the last three years. One of the 'benefits' of cancer treatment is that you develop closer relationships with the people who care for you.

While my medical team may sometimes have been irritated by my questions and probing, it was also clear that they appreciated my efforts to understand, make informed decisions and be as active as possible to help my recovery process.

This post was inspired by comments made by my medical team. One of them put the patient-team relationship in context, and made a lovely comment on the commitment of medical staff to our wellbeing:

> ... *I was happy to see your advice about the Internet to patients. One of our physicians has a good analogy when dealing with patients who are basing medical decisions on information from the Internet for family or friends. When you get on a plane for a trip, you don't ever think it is appropriate to go to the cockpit and start questioning the pilot on how he flies the plane. You trust that the pilot and team know what they are doing.*
>
> *Patients are diagnosed with complex illnesses and turn to the Internet for answers. These patients take up a lot of time questioning the diagnosis, the plan of treatment and why decisions are made. You would never turn to the Internet to question the pilot on his flying technique.*
>
> *Our specialists understand the complexities of your illness and work hard to ensure the best outcomes for the patient. On the other hand patients are their own best advocate and should be able to openly ask about concerns they have. ....*
>
> *None of us feel good when patients succumb to an illness. None of us profit from patients who don't live. I go home every night to my children and hope that I have done the best job I can do to keep my patients healthy and safe.*

Preparing for a Long Hospital Stay

Planning a lengthy hospital stay is like planning an extended vacation or business trip. The difference is that transitioning to hospital life means giving up control, having limited choices, and being dependent on others. Depending on your treatment and possible complications, you may end up spending a fair amount of time in the hospital (I spent close to a total of two months there for both my auto and allo stem cell transplants, with roughly half of that in isolation).

Get your life in order

When you are faced with cancer treatment, the cliché of getting your affairs in order (medical-speak for possible death) applies. This means having joint bank accounts, an up-to-date will, a personal care power of attorney with a 'Do not resuscitate' clause if that is your wish, and any other instructions that will make it easier for family members should the unfortunate happen.

On the emotional side, if you need to make family or other reconciliations, do it now rather than later.

Finances

Whether or not you have good healthcare (U.S.), a drug plan (Canada) and other benefits (e.g., sickness and disability plans) will make a difference. Understand what is covered and what is not, the expected impact on your savings, and how you could cover the cost of treatment. I was fortunate on all counts, with minimal financial worries, but others may not be so lucky.

In Canada, hospitals make money from parking, the cafeteria, communications and other services. Explore ways to reduce these charges by using nearby street parking and internet connectivity, for example.

Ensure connectivity

Most hospitals provide a WiFi connection, hopefully free. I find that e-mail is the most convenient way to stay connected, as it is less intrusive and requires less energy than phone calls. If you do not have a laptop or iPad, get or borrow one if you can, as the days are long without one. Unless you need (or want) to stay connected to your workplace, try to get away with only one device to use and charge.

Entertainment

iPods are great to drown out the background hum, both during day visits and longer stays as an in-patient. My laptop allowed me to watch DVDs (better choice of programming than commercial TV) to help pass the time, and after my relapse, the hospital had a number of large screen TVs with DVD players. This made using the iPad alone more than adequate. I read a lot as well, taking advantage of the quiet time when I had the energy.

Know hospital policies on visitors and food – and check for flexibility

Different cancer and stem cell transplant centres have different policies.

In terms of visitors: while all must be infection-free given the low immunity of patients, visiting times and the number of visitors allowed vary and there is some room to negotiate. A nurse once gave me a hard time about having an additional visitor; I just gave her a 'please' look and she backed off.

The same is more or less true of food. Hospital food is bland at best; home cooking is better. If you can eat, your family can bring food, and if your cancer centre allows it, try to have one home-cooked meal per day. It helps morale, trust me.

Have an 'exercise' routine

This depends on your condition and whether or not you are in isolation, either to protect you or others (e.g., I had a infection a number of times).

If you are not in isolation, try to get in the habit of walking the 'loop' around the ward a few times a day. In my ward, 10 'laps' was about a kilometre (1/2 mile) and a number of us would exchange greetings as we did our laps.

If you are in isolation, your hospital may have bike machines or similar equipment that provides an opportunity for some movement.

Remember – listen to your body. Push yourself to move a little bit, but not too much.

Get to know all the staff

For longer (or repeated) stays, you have the opportunity to get to know staff, and they to know you. Be nice to them – at all levels, including cleaning staff – and they will be nicer to you. A simple 'please and thank you' can go far.

Go with the flow

Read Insider tips to surviving your hospital stay, the best and funniest advice there is. Example:

> Be patient. There is no clock in a hospital. Nobody knows when any of your tests are scheduled to be done. Not the cleaning lady. Not your nurse. Not even the doctor doing the procedure knows when you're up. You'll know when you're up when they cart you away. Believing anything otherwise will just make you frustrated.

Remember, your objective is to be treated and get out as soon as possible so that you can spend the rest of your recovery as an out-patient, in the comfort of your home. 'This too shall pass' was my saying to get me through the difficult periods.

RETURNING FROM A LONG HOSPITAL STAY

Just as a lengthy hospital stay requires planning, so does the return home. While your condition and strength will shape the best approach for you, my experience following my stem cell transplants may be helpful should you find yourself in this situation.

Before you leave, get the information you need

Most hospitals are pretty good at providing written information sheets on follow-up care, related instructions, warning signs, and when and who to call. Read them and have your caregiver read and understand them. If these documents are unclear, ask members of your medical team for help (nurses are generally the best on practical questions).

Post the information in an easy to access, visible place for when invariably some complication requires you to call.

Recognise your weakness

The nature of the treatment, and the likely limited opportunities for exercise in the hospital, mean that you will be weak when you return home. In my case, this was particularly acute after I spent time in isolation due to a infection – even going up and down stairs was a challenge.

Recognise other limitations

Chemo, radiation and in my case, transplants, are hard on the gut, and your need to be closer to a bathroom may be an issue. Ensure that you have a 'bucket' in the car in case you experience nausea.

Get moving and restart your exercise routine

The major constraint for me, post-transplant, was the need to be close to a bathroom because of diarrhea and other stomach issues. My general weakness was also a challenge. Longer walks were out of the question, so I started walking around the block as soon as I could, as well as trying short stints on a bike machine.

As my situation stabilized, I started building up to longer walks. The section on Building Back One's Strength provides some suggestions for this.

Journal your condition

After a while, the ups and downs of recovery begin to blur. Keep a journal – on paper or electronically – that tracks how you are doing. This will provide you with a sense of whether things are getting better or worse, remind you of the responses to your questions at clinic visits, and help you formulate further questions for your medical team.

All you need to capture the important details is a few minutes per day. Of course, the scope of your journal can be broadened to include emotional and other issues should that be helpful (it was for me), but your medical team will be in a better position to help you even if you just record the minimum.

Manage your time with family and friends

You have to take the lead on how much socializing you can handle. Let family and friends know when you are ready for visits and whether you prefer e-mail, writing blog updates, or the phone. My personal preference when I am weak is for e-mail and my blog, although I used the phone for close family. Do whatever suits you, recognizing that as you build up your strength, this will change.

Set up your space

If you have a large enough house or apartment, sleep in your own room. The combination of my stomach problems, plus my need to drink a lot of fluid to protect my kidneys (which resulted in frequent bathroom breaks) made a separate room less disruptive for everyone.

During the day, I camped out in our den, so that I was close to my family but in a quiet area. Again, as life returns to normal, this isolation becomes less necessary.

While no one approach fits everyone, thinking about these issues and discussing them with your caregiver should make your return easier. Remember, your goal in coming home is to speed your recovery and, as much as is possible, minimize the need for return visits to the hospital.

BUILDING BACK ONE'S STRENGTH

We all grapple with what kind of recovery and rehabilitation program we should follow after cancer treatment. While your general health, age, treatment and other factors determine what is will be possible, the key thing is to find a program that works for getting you as active as possible.

In addition to keeping in touch with friends and family, which is so important emotionally, my experience with two transplants taught me some things that you may find helpful.

Know what you like to do

This is trite, but if you like doing something, you will do it. Before cancer, what was your exercise routine? What were your hobbies? Your interests?

Assess these in light of what you and your medical team think is realistic. You will likely need to scale back and allow for more time to rest.

Develop a routine – but do not be slavish

I found it easier to make a general routine of regular sleep (including naps), time for working on my blog and other projects, and walking. While clinic visits and events will interfere, this gave me some structure and focus.

Start with walking

The easiest form of exercise is walking. All the evidence suggests that half an hour of walking each day gets you most of the benefits of exercise. Walking can be done alone or with family and friends, which means more connection time. It is easily to scale up or down: when I am weak, I take short walks to get me out of the house, but when I am stronger, I go for longer walks for more exercise.

Runners can scale this up as their strength allows. As I recovered, I got back into cross-country skiing and biking.

Others may prefer stretching, yoga or Tai Chi to get back into shape without overly taxing the body.

Pace yet push – and allow for the bumps in the road

Find a balance. There will be some days when you do not feel well enough to do much. Accept that. When you feel better, push yourself a bit to do a bit more, recognizing the importance of building up strength in the longer term.

When you go through a 'bump,' be philosophical about it (unless your medical team 'suggests otherwise'), recognizing that 'this too shall pass.'

30

For example, I worried about gaining too much weight, only to have a bout of stomach trouble that caused me to lose most of it – and kept me from my walks. Building a 'reserve' was a good thing!

Find a project

If you do not have to go back to work early, pick a project to get your mind engaged and reduce 'chemo' brain. In my case, it was learning a language after my , and preparing a family tree after my . This gave me focus, retrained my brain, and gave me something concrete that I had achieved during my lengthy absence.

When I thought about my recovery, I realized that I had become 'cocky' about my progress and was taking it for granted. My stomach trouble reminded me (forcefully) of the need for humility and acceptance, and that the journey will not be straightforward. While the points I have laid out above continue to guide me, they are now tempered with more realism about what is doable – something that each of us has to work out.

Be as active as you can be!

Chapter 3

Support: A Compact

We are in this together: living with cancer, caring for someone with cancer, or as family, friends or colleagues who care. How we support each other throughout the journey makes a difference to all of us.

There has been a great deal written on what to say and what not to say to someone with cancer. Some of my favourite pieces are by Deborah Orr (here), Suleika Jaouad (here and here) and Bruce Feiler (here). Many of these suggestions apply to any difficult circumstance, not just cancer.

We are individuals, and react differently to what people say or do not say, do or do not do. The experience of cancer makes us more sensitive, and we need to look past some of the clichés that family and friends may use to deal with their own discomfort. We need to think back to when someone close to us had a difficult experience, and how well – or poorly – we handled it and provided support.

Most writings focus on giving advice to family and friends, with less emphasis on the person living with cancer. As with any relationship, however, the patient and those close to them have a joint responsibility to make it through together. With this in mind, I have come up with the following joint suggestions.

Recognize the awkwardness

Having cancer and telling people is awkward. It is also awkward for family and friends, who do not know what to say. Accept this, and get over it. Serious illness is a part of life that touches everyone sooner or later.

Be there

If you are a patient, figure out what kind of contact works best for you: e-mail, phone, or visits. Find a way, whether through family, friends, blogs (my approach) or other social media, to let people know that you would welcome contact. I personally found e-mail to be the easiest when times were rough, as I could read and respond to messages at my leisure, whereas phone calls and visits required more energy. As I got better, of course, calls and visits were welcome and more frequent.

If you are not the patient, take the patient's lead on how he (or she) likes to keep in touch, and whether visits are appropriate. Let the person know that he is important to you, and that you care for him and his family. You do not need to make a big fuss out of this, but just enough to let the patient know that you are concerned.

Nothing bothered me more than falling into a 'black hole' and being forgotten, which made me realize which friendships were meaningful and which were not.

Try to avoid the general question, 'Is there anything I can do to help?' It is more helpful to make a specific offer, like, 'Can I drive you to the hospital/clean your house/take your kids to school?' If you are a patient, have a concrete suggestion on hand should someone make a general offer. My request was often that people keep in touch or that we plan a walk together, as emotional support was what mattered most to me.

Be open and honest

It is all too tempting – for everyone involved, patient or otherwise – to downplay cancer and the risks of treatment. At the initial stages, people with cancer are in shock and, often, denial. Many are not comfortable sharing. Others may be, or may grow more comfortable. Both patients and those around them need to find the balance that works for everyone.

For patients, this is particularly true with your children and loved ones. Sharing with colleagues at work has its own challenges, depending on the nature of the workplace and relationships. On the whole, it is better to be open and honest, at least in terms of the big picture (e.g., my cancer is aggressive, treatment will be difficult, odds are good/not good). I probably shared more than most in my blog – partly to help others undergoing similar journeys, partly as a way working through the issues for myself.

If you know someone who is going through treatment, avoid false optimism. While it is a normal tendency to say 'You'll be alright,' or 'your worries are unfounded,' that may or may not be true. The person with cancer will have a much more realistic assessment than you. Softer variations on these expressions may go down better, but in my case – aggressive lymphoma, with 'challenging odds' – I just found it irritating. What could I reply, 'It won't be OK'?

If the patient starts discussing her worries (which are normal under the circumstances), hear her out and do not dismiss her. Acknowledge the patient's emotions by saying something like 'This is rough, does talking it through help you deal with it?'

Also, through most of treatment and initial recovery, cancer patients look awful (don't tell us, we know!). However, after recovery, when we have our normal complexion back (if not all our hair), it is OK to tell us we look good. This is another sign that we have emerged from the 'kingdom of the ill.'

Be aware and sensitive

When people undergo something difficult like cancer treatment, they and the people around them tend to be more sensitive – patients, because of their existential questions and brutal treatment, and others because they are faced with their own 'but there for the grace of God go I' mortality. Both sides need to be aware of this sensitivity, in the big and small aspects of their interactions.

Just 'being there' largely covers the big aspect of being sensitive. Tread carefully, however, on questions about survival odds, test results, mortality and so on, unless you are invited to discuss these. One of my most intense discussions was with a colleague in the final stages of cancer. We both knew that we did not have much time, and went right into the existential. With other friends, the progression is more gradual, although I do touch on the most serious topics with my closest friends.

Some of the small parts of being sensitive to each other:

- Short phone calls and visits are better than long ones. Know when to leave. If in doubt, go shorter, or ask. Some of my close friends were very good at reading how I was feeling, and I became better at saying, 'thanks, but I'm fading now.' Take the patient's lead: it's their dance, after all.

- People have mixed opinions about sayings like 'I feel sorry for you' or 'My thoughts and prayers are with you.' I never resented these expressions as they are a way for people to express how much they care for you. Others did. Deborah Orr suggests a better phrase: 'I so wish you didn't have to go through this ghastly time.' For me, however, 'it's the thought that counts' is an important expression in this context.

- Be flexible. Patients have good days and bad days. When planning visits, walks, or events, add, 'If you're up to it on the day.' Remember that this is about the patient; they have more latitude to cancel than you do.

- Be careful with black humour. Some love it (I do!), others do not. If you are not sure, it is better to err on the side of caution (for example, remarks about new 'hairstyles' – i.e., baldness –may work better with men than women).

- Do not recommend alternate treatments or doctors, unless invited. If you really feel that you have some unique information that has science behind it, still ask permission before giving advice.

Be forgiving – do not try to be perfect

None of us get it right every time. We learn from our missteps.

As patients, we need to be forgiving, recognizing that our family, friends and colleagues are expressing their love and care for us, no matter how clumsy they may be at times. Again, even poorly expressed caring is much better than being forgotten and left alone, so we need to appreciate it.

If you are family, a friend or a colleague of the patient and blurt out something inappropriate, just say 'Oops,' apologize, and move on. In most cases, this is enough to get back on track. If you are unsure of whether you said something inappropriate, just ask.

One of my closest friends, who called and walked with me on a regular basis, made a comment that resonated with me. It was along the lines of, 'By understanding what you are going through, I will be more understanding should I or someone else close to me wind up in a similar situation.' This was not cold 'utilitarianism,' but rather his deep understanding of our common humanity – and that dealing with serious and possibly terminal illness is part of our common humanity. My experience will help him become a better person while he supports me, and we have become closer as a result.

Above all, be there. The smaller things are just that: small. They are not important. The overall message of love and care comes through and both sides emerge closer and stronger than before.

Chapter 4

The Journey Begins

Treatment finally starts one Friday afternoon. The five months of chemo are as intensive as is possible without killing me.

DIAGNOSIS: MAY-JUNE

June 29, 2009

This post is a context piece before I started to write updates to my staff at work.

I felt a lump in my abdomen in early May and discussed it with my family doctor in late May. A series of subsequent referrals and diagnostic tests (ultrasound, CT scan, ultrasound guided biopsy) led to a confirmed diagnosis of Mantle Cell Lymphoma (MCL), Stage III.

Uncertainty is stressful, but the certainty of MCL, given the bleak prospects outlined on the web, was even more so. Not quite myself – I am usually more of a 'glass is half full' kind of guy, but the reverse seemed true. The highlight of this period was seeing Leonard Cohen in concert. His line, 'There is a crack, a crack in everything, that's how the light comes in' became a mantra and a metaphor for what this diagnosis meant for me and my family.

During this time, family and close friends were aware that my illness was likely lymphoma. At work, my boss and immediate team (my deputy and my office) were also made aware. After the formal diagnosis, I broadened the circle of those who new in waves, starting with my direct management team, and then extended management team, Director General colleagues, and a number of other close colleagues. These were some of the hardest discussions of my career. Even though I presented this as 'a sidestep in the journey of life', and, the ultimate 'learning experience' (with some trace of irony as I graduated from an executive development program focused on learning at about the same time), internally I was not quite so sure.

And in the meantime, it was a typically busy June in government. I had to lead my team to deliver on a number of major policy discussions and other priority initiatives; exhilarating and fun work that had to get done, despite the dread and fear dragging on inside me.

My all-staff message on June 29 was as follows:

> Dear colleagues,
>
> This is to let you all know that I will be absent for a number of months, due to treatment for lymphoma, starting shortly after July 6. I have asked my Deputy Director General to act during that period, and know that he can count on the same high level of support that you regularly provide me.
>
> While I will miss working with you and the day-to-day issue management, I will monitor my email and be available, treatment permitting, to support your management team on particular issues as required.
>
> Thank you for your understanding.

Andrew

Chers collègues,

Je tiens à vous aviser que je serai absent durant un certain nombre de mois, car je dois subir un traitement contre le lymphome, commençant peu après le 6 juillet. J'ai demandé à mon DG associé d'assurer l'intérim durant cette période. Je sais que je peux compter sur vous pour lui offrir le même niveau de soutien élevé que vous m'accordez toujours.

Le travail avec vous et la gestion des enjeux quotidiens me manqueront, mais je surveillerai mes courriels et je demeurerai disponible, si le traitement le permet, afin d'appuyer votre équipe de gestion dans le cadre d'enjeux particuliers, au besoin.

Je vous remercie de votre compréhension.

Andrew

TREATMENT PLAN

My treatment plan was for the Rituxan Hyper CVAD protocol with an autologous stem cell transplant. This took place on the following schedule and sequence:

Round	Dates	Treatment	Purpose
1	July 3-7	Cyclophosphamide, Dexamethasone, Rituxamab, Doxorubicin, Vincristine	Dissolve tumours and reduce lymph gland swelling
2	Jul 29 - Aug 2	Methotrexate, Cytarabine, Rituximab, Neulasta	Attack any lymphoma in the Central Nervous System
3	Sep 11-21	Cyclophosphomide, Lasix, Dexamethasone, Rituximab, G-Csf	Stem cell harvesting conditioning chemo (high intensity)
	Sep 22	Stem cell harvesting	Actual harvesting or collection of stem cells from my blood
4	Oct 2 - 12	Cyclophosphomide, Rituximab, Doxorubicin, Vincristine	Continue to dissolve any remaining tumours and further reduce lymph gland swelling
5	Oct 27 - 31	Methotrexate, Cytarabine, Rituximab, Neulasta	Continue to attack any lymphoma in the Central Nervous System
6	Nov 24-29	BEAM - Carmustine (BiCNU), Etoposide, Cytarabine (Arabinoside), Melphalan)	High intensity BEAM conditioning regime
	Nov 30	Stem cell transplant	Engrafting of my stem cells back into my body

SUMMER 2009 – LEARNING MY NEW ROLE

Week 1 - July 10, 2009 - My First Round

Just to let you know that am doing reasonably well, despite some ups and downs last week that required me to go back to the hospital. So I have a 'suite' with a view, full internet/Skype connectivity, and with my energy is coming back. My family keeps me fed, both literally (hospital food leaves something to be desired, to be diplomatic) and culturally (books, magazines, DVDs). Excellent care and monitoring, and a nice mixture of indicators – quantitative (counts, vitals, and the like) and qualitative (how I feel, which I have to learn to feel and interpret, and share this with the medical team).

Quite the learning experience.

I asked my colleagues at work to send me the occasional document/report of interest – as I am feeling well enough to get bored!

Week 2 - July 20, 2009 - Side Effects

This week included the usual ups and downs and hiccups. Had a few good days at home then back in the hospital again – hopefully this is the last of the hiccups and future cycles will go more smoothly.

Doing some great reading (*Ascent of Money* by Niall Ferguson, *Washington Diaries* by Allan Gotlieb, will start some fiction soon).

Learning experience – at the individual, group and system levels – continues, and my team sent me some very nice messages and cards.

Too nice to be inside – amazing how the weather looks better when you have to stay in! – but I am nevertheless doing well.

Week 3 - July 27, 2009 - Recovery

Just to let you know that I have been spending the last few days comfortably at home, resting, going for walks (weather permitting!), catching up with friends and family, and getting ready for cycle 2 this Wednesday.

I now have my new look – as one of my friends says I now look like an Australian swimmer, with my bald head!

I have really learned to appreciate and take advantage of the good days, and the simple pleasures of being with my family, staying connected with friends, walking, and eating good food.

Week 4 - August 2, 2009 - Round 2

Overall not a bad week. Some good time at home going for walks and catching up with friends, and the second round of chemo is done. Should be back home soon – just under observation (last round I went home too early...).

Catching up on reading (*Love in the Time of Cholera* by Gabriel Garcia Marques, *Origin of Species* by Nino Ricci), and really trying to use my time to broaden my sense of awareness – making this time not only a learning experience but a bit of a sabbatical, strangely enough.

Sounds like you all are busy and getting things done – keep it up but also keep up your holiday plans and balance.

Week 5 - August 10, 2009 - Further Recovery

A good recovery week from chemo round 2. My side effects have been manageable, and I am glad to be at home.

My energy levels will improve following a blood transfusion taking place as I write – and I am really curious to feel the difference. I do not expect to transform from Clark Kent to Superman, but it should make me more active.

In terms of reading, found helpful the emphasis on awareness/presence in *A New Earth* by Eckhart Tolle (as well as his distinction between acceptance, enjoyment and enthusiasm), and *The Use and Abuse of History* by Margaret MacMillan, while relevant for my team's work, is also a wonderfully insightful read and note of caution.

Week 6 - August 17, 2009 - Quasi-Vacation

This is my quasi-vacation week. No treatment scheduled, no major side effects, and at last summer weather! Lots of good walks, but less reading (*The Tipping Point* by Malcolm Gladwell, interesting examples of group phenomenon but light, and half-way through *Moral Disorder* by Margaret Atwood, which am enjoying). Even made it to a movie last week: *Julie & Julia*, a fun movie if you like France, French cooking, food, and Meryl Streep (which I do). Some very nice visits and calls from family and friends.

Have about another week before the next round of chemo so intend to enjoy the respite. I am really learning to live in the now: when 'the now' is rough, thinking 'this too shall pass' helps, when 'the now' is good, enjoy!

Hope you are all well and at least some of you have planned holidays during this actual summer weather.

Week 7 - August 24, 2009 - Quasi-Vacation Continues

My quasi-vacation from treatment continues. I have a respite until September 5th, when the conditioning regime for stem cell harvesting begins. The medical team accommodated my request that I be able to take my son to Toronto next week, to get him started at the University of

Toronto, or U of T (one of those family milestones that one does not want to miss, as it will be his first year!).

I have been walking for about two hours a day and the improved weather helps a lot. I had many good visits from friends (including a number from overseas). I also finished the Atwood book (a good read) and have almost finished *Outliers* by Malcolm Gladwell, which am enjoying and finding more interesting than *The Tipping Point*. It is a good illustration of how innate talent is helped and supported by people and circumstances, and is relevant relevance to my workplace in understanding some of the informal (and formal) systemic aspects of society that impact individuals and groups, with discriminatory effect.

I saw a great movie, *The Hurt Locker*, about a bomb disposal unit in Iraq (one of the better Iraq war films, and really strong writing and directing, which maintain the tension and interest throughout), and watched another one for escapism (one of the Harry Potter series), given that when our kids were into the books, I read them all!).

I hope all is well with you as summer draws to an end and we approach what will be a busy fall at work.

WEEK 8 – MY 'CHEMO' HOLIDAY

August 31, 2009

It is hard to believe that about two months have passed since I started this journey.

My 'chemo holiday,' as my irreverent brother calls it, continues, again with walks and visits as the main focus.

I only read one book this week, The Last Lecture by Randy Pausch. While moving, it came across to me as a bit superficial, although I liked the aphorisms on 'how to live your life' – there were some nuggets there.

In terms of movies, I went to see Inglourious Basterds by Quentin Tarantino (my son is a fan), and it is one of his best films ever. While ultimately I find his work too focused on cleverness and style, and thus ultimately lacking in meaning, there are some amazing scenes in this movie that are wonderful examples of filmmaking craftsmanship.

Our kids, along with some of their friends, invited us to a premiere last night of their summer film project, Detective Inkwad and the Lisp. It was fun seeing how their filmmaking and acting talents have progressed over the years (a wonderful titling sequence with a New York background and a great shoot out scene were my favourites).

I had a good session with the stem cell harvesting/regrafting medical team about the next stages of treatment. Suffice to say that this really is the 'rocket science' part of the treatment, and the next step is the two-week stem cell harvesting cycle, starting on September 8th with some chemo. This should be another interesting 'learning experience'. One of the good things about the team in terms of communications is that they are very good at not overwhelming me with information, but rather take a staged approach to allow information to sink in and for questions to be raised. Repetition and reinforcement work.

I thanked my staff for the generous gift certificates they gave me. I have been enjoying good healthy snacks and food from Wild Oat and Kardish (local health food stores). With the Best Buy card, I updated the iLife suite on my Mac to take advantage of the new features on iPhoto, particularly face recognition. As a result, I have been spending a fair amount of time reviewing and updating our photos – part of the problem in the digital world is the sheer number of pictures, so time to organize and prune our collection is time well spent, and the new software speeds up the process.

Our main focus this week is taking our son to Toronto to start university, which brings with it a mix of emotions as he begins this next stage of his life.

To those of you with kids going back to school this week, *bonne chance avec la rentrée*; to the rest of you, enjoy the last week of summer, despite the coldish mornings.

WEEK 9 – OFF TO UNIVERSITY

September 7, 2009

We had really good visit to Toronto to 'install' our son in residence at U of T. It was a bit harder on us as parents than on him (always harder on those left behind), but he felt a mixture of nervousness and excitement, and the first few days were harder than he expected. He is settling in well, but our house seems a lot quieter and we miss his presence. On the positive side, our daughter has become more talkative and engaged, no longer worried about what her older brother might think!

No serious reading this week because of the Toronto trip. I went for a lot of walks to take advantage of the weather, and even did some yard work!

My 'chemo holiday' comes to an end tomorrow when I start my third round of chemo, which will be followed by stem cell harvesting. The treatment will take place on an out-patient basis this time, which is so much better than staying in the hospital. This will be good reading time.

WEEK 10 – BACK TO REALITY – STEM CELL HARVESTING

September 13, 2009

My 'chemo holiday' has come to an end. The first part of treatment went well. The second part started well, and included an all night session of watching movies with my daughter as I had to drink fluids throughout the night (we kept to light action movies: *Hero, Superman, You Only Live Twice, Bourne Identity*). However, I was given a stronger dose of chemo than last time and experienced more severe nausea and vomiting. I ended up back in the hospital for a day to get over that and get my electrolytes back in balance. I am now back at home and able to go for walks. The whole thing was an unpleasant learning experience (i.e., next time I will get chemo as an in-patient, not out-patient), but a short one! This week, the focus is on immunotherapy, so it should be relatively easy.

I read a really interesting book by Vladimir Nabokov, *Invitation to a Beheading* – a Kafkaesque and surreal story of someone in prison for an undescribed crime, and the characters that surround him. I am currently reading *The Black Spruce* by Joseph Boyden, which I am enjoying tremendously (also really liked *Three Day Road* – both books, and *A Fair Country: Telling Truths About Canada* by John Ralston Saul, all of which are helping me to better appreciate the aboriginal element of our society).

I am hoping that the weather holds so I can continue my walks.

My team is in the final stages of office move preparations and I wished them well. Moves are never fun, and quite a logistics exercise, with a more convenient location close to our colleagues.

WEEK 11 – RECOVERY

September 20, 2009

This week was generally good. No major side effects apart from fatigue and some bone pain (from the medication stimulating the growth of my stem cells). I was able to do lots of walking – still blessed by great weather – and otherwise take advantage of the fresh air. Wrapping up the stem cell harvesting cycle made this week a busy one, but I got plenty of reading time as a day patient.

I finished *The Black Spruce*, which I highly recommend; I also read *The Alchemist*, by Paulo Coelho, a charming parable on realizing dreams, overcoming obstacles, the interconnectedness of people and things, and how the journey is the destination. I just started *Payback* by Margaret Atwood, and realize that I had forgotten what a good essayist and lecturer she is. I keep updating my LinkedIn profile with the Amazon 'Reading List' app to keep track of my reading – for those of you that have not already tried LinkedIn, it is a good professional social networking site that more and more people within government are joining.

My team moved offices (finally) to the Ontario side – would have liked to have been with them for the move, but I have been spared the actual pain of moving!

WEEK 12 – HALFWAY THERE!

September 27, 2009

This was a great week. Stem cell harvesting went perfectly (I was even able to do it in one day rather than two, which reinforced my focus on results!) and was followed by a really nice series of visits with people, to take advantage of my immunity being relatively strong. It was great to visit our new offices and see some of my staff, as well as to attend the get-together for my boss's farewell with my colleagues. The highlight was having our son back from Toronto, and seeing how he continues to grow and develop.

Psychologically, the half-way point and stem cell harvesting had more of a positive impact than I expected – this must reflect my overcoming some of the underlying worries that I had.

I finished Atwood's *Payback*, which I highly recommend, as it gives one a broader understanding of the social and cultural underpinnings of debt, with her wry and ironic wit making it quite funny in places (apart from the last chapter which felt a bit heavy-handed). I have almost finished *Why Your World is Going to Get a Lot Smaller* by Jeff Rubin. While it has not convinced me to buy a hybrid, it does make a convincing case that the medium- to long-term trend is one of increased energy prices – although I am not sure the adjustments (reverse globalization, changed patterns of urban development) will happen as quickly or as easily as he implies.

My next round of chemo should be scheduled for later this week or early next week.

WEEK 13 – BACK TO REALITY

October 4, 2009

I am back to the reality of chemo for cycle 4 over the past three days. It went well overall, and I managed to get through it on an out-patient basis. The side effects were manageable, and I enjoyed being at home with family and able to go for walks, albeit slightly shorter ones. I had some nice visits before the chemo started as well.

Good reading this week, with a Mid-East focus. *My Prison My Home* by Haleh Esfandiari tells the powerful story of her imprisonment and interrogation in Iran, and the integrity, discipline and strength of character that allowed her to be one of the few who emerged with dignity intact (disclosure: Esfandiari is a family friend and we were in Iran when her troubles began, which makes her story that much more immediate to us).

I also read/started *The Much Too Promised Land* by Aaron David Miller, a fascinating insider account of 20-some years of American Arab-Israeli diplomatic efforts. He captures well the dynamics, personalities and sensitivities on all sides, and it is interesting to view the Obama admin's approach in light of the lessons Miller learns from previous administrations.

Movie-wise, I saw *The Informant* by Stephen Soderbergh, which was well crafted and edited, and featured some great character sketches.

I have also been exploring the online consultation forum in Ottawa for a redevelopment of our old fairgrounds and football stadium. It was interesting to see how online consultations work, the widely diverse opinions, most expressed politely, and curious to see how these get summarized in the overall report.

My focus next week will be on recovering strength.

I hope you all have a good Thanksgiving weekend.

WEEK 14 – FEELING CRUMMY BUT TWO-THIRDS DONE!

October 12, 2009

I had forgotten how tough this particular cycle was (Hyper CVAD 2A – the same 'cocktail' and protocol as cycle 1). To use that wonderfully precise but unscientific word from one of my favourite doctors, it was a 'crummy' week, and my energy was low. In the end, I did have to go back to the hospital to deal with some complications. Nothing like cycle 1, but a reminder of how powerful the meds are.

While I was able to start *The Evolution of God* by Robert Wright (a very good read contrasting how religion and the concept of God have evolved across societies and the ages), I was not able to get through as much as I would have liked.

It was great to see our son for Thanksgiving, although a bit amusing that my actual dinner was in the isolation ward, with him and my wife in isolation gear (think Darth Vader in hospital pastels!).

This week should be another recovery week; the next cycle will start in about three weeks.

I hope you all had a good Thanksgiving break with your loved ones.

WEEK 15 – A REMINDER

October 16, 2009

A 'this too shall pass' week, with a reminder about how much we take for granted.

Low immunity and a common cold meant that I stayed in the hospital for a number of days, on a day-to-day basis, until the doctors were comfortable that my 'counts' were back up. Due to my symptoms, I was automatically under the protocol – full isolation, etc. One word of advice, having had the H1N1 test and having been in isolation: do all you can to avoid it, and follow all the general precautions to minimize the risk of flu to yourself, family, friends and colleagues.

Being in isolation for a number of days made me think back on some of my 'prison' readings from this summer (Nabokov's *Invitation to a Beheading*, Esfandiari's *My Prison, My Home*). After a few days, I was feeling somewhat stir-crazy, and thinking back to these readings provided me with needed perspective. My brother helped as well, reminding me that I had visitors, internet, books, my Blackberry, and good care – and no need to do the dishes – so I should get over it!

I finished *The Evolution of God*, which I enjoyed. However, as one friend pointed out, Wright confirmed my secular biases in terms of his overall optimistic view of the universality and progressive nature of religions, so I will need to find some additional readings to reflect further on the differences and commonalities among religions.

I am reading *The Power of Now* by Eckhart Tolle, building on my earlier reading of *A New Earth*. It is somewhat repetitive, but I am still drawn to the core messages of being connected to the current moment, of managing clock versus psychological time and of acceptance ('this too shall pass'), and the importance of finding ways to connect to something deeper, whether through prayer, meditation, or reflection, are all helpful reminders.

I was finally able to get out of the house again and restart my walking routine, and enjoy the last few days of fall with its intense, vibrant colours. This connection time, with nature and with my wife, is such a central part of my routine and getting through the treatment journey.

I will be seeing my doctor Monday to schedule the next round. I have a sense that the last few months will drag a bit – weather and the accumulated impact make a difference – but every day means progress, and I should have a few more good weeks for walking and being outside.

WEEK 16 – RECOVERY

October 24, 2009

This was a good week in terms of regaining strength and balance. I went for many good walks with my wife, as well as some with friends, and I am enjoying the last of the fall weather. I also had several good discussions with colleagues at work, which help keep me connected with the 'real world.'

I have been reading *Shalimar the Clown* by Salman Rushdie, his post-9/11 novel on terrorism, but like all his novels, a wonderful and engaging panorama that plays itself across families and continents. I have always enjoyed the sheer power and playfulness of his writing, ever since *Midnight's Children*.

With the advent of shorter days, we have started to watch more DVDs. *Lemon Tree* is a good Israeli film that captures well the day-to-day dynamic and imbalance between Israelis and Palestinians, as well as some good character sketches. *The Queen and I* is a charming film about a leftist Iranian filmmaker, who protested against the Shah before the Iranian revolution and who develops an appreciation for and warmth towards the former *Shahbanou* (Empress) of Iran. The *Shahbanou* comes across as much more down to earth and warm than one would expect. On the lighter side, we saw *Where the Wild Things Are*, since the book was one of the favourites that my wife and I used to read to the kids, and I was curious to see the screen adaptation. Funnily enough, I viewed the monsters as a bit of a metaphor for all the chemo and related meds piling up on me, and in the end making me stronger!

We have all had our flu shots, with H1N1 planned for this week (one of the 'benefits' of being high risk!).

I have started reflecting on the 'lessons learned,' both practical and deeper, in this journey, and have also started the writing process (a week without 'chemo brain' is to be enjoyed – and taken advantage of). I am focussing on three elements: dichotomies/dualities or how I viewed myself (e.g., acceptance/anger, surrender/control, individual/group, being/thinking), reflections on what will shape me in the future (e.g. around themes of time, people, sharing, blessings, being in the moment, engaging), and lastly some practical tips for dealing with the healthcare system. This will continue to evolve, but almost four months in, some ideas are taking shape.

I had a good session with the doctor and scheduled round five for Monday. Judging by my previous journal entries (more reliable than memory!), this should be a relatively easy cycle, although it is in-patient for a few days.

WEEK 17 – ROUND 5 DONE!

October 31, 2009

Four months already. I surprised myself by striding, rather than walking, into the hospital Monday for round 5, reflecting on how much stronger I felt, both physically and mentally, than when I started on July 3rd. I am not out of the woods yet, and rebuilding my strength will take time after my final round, but I have a clear sense of being on the home stretch.

This round was actually one of the easier rounds (Hyper CVAD 2B), although it is in-patient given the nature and timing of the meds. It was kind of funny to be in my usual ward, seeing many of the same nurses and doctors, repeating a cycle, and reflecting further on the journey and how far I have progressed. Certainly seeing the other patients, much more sick than me, gave me perspective in terms of my relative health and prospects.

I had less of a bounce in my step as I left the hospital on Friday after four days of chemo, but it is good to be home for the weekend. I took a short walk outside in the evening and it felt delightful to get back into the home routine. I have been dealing with slight crumminess, chemo throat and irritability, but these side effects are manageable. As usual, complications tend to arrive the week after, and my biggest concern is to avoid infections as my immunity goes down this week.

My family and I got our vaccine on Monday, the first day it was available. It took four hours (seven for our son in Toronto), part of the normal confusion of any first day, but it is still a bit strange after all the exhortation for people to get the shot that there was less capacity than needed to meet the demand. All of us only had a sore shoulder for a day or so with no other side effects. This year is my first time ever getting flu shots; given that H1N1 does appear to be spreading fairly quickly, I would encourage you to get yours as soon as possible.

WEEK 18 – BOUNCING BACK (WITH SOME HELP)

November 8, 2009

This was a good recovery week. I am back my walking routine (the weather has been cooperative), and most of the side effects were gone by early in the week. However, my blood counts are very low (this is to be expected), so I had a 'booster' on the weekend to bring up my red blood cell and platelet counts (the nurse gave us a salutary scare on the risks of low platelets – dramatically so – and reminded me to be extra careful).

I had a good session with the doctor on next steps. As she mentioned, there is a bit of an assembly line here, and I need to be thoroughly through the current cycle in terms of blood counts coming back up, etc., before I am passed on to the next 'station' for the stem cell regrafting. The likely timing for this next stage is the end of November or first week in December. The treatment will be out-patient: six days of intense chemo, followed by a vulnerable period of two weeks. I am not exactly looking forward to this, so I got the Beatles collection (in the original mono version) to provide what I think will be some needed cheer and bounce.

My reading this week has been *The History of God* by Karen Armstrong. Although written before *The Great Transformation*, it complements it nicely with its focus on Judaism, Christianity, and Islam, and their evolution as religions to suit the needs of changing societies up until the modern period. Again, a lot of commonalities emerge, particularly distinctions between more literal and spiritual interpretations; individual and community; the importance of ritual, rationality and spiritualism; and relations with other religions.

Film-wise, *Adoration*, directed by Atom Egoyan, is a complex, multi-layered film that moves between fantasy and reality, and shows how these intersect with existing family tensions. I am not sure that it worked perfectly, but it held my attention. Less successful was *L'Heure d'éte* (Summer Hours), which captures the family dynamics following the death of a mother and the process of disposing of the family home and associated objects.

I have been transferring our old family tapes to DVDs. Like everything else, direct transfer is easy, whereas selective editing and playing around with iMovie/iDVD makes it more complex but yields a better result – and of course it is fun to revisit the time when the kids were small.

A few weeks back I mentioned the 'lessons learned' pieces. I have posted the first one, Navigating the Healthcare System, for comment and feedback, and to refine my thinking and reflection. Hope to post one piece per week over the next few weeks.

It looks like I will have a fairly good 'chemo holiday' over the next few weeks, despite all the various appointments required to get me ready for the next and final cycle, but I will need to remain careful not to catch anything.

Our son will be home for his mid-term break next week, and it has taken a difficult bit of planning to align his break plans, the time needed for H1N1 inoculations to work (10 days), and my recovery from low immunity – but it is all coming together and should be a good visit.

WEEK 19 – ENJOYING THE WEATHER

November 15, 2009

Glorious weather and a good recovery overall this week. I needed a further 'booster' of red blood cells and platelets, but over the low immunity phase. I went for lots of long walks in the first part of the week, but had a bit of a cold during the latter half, which forced me to live mostly indoors.

I met again with my doctor to confirm that I am on track for the stem cell regrafting. This time she was with students, making for an interesting lesson on terminology and audiences. When explaining my mantle cell lymphoma to the students, she was particularly direct, noting that it was a male disease, incurable, with treatment aimed at remission. She then asked whether I was planning to return to work, intimating that remission may not be as long as other doctors had suggested to me (80 percent long-term success).

Factual to the students, with the sensitivity of a stone for me as a patient! I was taken aback. My wife and I, upon reflection, came to the conclusion that this must be the way doctors and students speak to one another, without taking notice of the fact that a patient is in the room. I will raise this concern with my doctor next time I see her, but the incident reminded me of how important it is to always consider how one's words may land and be aware of who is in the room.

I had a wonderful visit with my son, who was home for his mid-term break. We spent good 'hanging around' time together, which included some movie classics (*Patton*, *Chinatown*, but couldn't go with him to see *Lawrence of Arabia* on the big screen – sigh), and belated celebration of his 18th birthday. Hard to believe that he has reached this milestone already, even if it is a bit of a cliché for me to say that. I also had a good time working with my daughter on some Cappie (high school theatre awards) and school issues, recalling my old activist days in high school, and supporting her and her friends' efforts to influence authorities.

I read some good books this week. First, *Abolition of Man* by C.S. Lewis, a trenchant series of lectures on relativism and enduring values, with some wonderful references from a range of religions, including that of ancient Egypt (but not Islam), on common values across religions (it reminded me of *The Closing of the American Mind* by Allan Bloom in some aspects). Second, *The Road* by Cormac McCarthy is wonderful – rich yet terse writing, a particularly bleak post-apocalypse account of the world, and a great depiction of the love and loyalty between a father and his son. I am curious to see how they adapt the book for the upcoming movie. I also (belatedly) saw *Entre les murs* (The Class), which captures the multicultural classroom dynamic and tensions in France very well.

I have posted the draft of the second of my reflections pieces, Dualities, covering my reactions to dealing with lymphoma, and again asking for feedback. I received a number of good comments regarding the Navigating the Healthcare System post.

This next week will be a further recovery week, and I hope that the good weather will continue.

Week 20 – Getting Ready

November 22, 2009

This was a very good week, full of walks thanks to the nice weather and the fact that I finally threw off my cold. I was even able to gain some weight.

I had a good session with the doctor and senior nurse responsible for stem cell regrafting. In contrast to last week's experience, this doctor was both thorough and empathetic (all the nurses were excellent in this regard).

As I mentioned previously, this is the rocket science part of mantle cell lymphoma treatment, which even has a daily 'count down' for the conditioning regime (protocol) to prepare my body for transplant. This is all on an out-patient basis, under close supervision, with daily checkups. This will be my strongest chemo so far – the doctor noted that the chemo is at the limit of what I can tolerate – and will essentially wipe out any remaining tumours and 'reboot' my bone marrow, with likely side effects in the mouth and digestive track.

As always, the main effects will happen after the chemo when my immunity and other blood counts drop. All done by Christmas (just!) to allow me to enjoy the holidays with family. Rebuilding my strength and energy is about a three- to six-month process; needless to say, I plan to try to bring that closer to three months with my usual focus on results. Nonetheless, as with all cancers, the overall success is only known after three years or so, and I will have that hanging over me for some time.

I did some interesting reading this week – Dorothy Harley Ebers's *Encounters on the Passage: Inuit Meet the Explorers*, a wonderful account of the glory age of Arctic exploration, told from both the official paper accounts of the explorers and, more interestingly, through the oral history of the Inuit. I only wish this had been out before I went to Nunavut in 2006.

Two classic films this week: *Rear Window*, directed by Hitchcock, a tightly framed – literally – suspense; and *Dr Zhivago* by David Lean, an enjoyable film but perhaps not the best one to watch with winter coming – one can almost taste the snow!

My last part of the reflections triptych, Lessons Learned, is now up in draft form, for comment and feedback. I will come back to these in the new year, when I have some distance from my treatment, and refine my thoughts as appropriate.

One of the interesting things I am noting about the blog is that more of my readers seem more comfortable with the directness – and privacy – of email, calls or walks than with the public and shared nature of the comments function. I am not sure whether this reflects general comfort or discomfort with social media, government practice/preference to be anonymous, or some other factors. Either way, any feedback and comments are welcome.

As next week is a treatment week starting Tuesday, I will have lots of time at the hospital, and hopefully energy, for reading. More apprehension this time than for previous rounds, but it is the last round, so almost done!

Chapter 5

Transplant and Beyond

With the tumours and other signs of lymphoma gone, I enter the final stage of my treatment. I then recover, go into remission, and return to work.

WEEK 21 – SO FAR, SO GOOD

November 29, 2009

It has been a steady week of daily visits in the morning for my chemo, a leisurely reading of the newspaper, cheery Beatles music, and then a return home to rest and recover. I experienced minimal side effects at the beginning, though they started to make themselves felt on the weekend, and we have been able to keep up our walking routine. My last chemo is this Sunday morning, so I am feeling a bit tired and wiped out, but pleased that this stage is over.

Time Period	Expected Experience
Nov 23 - Dec 7	Side effects should be starting to bite towards the end of this period but overall should be manageable.
Dec 8 - 23	Low immunity, high risk of infections. The Clinic rule is to call and come in quickly so they can nip anything in the bud, rather than waiting.
After Dec 23	Recovery period just in time for Christmas.

One of the nice things about the particular ward I am in (leukemia and bone marrow transplant) is that all rooms are private and the staff have more time to chat and explain. My wife and I had really good discussions with the pharmacist, who broke my schedule down into two-week chunks (while also noting that I should take things day-by-day).

My other visits this week:

- Dietician: only eat well-cooked and well washed food for the next three months, plus protein and other supplements to help get through any weight and appetite loss through the next month or so; and,

- Social worker: checking to see if there were any issues (we had seen her colleagues from the other clinics) so I ran her through how we are doing and the strong support network I have, and mentioned my journal and blog as means to capture and cope with the journey. We agreed to further contact if required.

I have not had as much energy for reading, but I started *Crossings and Dwellings: A Theory of Religion* by Thomas Tweed. It is a bit heavy on the theoretical side, but includes some interesting insights on the role of one's own perspective in perceiving religions, and how religions both reinforce the particular (dwellings) and help one transcend it (crossings). I will see if the book becomes more engaging. I read a good op-ed by Nicholas Kristof, The Religious Wars, which compares a number of books that make the case for less literal and more universal approaches to religious traditions, while also recognizing the force and power of religion and faith.

Film-wise, we went from the steppes of Kazakhstan (*Tulpan*, an interesting film about frustrated love and the simple life of goat herders) to the runways of Paris and Rome (*Valentino: The Last Emperor*, a wonderful documentary of the legendary designer, capturing his obsession and that of his team in the creative and business process). *Quel contraste!*

Monday afternoon I get my stem cells back. Since they are mine, my doctors do not expect an adverse reaction. However, I still have to contend with my reaction to the chemo, which will continue to kick in later in the week. This will be quite a 'this too shall pass' period, but we are greatly comforted by the strength and care of the medical team in explaining to what to watch out for in order to minimize risks and side effects.

WEEK 22 – REBOOTED... AND WIPED

December 6, 2009

Monday, November 30 was Day 0, when my stem cells were infused. Somewhat anticlimactic, and a bizarre combination of a sense of both accomplishment (the end of the treatment phase) and anticipation (dread) of the side effects. Celebrations would be premature, and any glass of champagne will have to wait for Christmas when all is done.

My immunity plunged on Day +1, and the side effects came in a rush on Day +2. The nurses refer to this stage as 'the wall'. I had been expecting a more gradual process of feeling increasingly crummy, but the crumminess arrived all at once: extreme fatigue, infection, loss of appetite, nausea, etc. Very much a different order of magnitude than in previous rounds. I was given two 'boosters' of red blood cells to give me more energy, and later in the week, platelets to ensure no bleeding risk. The medical team reassured me that all this, while unpleasant, was expected and normal.

By Day +5 (Saturday), I was starting to have sense that I was pulling out of the initial 'wall'. Nurses were reminding me, gently – and sometimes not so gently – to get on with it and make more of an effort to move and eat. So while the 'wall' was quick and sudden, recovery is more gradual, though noticeable – even despite not being out of the woods yet. On the good news side, the daily monitoring allows the medical team to nip problems in the bud, before they become bigger infections and fevers. I was thus still able to to remain a day patient". In sum, I am already in the second two-week stage, which hopefully means I will pull out of this one quicker as well. Not as much energy for reading and watching these days – sleeping is my main activity!

I finished the Tweed book, *Crossings and Dwellings*, just in time. Chapters 4 and 5, which feature the comparative work, are interesting, but overall too theoretical for my taste. A friend sent me the attached article by Roger Scruton, <u>Forgiveness and Irony: What Makes the West Strong</u>, where he argues that citizenship depends on a sense of forgiveness (grants the other the freedom to be) and irony (recognition and acceptance of otherness). Good food for thought, and another take on the literal versus the more spiritual approaches to religions. Quote:

> 'Forgiveness and irony lie at the heart of our civilization. They are what we have to be most proud of, and our principal means to disarm our enemies. They underlie our conception of citizenship as founded in consent. And they are expressed in our conception of law as a means to resolve conflicts by discovering the just solution to them. It is not often realized that this conception of law has little in common with Muslim sharia, which is regarded as a system of commands issued by God and not capable of, or in need of, further justification.'

I also, to my surprise, found the energy to read *E=mc2* by David Bodanis before the week was over. It is a light but charming book on the discoveries and discoverers behind the famous equation.

I also watched *Il Divo*, a fascinating account of Italian politics and the Prime Minister during the 80s and 90s, Giulio Andreotti.

Next week will be one of gradual recovery, as I also get the growth medication to boost my white blood cells. One of the ironies of this particular treatment is that while the actual protocols, sequencing and interventions are remarkably sophisticated, the actual bodily reactions and responses are highly predictable and almost mechanical. A 'this too shall pass' approach, tempered with the need to take things day by day, works well; I have, however, been grumpier and more hermit-like than during previous rounds, which reflects the depth of the side effects.

WEEK 23 – WAITING OVER, BUT...

December 13, 2009

A roller coaster of a week – I waited for my counts to increase and spent most of my time at the hospital.

The focus was the 'waiting game' for my counts to increase. Any time after Day +8 (Tuesday), my white blood cells and neutrophils were expected to increase with the help of a special medicine, Neupogen. Once they get started, I was told, the counts normally increase quickly, helping to address the mucositis and gut problems affected by chemo, bringing these and most other side effects to an end.

I sat and waited (literally) as daily blood counts were taken, and impatiently awaited the results. Intellectually, I knew the results were predictable; emotionally, seeing the first uptick would mean a lot, as it signifies the end of treatment, and the beginning of recovery.

The results arrived Thursday, and I felt immeasurably better and relieved! It worked!

Then on Sunday, my counts dipped. I was in a bit of a funk until the doctor explained that the occasional dip is normal, and the growth in counts is not a linear process. It would have been nice to know that beforehand. Nothing in life is linear!

At least getting admitted to the hospital was easy. In previous rounds, the routine was to contact the hematologist on call, discuss and sometimes debate a bit whether I should come in, and then go to emergency. BMT (blood and marrow transplant) patients, in contrast, go 'business class.' One call, and then directly into the ward – no fuss and no bother. No time spent in emergency, where I could easily catch other microbes. It makes such a difference to be whisked through; in speaking to the doctor, I learned that she wishes they could do the same for more chemo patients to minimize risk and increase emotional well-being.

Once at the hospital, I was back in my 'suite' and comfortable, albeit under isolation. I had a rudimentary bike machine so that I could get some exercise, which helped. Overall, I was feeling a lot less crummy than last week. The main discomfort was having a cold, cough and sore throat, all of which are relatively minor, and all of which diminished as the week went on. I was initially released on Friday, and had a wonderful winter walk on Saturday morning, but the fever came back – along with bone pain (from blood cell growth in the bone marrow) – on Saturday night. As a result, I am back in the hospital writing this blog. This time I am a bit less sanguine about being here!

Reading wise, I read the classic *Mere Christianity* by C.S. Lewis. Based in part on his lectures to World War II airmen about to be sent off on dangerous bombing runs, it helped me to better understand Christian beliefs, expressed at a time when the contrast between good and evil was being drawn out clearly. I understood that I needed to find equivalents for other religions and asked my readers for ideas.

I also watched some old Chaplin shorts. I find they are the right antidote to the institutional setting of the hospital.

Looking back to when I started my treatment some five months ago, I found an almost perfect symmetry between my first round and last rounds. Both rounds gave me similar side effects: C. dificil and pneumonia (though they were much more attenuated this time, and both were caught and treated earlier than in the first round).

There is, of course, a major difference: apart from those small hiccups, I am done!

WEEK 24 – RECOVERY, AND THANK YOU

December 17, 2009

It's over, and better yet, feels like it's over!

Tuesday I came home, and Thursday, after hospital day visits and check-ups, my status switched from active patient to clinic follow-up (initially on a weekly basis). My blood counts are recovering nicely, and the side effects are gradually diminishing, although I still have no sense of taste. My energy level is still very low, but that will come back slowly.

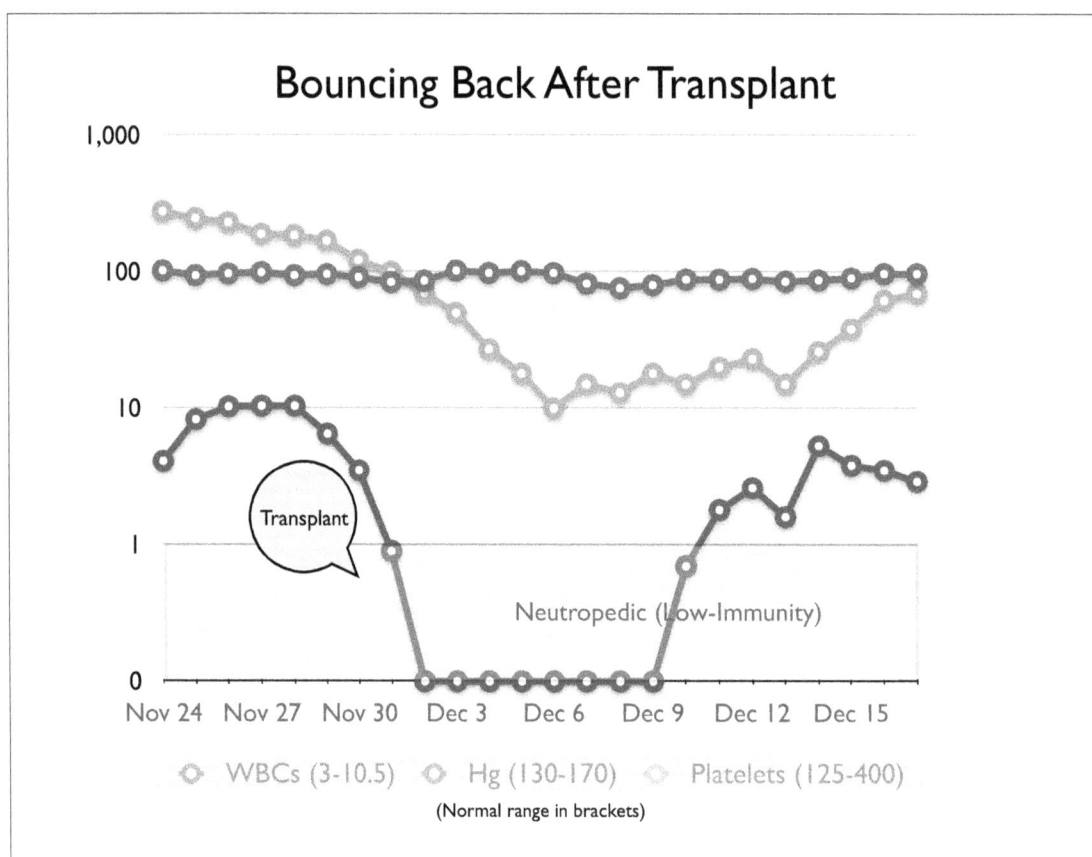

I am really looking forward to spending the holidays with my family (our son arrived Friday), especially given that we can all breathe a sigh of relief. Since my immunity will be low for the next few months, I will remain a hermit in terms of visits and public places, but should re-emerge in March if all goes well.

There was a good article by Julie Mason in *The Ottawa Citizen* on the metaphors of fighting cancer (In Search of a Better Metaphor), which resonates with me as I come out of treatment.

My book this week is *Holy Terror* by Terry Eagleton, an intriguing political, philosophical, theological and literary account of the origins of terror, and of how thin the veneer between civilization and violence can be. A bit challenging for the 'chemo brain' I've been experiencing these days, but lots of provocative and interesting thoughts to reflect on.

Video-wise, a quiet and easy week: *Apollo 13*, which brought me back to my childhood, when I was fascinated by space, and *The Wire*, an almost-too-gritty look at the Baltimore Police Dept and the community they serve.

Some thank-you's for all the support provided over the past months:

- to my immediate and extended family, particularly my wife and kids, for giving me the reason and the motivation to pull through;

- to friends and colleagues who sent cards, called, took me for walks, sent emails, posted comments, included me in their prayers, or otherwise expressed themselves and kept my spirits up;

- to my medical team for their care and attention throughout the process, with particular thanks to the nurses whose warmth and caring made all the difference while I spent all too much time at the hospital;

- to my employer for ensuring I could take the necessary time off to focus on my treatment, and for having a generous sick leave and medical plan, and to my staff and colleagues for their personal support; and,

- to all of you readers, whether you expressed yourself or not, for following my journey; I hope it has been a learning experience for you as it has been for me (and I can assure you that it is better to learn vicariously than to go through it yourself!)

I intend to keep up with the weekly updates but will not send out reminders during the holidays. I am not quite sure how the blog will evolve as I go through the recovery phase, but expect that it will develop organically. Stay tuned.

In closing, thank you again for all of your support during my journey to date, and my best wishes to you and your families for the holiday season.

WEEK 25 – THE HOLIDAYS

December 27, 2009

A good week. We are getting back into our walking routine and enjoying the holidays. My taste buds are still weak, so the holiday foods aren't quite the same as in previous years, but the general ambience helps me reconstruct the flavours in my head.

I had my first clinic visit since the transplant, which went well. No news is good news if they don't call you back with your blood counts, and they didn't. However, I will get the counts after the holidays at my next visit, and will start charting them again. I have become a bit obsessive, as the counts are the main objective measure of how I am doing!

We had our blended holiday celebration this week, starting with the celebration of Shabeh Yalda. A Persian celebration of the longest night of the year and the eve of the Winter Solstice, it commemorates the birth of Mithra, the Sun God, who symbolized light, goodness and strength on earth. We all listened to Iranian classical music, read some Hafez (one of the famous Persian poets from the 14th Century), and ate traditional Persian dried nuts and fruits.

Later in the week, another celebration of a birth and renewal. Christmas, for which we were joined by my brothers, was an equally joyous occasion, as we enjoyed being together, sharing food and gifts, and being thankful for what we have.

Movie-wise, I watched a number of classics this week: *It's a Wonderful Life* by Frank Capra, my favourite classic Christmas movie, with its message of the impact we have on others; *Dial M for Murder* by Hitchcock, a cleverly written and filmed mystery; another Hitchcock, *The Man Who Knew Too Much* (fun, with some great suspenseful moments, but a bit more drawn out than is common today); *The Big Sleep*, based on a Raymond Chandler story (starring Humphrey Bogart and Lauren Bacall, it was a bit complicated, but lots of fun); and *Judgement at Nuremburg*, about the pressures and ambiguities facing a judge in the Nuremberg trials of mid-level Nazi officials.

I took a break from serious reading, and on my son's (the Tarantino fan in the family) suggestion, read *The Kill Bill Diary* by David Carradine. It is a wonderful, light read that captures the highs and the detailed work of movie making, as well as the sheer obsessiveness and drive required to push a movie forward, get the vision right, and pull it all together. Not an easy industry! I received a number of good books for Christmas, so stay tuned.

Next week will be more of the same: going out for walks, working out on the bike machine, and gradually building up my energy, all while enjoying the time that all of us have together.

WEEK 26 – THE HOLIDAYS CONTINUE

January 3, 2010

Another good rebuilding week. I am gradually increasing the frequency of my walks and other exercise to build up my strength, and am enjoying the time with the whole family together. By the end of the week, I was shovelling some snow, driving once again, and able to stay up later.

Even my taste buds seem to be showing a bit of improvement, as meals are becoming more tasty. While I didn't have the energy to stay up until midnight for New Year's Eve, I did have a wonderful family dinner (partially prepared by me, another sign of increased energy). Needless to say, we are all looking forward to an easier year than the last one, but remain conscious of the twists and turns that life brings.

Lots of movies this week, and a rather eclectic mix. Pixar's *Up* starts off with some brilliant film making but then goes into the standard formula for the rest of the movie; Spielberg's *Close Encounters of the Third Kind*, a gift from my daughter, still looks good after all these years, and has a more leisurely sense of pacing than is found in today's movies; Kubrick's *Paths of Glory*, a classic anti-war film set in World War I, with a terseness and directness in the story telling; Coppola's *The Godfather*, another classic that wears well, thanks to the strong screenplay, atmosphere and cast; and for pure fun, as well as to test whether Blu-ray is much sharper than DVD (somewhat, but not as big a jump as the transition from VHS to DVD), *Harry Potter and the Half-Blood Prince* and *Star Trek*.

Reading-wise, I continued the movie theme with *The Film Club* by David Gilmour, a gift from my son, and a good father-son relationship story about how a father educates his son by watching movies with him (Gilmour is a former film critic). I also read *The Year of the Flood* by Margaret Atwood, which tells the same story as *Oryx and Crake* from a different perspective (that of the 'Gardeners,' the sect that live with minimal impact on the environment). I found it an easier read than *Oryx and Crake*, but it portrays the same depressing dystopia.

Next week I have another clinic visit, so we will see whether the improvements I feel are reflected in my blood counts. This is a strange new phase; without the regular schedule of treatment (thankfully over!) to 'occupy me,' the focus becomes more of a waiting game for test results. I feel relief that I can get on with my life again (thankfully), although with some uncertainty at the back of my mind.

Another transition, accentuated by the end of the holidays and the the kids' return to school. My challenge over the next few weeks will be to find a new routine that moves me along in the process of transition, physically and mentally, and prepares me for my return to work in a few months.

Best wishes to all for the New Year.

WEEK 27 – FINDING MY PACE

January 8, 2010

Over half a year has passed since I started this journey. I am happy that the hard parts are over, and am enjoying the rebuilding phase. A quieter week at home, as our son is back in Toronto for university and my mother-in-law, who helped us so much over the past months, has left as well.

I had a good session at the clinic this week. My counts continue to go up (platelets already normal; white blood cells and haemoglobin take longer to reach normal but are up). The doctor was pleased with my progress and my 'exercise program' of walks, shovelling snow, etc., and indicated that if all goes well, there should be some relaxation of my 'hermit' restrictions in a few weeks (e.g., able to go to movie matinées, etc.). After my next visit in two weeks, I will move to monthly visits (less is more!).

I have started my new routine to get myself back into mental and physical shape. My main project is to learn Farsi properly, and I am having fun, for a few hours each day, with the Rosetta Stone course. I am enjoying the process of re-learning Arabic script (it comes back more quickly than I expected) and refreshing my Farsi (it was so much stronger when the kids were small). It is also fun to see how software-based language learning has progressed – none of this existed when I learned other languages. The software uses an intuitive, native-language approach to learning, a challenge for me given my more analytical learning style. Nonetheless, I am learning, and the course is supplemented with helpful pronunciation and grammar hints from my wife!

I have been trying to spend a fair amount of time outside, whether by walking, shovelling snow, or (as of next week) cross-country skiing, as this really helps the rebuilding process. I have progressed from short to longer walks, and while I am far from 'buff,' at least I am feeling some of my muscle tone coming back. Slow but steady progress.

I am also increasingly getting re-involved with the office and with work files. I enjoy the interaction and the chance to see whether and how files have advanced or not. By the time I return physically to work, I should be reasonably up-to-date. This will make things easier for me, as well as for my team.

There was less time for reading this week, but I am working through *A Generation of Seekers* by Wade Clark Roof. An account of the American boomer generation's religious and spiritual journey, it examines how this generation has redrawn the balance between individual and institutional approaches to religion, and argues that class and education are among the bigger dividers in the approaches people take.

We rented *Food, Inc.*, Eric Schlosser's doc on what industrialized food production has become, and the issues that this transformation raises. It does make one reflect more on what one eats, from both a social and ethical point of view, and on how to rebalance one's diet towards more organic and locally grown produce to the extent possible. Not to be viewed before eating, however!

I also watched The Fog of War, a doc about Robert McNamara, the Secretary of Defence under Kennedy and Johnson and the former President of the World Bank, and particularly his reflections and lessons learned. The list:

1. Empathize with your enemy

2. Rationality will not save us

3. There's something beyond one's self

4. Maximize efficiency

5. Proportionality should be a guideline in war

6. Get the data

7. Belief and seeing are often both wrong

8. Be prepared to re-examine your reasoning

9. In order to do good, you may have to engage in evil

10. Never say never

11. You can't change human nature

My two favourites of the lessons? That belief and seeing are often wrong, which leads to the following rule, that one should be prepared to reexamine one's reasoning.

The complete list of lessons is as relevant now as it was then, whether to recent and current conflicts, or to any other complex decision-making processes. The challenge is to apply these lessons when under pressure, particularly group pressure and groupthink. Well worth seeing and reflecting on.

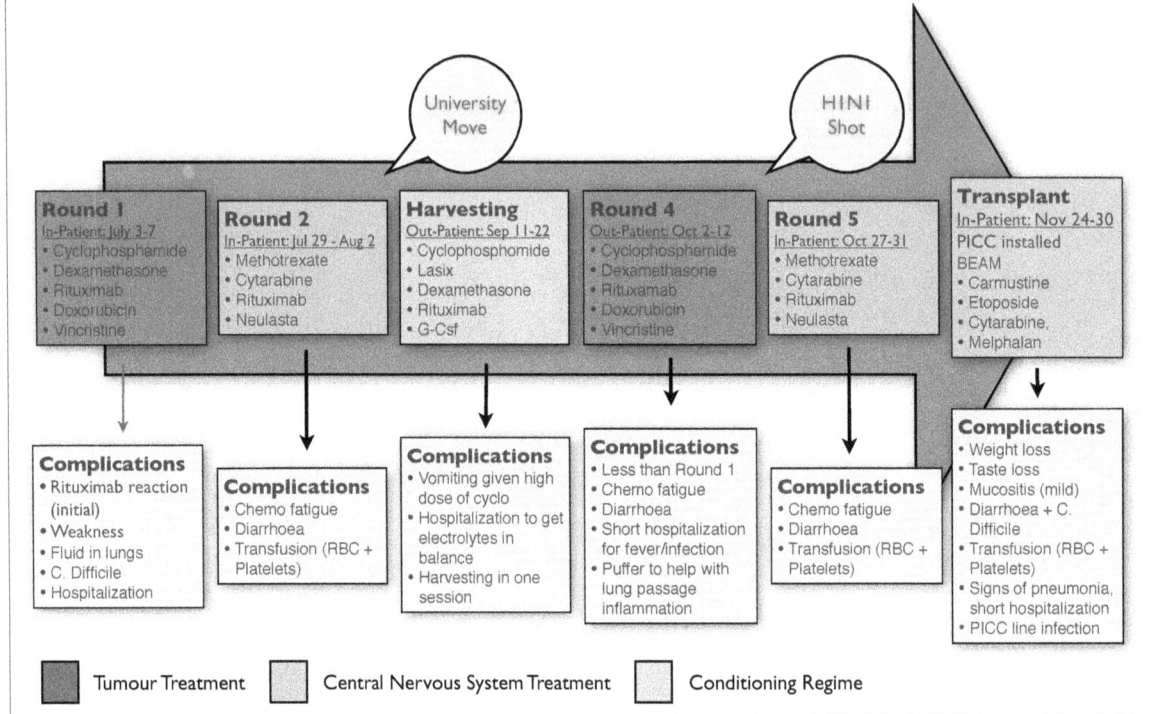

Looking Back:
R Hyper CVAD + Auto SCT

RESTARTING THE CLOCK

January 17, 2010

One of the things that has been at the back of my mind for some time is the question of when it is right for me to 'restart the clock' for my return to 'normal.'

From the medical team's perspective, Day 0 (the day of the stem cell transplant) was the logical time, but given the nature and time span of the recovery process, that seemed premature. Using my planned return to work date in March or April seems a bit too narrow in focus, and the start of the solar new year, while a powerful symbol of rebirth and regeneration, seemed a bit too cute.

Fortuitously, I turned 52 this weekend, and while coincidental, it does seem like a good time to turn the page and focus on the future. Though my physical and mental strength are still being built up, in many if not most respects I am well on my way back to normal. My lymphoma journey, in many ways, has come to its end, as my focus turns towards reintegration into the workplace and my regular activities.

Where my blog is concerned, I have less to write of broad interest as I continue with my new routine of physical and mental conditioning, which includes increasingly becoming familiar with work files. Rather than blogging on a weekly basis to recount my new routine, it seems time to stop the regular updates. Instead, I will just write the occasional post, after the regular clinic visits, to capture the lymphoma journey aspect of my life.

The reflection pieces remain particularly important to me as 'touchstones,' given that there will always be thoughts at the back of my mind regarding possible relapse. Hence the need for me to use my time here wisely and with purpose.

Many thanks to all of you who have read the blog, and have provided me with feedback, encouragement and support throughout the journey. I look forward to seeing you in the next few months as I return to work and regular activities.

CLINIC VISITS – ON TRACK

February 21, 2010

Since I last wrote about a month ago, have had three visits to the clinic (19 Jan, 2 Feb, 16 Feb) and continue to build up my strength. My blood counts continue to improve (white blood cells are now in the low normal range, haemoglobin close to normal), I look healthier (even my hair is well on its way to coming back), and my general energy level is up as well.

My medical team is very pleased with my progress – almost three months since the stem cell regrafting – and, touch wood, there have been no hiccups or complications to date. I am able to relax some of the precautions a bit. I can now go to movie matinées, so I have started to catch up before the Oscars (*Up in the Air, Invictus,* and *Avatar* so far).

I will have a CT scan later this month to confirm formally that everything has cleared up.

My physical and mental conditioning continues, through long walks, language study, and the process of becoming more and more familiar with work files. I am on track to return to work in the latter half of March, and had a good meeting with my boss and management team to help prepare for my return.

In the meantime, I am enjoying the last few weeks of this 'relaxed' life, but looking forward to my return to work and all the interaction and interest that it will entail.

BACK TO WORK - BUT ONE LITTLE THING

March 28, 2010

I have returned to work this week on a part-time basis (three days per week, six hours per day). Great being back with colleagues and friends, and having the sense of being back to 'normal.' I had, of course, forgotten how busy the place was – my team had sheltered me during my absence. I was suddenly confronted with receiving several hundred emails a day, juggling a number of issues, and the usual approving of policy documents and media material.

The subject matter and related public debates remain as interesting as ever. From an energy level, I found that meetings were the most demanding, given the need to be on my toes and read the room and issues in real-time.

Had a good all-staff meeting to see everyone (and for everyone to see me and my new head of hair!) and thank them for their hard work and accomplishments, giving particular thanks to my replacement, who led the team so effectively.

Sharing some of my reflections with the team, particularly those on the importance of people and time, I let them know that I will retire when eligible in 2013 given the nature of my lymphoma. It was a funny feeling; for so long, I have been on an upward trajectory. Then life intervenes, a decision needs to be taken, and I have to stop, concentrating instead on coaching and mentoring the next generation. Filling out the standard 'talent management' forms drove home the point. As an official, seeing my retirement plans in black and white took my breath away for a moment, but I quickly composed myself and reaffirmed this as the right decision for my family and I.

Given that much of what occurs in the workplace has elements of the absurd (this is especially the case in government – think *Yes, Minister*), I asked my team to call me out should I show unhelpful signs of irreverence or cynicism. Hopefully, my new perspective on the importance of people and time will be helpful for leading my group and helping them deliver on government priorities, and will improve the way we work together and with others. If not, my call for feedback will remind me again that I need to focus on the group, not on myself.

My monthly clinic visit was mixed. On the bright side, both my white blood cell and platelet counts are normal, and my haemoglobin is the highest it has been (getting close to normal). On the worrisome side, while my CT scan showed that my lungs are clear, there remains a small tumour in the abdomen. The doctors are not yet sure whether this is simply scar tissue or something more serious, so I will be off to do a PET scan in the next few days. If there is activity, then I will need some radiation treatment, which is relatively easy: 10 minutes a day for five days, minimal side effects. Hopefully this is just a false scare, but it is another worry that neither I nor my family needed just when we thought things were back to normal.

Despite this news, I had a wonderful and funny chat with my doctor, who in light of my being back to work, and my business and pleasure travel plans, said with a smile that I was 'going to be a difficult patient.' She also noted, however, that I was not given a stem cell transplant just so I could 'sit at home and mope,' and that if being back at work was good for my psychological well-being, fine – but that I should take my time ramping up and not overdo it. Good advice!

ALL CLEAR

April 18, 2010

On Monday, my doctor called with the PET scan results and confirmed I was all clear. In medical speak, a negative is a (big) positive!

She normally doesn't call in results, but given that the clinic was overly busy, she made an exception and saved me a day of worry. My wife and I just gave each other a very big and relaxed smile on hearing the news, the accumulated worry at the back of our minds instantly dissipating.

Going through the actual test (like a CT scan but a 'double doughnut'), lasting about 35 minutes, brought back all the memories and worries of the period when I was first being diagnosed. It's funny how the diagnostic phase, for me, is always worse – the uncertainty, the 'what if' questions – than knowing the actual results and getting on with the treatment. Being back at work helped push that concern back into the background; not only does the devil 'find work for idle hands' – so does worry.

Now that I know that I am 'all clear,' I can focus on life and living, with only the general background worry of when my lymphoma could come back.

I have been back at work for about a month now, close to full-time. My energy level has almost returned to normal, but I try to pace myself and manage my time carefully to ensure that I benefit from the energizing aspect of work.

It is interesting to observe what has changed and what has not. There is a much greater emphasis on thorough performance management, a good systemic change reflecting the new Deputy Minister's priorities. The people and issue dynamics appear largely unchanged, and remain as interesting and varied as ever. As always, much of what we do is overly focused on content details and on form or process, and not focused enough on overall objectives and outcomes (the system level). One role I am playing, sometimes effectively, sometimes not, is that of stepping back to the objectives level to help guide the content-level details and processes.

While I have all the patience in the world (and bemusement) for the organizational dynamics and behaviours that form the theatre of life, I have less patience for certain unhelpful behaviour patterns at the individual level, and will have to find positive ways to influence and help address these. When all else fails, I take some deep breaths to collect myself, or go back to the zen 'this too shall pass' thought that often kept me going through chemo.

My reading is now back to issue papers, articles, Powerpoint presentations and reports, some interesting, some less so. I am keeping up with movies, the most recent ones being *An Education* (not entirely believable, but a well-crafted coming-of-age story), *Broken Embraces* by Almodovar (not his best, but wonderful moviemaking-within-moviemaking), and *Katyn* by Wajda (a very powerful retelling of the Katyn massacre, and one that helped me understand the importance of the event to Poland's identity).

CLINIC UPDATE – GRADUATION

May 9, 2010

On Tuesday I had my regular visit to the clinic, and this time I saw the head of the clinic rather than my regular doctor. A good sign, really, as part of the normal process is to see him at the beginning of the stem cell transplant process and at 'graduation,' as he put it (leaving me largely in the hands of other doctors in between). We chatted a bit, and I told him how much I appreciated his warning us of all the potential side effects and discomfort I might have. I also told him that I had gotten through the treatment comparatively lightly, and he replied with the trite but very true 'prepare for the worst, hope for the best' cliché.

I am approaching the six month mark, and am deemed to have come through well, with the lymphoma in remission. I now graduate to the 'long term' blood and marrow transplant (BMT) clinic, another step on the way to full recovery. While I will continue to be monitored regularly, and will have two to three CT scans per year for the next few years, the focus is and should be on living. The head of the clinic was (in contrast to his colleague!) quite pleased to see me back at work and doing my normal activities, and said that I really have no constraints at this stage. However, like most cancer patients, I need to be more careful about exposure to the sun, watch my diet, do exercise, and keep in mind other factors that increase health risk. These are all part of my lifestyle anyway; I just need to be more disciplined with all of them.

As I integrate more into the day-to-day pressures of work, I remain conscious of the need to make time for appreciation and reflection. Walking to and from work gives me a fair amount of that, particularly during the wonderful time of renewal that is spring – a chance to appreciate the colours and scents of all the vegetation, and the play of light on the fresh leaves, all of which give me almost a tingling sensation of life and being alive. At meetings, I concentrate much more on presence – being there – and am more disciplined with my Blackberry. I am also finding a new balance to how and what I delegate, both to manage my workload and to help coach and mentor my team.

I will take my first few business trips over the next month (another part of getting back to normal) at the same time as my team has a number of key government priorities to deliver. Managing this with balance is the next challenge!

Things have been fairly quiet on the movies front. *Coco avant Chanel*, while visually beautiful, was a bit sterile; but rewatching *Les Invasions Barbares*, the wonderful Denys Arcand movie about the love and friendship supporting a man dying of cancer, with wonderful asides on contemporary Quebec, reminded me of how important the support of my family and friends was – and continues to be – throughout my journey.

6 MONTH 'BIRTHDAY'

May 30, 2010

6 months ago, I had my stem cell transplant – my 'birthday' in terms of lymphoma. Like all birthdays, this is more of an abstract marker of time than an accomplishment: for me, the PET scan, the last clinic visit and my 'graduation' to the long-term clinic were more substantive. However, given that each new day is a gift of time to be with people and to do things, this 'birthday' does have meaning.

One person, having seen me in a number of settings over the past few months, told me that I have a real sense of enjoyment of 'being here' and clearly am making the most of the gift of time that my treatment has given me. At the back of my mind is the duality between the gift of time and borrowed time; my mood reflects whether or not I feel that I am using this gift of time well, in terms of being with my family or other people, doing something interesting and meaningful, making a positive impact, going for a walk or bike ride, or even completing more mundane chores like washing the car.

As a reminder to use time well, I am going back to my journal regularly to see where I was a year ago. One year ago exactly, I received the call, following a worrying ultrasound a week earlier, saying that the doctors thought it was lymphoma and ordered a CT scan, biopsy and blood work. I was then in the uncertain stage of not knowing what lay ahead, except that it would not be good. A few weeks later, on the same day as my staff retreat, my lymphoma diagnosis was confirmed; this week, I have another retreat, but this time I can focus on the team, rather than worry about myself. Progress!

I have a certain zen attitude in the workplace, where the dynamics are not under my control, and I increasingly view my role as being one of helping people and issues move forward with a minimum of noise, distraction and fuss. Always interesting to see how e-mail (and other) conversations develop, accelerate, diverge, and reconverge; in some ways, there is a lot of 'chatter' where one or two messages would have sufficed, but this is part of us being people. We need to converse and develop agreement.

I have been travelling more, meeting more stakeholders on a variety of files. I appreciate sense of possibility, and the range of life experiences and perspectives, that different people bring to the issues. These may not always be easy to manage, but therein lies what is interesting about people and society. I will be travelling internationally in the next few weeks, and therefore will have additional opportunities to and reflect on different approaches and perspectives as I work on the particular issues and files.

All-in-all, I keep coming back to my key reflections on the importance of people and the value of time as I continue the journey.

CLINIC UPDATE – DOING FINE

June 27, 2010

Another clinic visit, another series of small milestones. I am off one medication, and am being re-immunized with all the shots I had so many years ago as a child; part of my rebirth.

Reflecting an increase in the number of cases of lymphoma (sign of the times and the environment), the hospital has started another lymphoma clinic, specifically for stem cell transplant patients like me. As the new clinic's first patient, I have a head start to be the longest surviving one. Another goal to keep me focused on life!

I asked my doctor about a study by a Lyon-based team on the successful use of Rituxan after treatment to reduce return rates of lymphoma. Reassuringly, he was very familiar with the study and findings, but noted that it was for follicular, not mantle cell lymphoma (MCL). The hospital has provided this treatment (quarterly Rituxan and CT scans) for the past 10 years. While effective, the treatment has the side effect of adding to patient anxiety levels, given the frequency of CT scans.

I am always impressed by the extent to which doctors and members of the medical team are focused on their patients' psychological well-being in addition to treatment. It reminds me of what appears to me to be the converse situation, as described in a New York Times article on the MD Anderson Cancer Centre, where the obsession seems to be more on treatment and technology, rather than on quality of life.

My doctor reminded me, gently, that we only know how to treat MCL, and not yet how to cure it. While this remains a sobering background thought, my hope is to have as long a remission as possible, perhaps aided by the development of new and improved treatments by the time my MCL comes back.

From a day-to-day perspective: my energy levels are good, I have been getting lots of walks and exercise, and I am enjoying work and the time with my family. I had a great work trip to Europe, with interesting and varied meetings, some with old colleagues, some with new. I enjoyed all of these on both a professional and personal level.

A highlight was discovering the Vélib bicycle system in Paris, and cycling from place to place rather than taking the metro. It brought a real sense of freedom and discovery, once I got out of my North American, coddled worry about traffic and riding without a helmet (though I still rode defensively!). There were also some good opportunities to catch up with family and friends, who were all relieved to see me looking so healthy and well.

A year ago, I was in the process of telling family, friends and colleagues about my diagnosis, and my planned absence from work; all involved were in shock. This time, my family and I have been sharing that we are all off for a major holiday to Australia next week, to visit friends and discover a new (for us) continent. What a difference a year makes! It will be a real holiday to treasure and enjoy, after all we have been through together.

WHAT A DIFFERENCE A YEAR MAKES

August 29, 2010

Last summer I had my first cycles of chemo, experienced considerable side effects, and spent much of the summer in and out of the hospital. This summer, I am back to life and living with a great trip visiting friends in Australia. To top it off, I got my CT scan results this past week: 'as good as it gets,' according to my doctor.

In Australia, the lushness, diversity and variety of life of the tropical rainforest near Port Douglas and the Great Barrier Reef moved me more than the aridity and desolation around Uluru (Ayers Rock), even though previously I had always been fascinated by desert-like landscapes in the Middle East and South America. There is something about the vitality of life. Even in the desert, I felt a sense of wonder at how 'life will find a way' in an inhospitable environment, rather than at the landscape itself.

Of course, being with friends, and seeing our respective children renew and further strengthen their friendship, was equally life-affirming.

Overall, it was a wonderful holiday for all of us together, and a great way to celebrate coming through the treatment and worries of the past year.

I am discovering a new duality – being of this world and not of this world. I feel as if I participate and yet have distance, and am almost an observer. Tom Ford's *A Single Man* captured some of this dynamic of something lost, and somehow – through effective filming and editing – captured the distance well. I sometimes have to remind myself to 'drag' myself out of observing and back to being, but at the same time take advantage of a more detached perspective on things.

The same day as I received the good news about my CT scan, I visited a colleague who has just been diagnosed with cancer. I am coming out of the tunnel, and my colleague is going in; but both of us were able to share our fears and worries, as well as our blessings, and provide each other support in a way that reflects our direct personal experience. Also, this month one of my brothers had a serious operation, and I found myself helping to talk him through his worries. A chance to give back, after all the support people have given me, and another strong reminder to live fully and focus on what is important.

In the giving back spirit, I have found myself drawn into participating in the annual Light the Night Walk, organized by the Leukemia and Lymphoma Society of Canada. I generally feel uncomfortable about such kinds of events, preferring to make personal donations; for better or worse, however, lymphoma is one of my identities, which is drawing me in this direction.

As September starts, our kids are returning to school and university (and our parliamentarians to Parliament!), reminding me again of renewal, growth and getting back to the normal annual cycle of our busy lives.

ONE YEAR 'BIRTHDAY'

November 28, 2010

One year ago, I received my stem cell transplant; six months ago, I was back at work and deemed to be in remission. Looking back at my journal and the roughness of my treatment, I keep on marvelling at and appreciating life.

Apart from a hard-to-shake cold in September, my general resistance has been good, and I have had to take fewer absences than many colleagues. I had one scare with what I thought was a lump, but the CT scan showed that all is clear ('perfect,' according to my doctor). Likely just a small hernia, something to get fixed but nothing to worry about (all this after worrying, of course, for the few weeks between sensing the lump and the scan results, dreading that lymphoma may have come back far too quickly). My blood counts are good, apart from platelets being a bit low. I am now on six-month, rather than three-month, scan cycle, and will probably shift to MRI to reduce radiation exposure. As good as it gets!

Some real lows and highs over the past few months. The colleague diagnosed with cancer mentioned in my last post passed away quickly, about 10 days after I saw her. Everyone was in shock, over both her death and the speed with which it occurred, although some of us knew the grim odds. For me, a double shock: first, the shock of her death itself, and secondly, the sharp reminder of my own vulnerability, reinforced by the sense, through sharing with friends and colleagues our memories of her life, of pre-living what might take place should the same thing happen to me. I felt like Tom Sawyer at this own funeral; it was both weird and disturbing.

A few months later, another low: helping our daughter deal with the suicide of one of her classmates; feeling the grief myself as a parent; seeing how the school community, and the community of the victim's family, dealt with the grief, and with supporting her family. I was again reminded, all too vividly, of just how precious life is, and how important it is to savour each and every moment and support one another.

On the highs side, my wife and I took a wonderful 20th wedding anniversary trip to Paris, enjoying the city, the food, the life; it both brought back memories and built new ones. An opportunity to savour life in all its aspects, and one to be repeated. We also had a nice, short trip to Toronto to celebrate our son's birthday with him, and enjoyed being with him and seeing how he continues to grow and develop as a person and in his interests.

I am also getting better, during business trips, at finding some time for myself: to walk, to explore, to enjoy, and to meet up with friends. Even short catch-up opportunities are to be treasured. There is a real spiritual side to some of my walks as I imbibe the light, the feeling, and the history of some of the places work calls me to.

Overall, I have been having lots of fun at work as we develop new ideas, push them along, and bring them to the point of implementation.

My personal reading continues to suffer in favour of required work reading, but film remains. Two to highlight. First, *El Secreto de Sus Ojos*, a wonderful Argentine movie about memory, reality, loss and refinding. Beautifully crafted, and again a reminder of the preciousness of life. Since I lived in Argentina for a few years right after the military dictatorship, the theme of remembering and forgetting resonated particularly. Second, *Hereafter*, the Clint Eastwood film on people dealing with what might be next. Again, beautifully crafted in terms of how three stories are brought together (although others in my family were less moved by the overall theme).

QUICK UPDATE – BLOOD COUNTS

December 5, 2010

Blood count results in and up for all, including platelets where my doctor had some concern. Nice bit of good news as I head into the holidays.

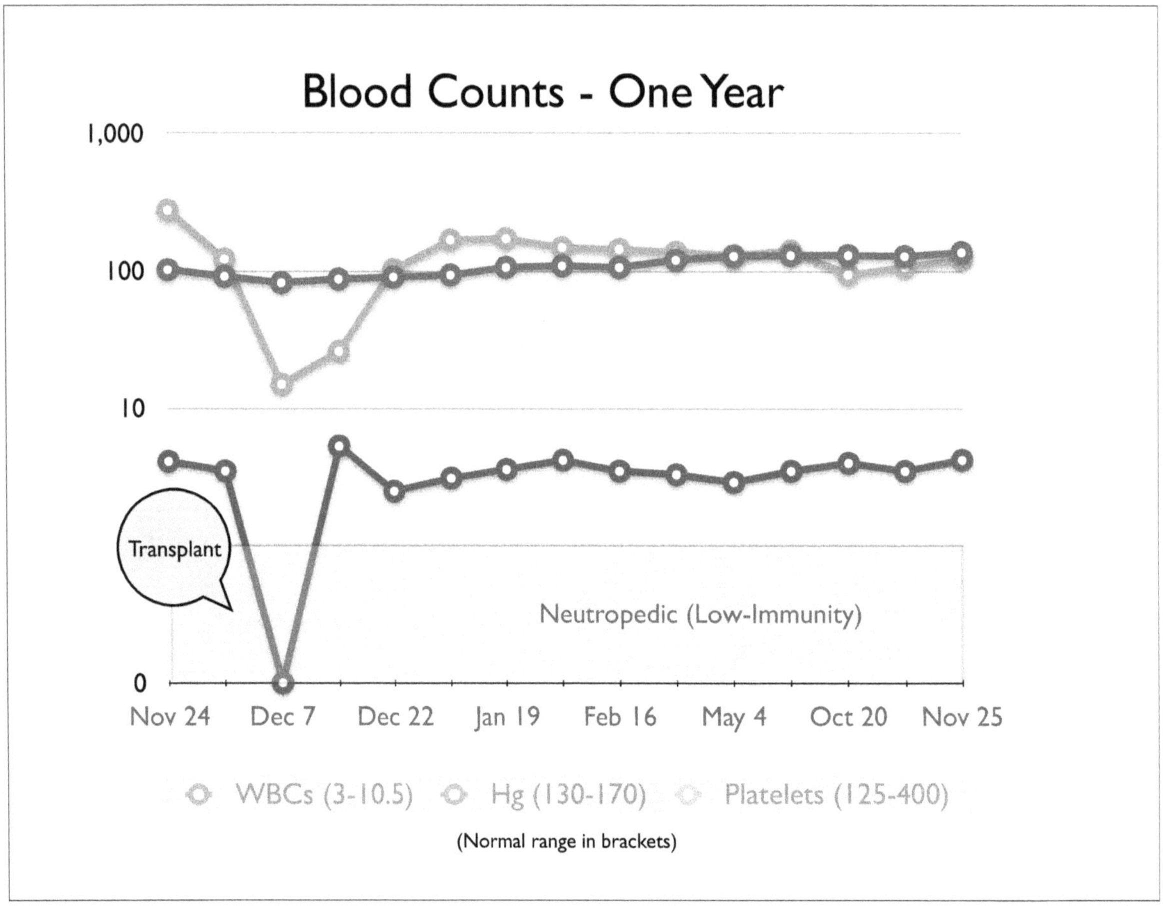
Blood Counts - One Year
1,000
100
10
0
Transplant
Neutropedic (Low-Immunity)
Nov 24
Dec 7
Dec 22
Jan 19
Feb 16
May 4
Oct 20
Nov 25
WBCs (3-10.5)
Hg (130-170)
Platelets (125-400)
(Normal range in brackets)

2010 IN REVIEW – BLOG STATS

January 2, 2011

An update from Wordpress on my blog in 2010:

'The stats helper monkeys at WordPress.com mulled over how this blog did in 2010, and here's a high level summary of its overall blog health:

The Blog-Health-o-Meter™ reads Fresher than ever.

A Boeing 747-400 passenger jet can hold 416 passengers. This blog was viewed about 1,800 times in 2010. That's about 4 full 747s.

In 2010, there were 12 new posts, growing the total archive of this blog to 40 posts. There were 7 pictures uploaded, taking up a total of 34mb.

The busiest day of the year was November 19th with 98 views. The most popular post that day was Week 8 – My 'Chemo Holiday'.

Where did they come from?

The top referring sites in 2010 were community.lls.org, mail.yahoo.com,mail.live.com, cancercompass.com, and en.wordpress.com.

Some visitors came searching, mostly for lymphoma, my lymphoma journey by andrew, lymphoma journey, www.mylymphomajourney.wordpress.com, and lymphomajourney wordpress.

Attractions in 2010

These are the posts and pages that got the most views in 2010.

1. *Week 8 – My 'Chemo Holiday' August 2009*

2. *About my Blog October 2009*

3. *Healthcare System November 2009*

4. *What a difference a year makes August 2010*

5. *Lessons Learned November 2009*

In closing, Happy New Year to all of you.

THANK-YOU VIDEO

January 9, 2011

A friend of mine sent us this video – great reminder of all the people who continue to 'Stand by Me' and wonderful message on the universality of music and the creativity and joy it brings.

Stand by Me

ONE LESS THING TO WORRY ABOUT

January 16, 2011

No worries. The small hernia that caused me a scare in November was looked at last week and no need for an operation. Less time in hospital is good!

Quick update on films I have seen and liked: *Social Network* (great screenplay, acting, and captures a story and culture that keeps on going), *Black Swan* (obsession), Inception (clever playing with reality), *True Grit* (wonderful sparse storytelling and look), *The King's Speech* (great dynamic between the King and Logue his speech therapist), and *Mao's Last Dancer* (inspiring life story of the growth, exile and return of a leading Chinese dancer).

And for books, finally read *Night* by Elie Wiesel, the classical Holocaust novel, and also had the privilege to hear him speak, an incredibly powerful and moving experience, given his use of words and the deepness of his reflections. And *A Very Brief History of Eternity* by Carlos Eire, an interesting history of how the concept has evolved throughout history (brief as it is), and the possible rapprochement between theology and cosmology, engagingly written with a fair amount of wit.

As another birthday approaches, along with the new year, looking forward to more 'no worries'.

Chapter 6

Dualities

We are often pulled in different, opposing directions, and take time to find the balance between acceptance and anger, surrender and control, individual and group, being and thinking, living and dying. How we find balance and what that balance is influences our attitude.

Throughout my journey, I was struck by a number of dichotomies, or dualities, as I reflected on my reactions and the reactions of those around me. Looking at my reactions through a framework of opposites or contrasts gave me a better sense of where I was on a continuum, and how my state of mind evolved over time. When I was having a good week, I was clearly leaning in one direction; during a bad week, I would lean toward the other. Recognizing the dynamic prevented me from veering into depression or, at the other extreme, Panglossian optimism.

My attempts at staying centered were challenged when I relapsed much sooner than expected, after only 14 months. It took me longer to get back in the same space, and that round of treatment was harder on me. Given my treatment options – do nothing and have further relapses and death within a few years, or go the high risk route of an allogeneic stem cell transplant – the stakes seemed higher.

Here I explain some of the dualities that I came back to most often, which evolved over time.

Acceptance / Anger

A lot of my cancer-related reading, and some comments by friends and family, focussed on anger being a normal reaction. How can this happen to me? Why me, married with two children, rather than my brothers, who are not? Do all my efforts to keep fit, eat well, and have a balanced life mean nothing?

Relapse made it worse – why could I not have the average 3-5 years before relapse?

However, I never really surrendered completely to anger, even during the difficult days coming to terms with my relapse and the brutal options I faced. Anger did not help me or my family and friends deal with what I ultimately had to accept and take as a given, fair or not. The darkness of anger, and its corollary, depression, simply did not resonate with what I had to do to get through the treatment, and my need to support family and friends in their support for me. Eckhart Tolle's discussion of acceptance was helpful here, as was the focus on acceptance in many religions.

Surrender / Control

A related duality is that of surrender and control. While much of the cancer literature features language like 'fight,' 'combat' and 'cure,' I found myself more inclined to surrender to the fact that I was no longer in control. I had to rely on my medical team for their advice and direction. I had to rely on family and friends for practical and especially emotional support. I also had to rely on my colleagues and workplace for support during my absence. I am used to being in control, so having my life in the hands of others shifted my perspective, and gave me a new appreciation for the importance of other people. Interdependence and the trust in others that it entails became key to how I saw my relationship with family, friends, colleagues and my medical team.

While overall I needed to surrender, I also needed to figure out where I could and should exercise control. Surrender was the big picture, but the devil was in the details. I was personally able to find control on a number of levels.

First, I engaged substantively with my medical team and made an effort to be on top of my 'file.' Post-relapse, I became even more involved. I provided more feedback when things were not moving quickly enough, made stronger and more pointed suggestions regarding treatment options, and insisted on getting a second opinion.

Secondly, and on the emotional and psychological levels, having some control meant using the time available to me during the treatment – and between treatments – to achieve something. For me, this was a mix of walking with my wife (wonderful time to connect with her, plus the comfort of physical movement and enjoying nature and being outdoors) as well as ensuring that I remained connected to my kids. It also meant coming up with a reading list, based on my own interests and suggestions by friends, to keep me intellectually engaged and alive, rather than spend my time watching videos. Travel, both during my remission (family holiday to Australia, Paris getaway with my wife) and between the 'salvage' chemo and my stem cell transplant (another Paris getaway with my wife) was also important for experiencing life and creating memories.

Thirdly, writing has been a way for me to make sense of it all. During my initial treatment, my writing took the form of a daily journal, in which I kept track of what I was going through, emotionally and physically. This was reinforced by my weekly updates to staff and colleagues, which then turned into my blog. In the initial phase of my relapse treatment, I focussed more on the blog, developing it further by finding and sharing health-related articles that resonated with me. The mechanics of the 'salvage' chemo, and the largely repetitive nature of the side effects, were less interesting, and the emotional and treatment option discussions were best captured in the blog. And similarly, I captured the various ups and downs (mainly ups – I was lucky) in my allo SCT and recovery period, allowing myself for some more in-depth commentary on books that particularly interested me.

Individual / Group

One of the first bits of advice I received was about the importance of looking after myself. In a very real sense, this was true – the lymphoma affected me, I was the one being treated, and I was the one whose mortality was in question.

Yet at the same time, it was not just about me. First of all, it was about my family, the impact that my journey was having on them, and how much we all relied on each other. It was about my friends, and it was also about my colleagues, with whom, again, I have a degree of mutual reliance and support.

My focus shifted from the 'me' to 'the group,' and what I could and should do to help them. The degree to which I could support them, by being open and sharing what I was going through, and focusing on acceptance rather than anger, would in turn help them provide more support to me – a self-reinforcing circle of support. For me, it was about myself with the group, not myself as an individual. Interdependence, not independence.

This became even more acute when I had to faced the options of doing nothing, and essentially having up to 2 years to live, or taking the high risk of the stem cell transplant in the hope of living longer. When my son asked me what I thought of these options, right after I received a brutal second opinion, my first thought was about the importance of being there longer for my family. Were I alone, doing nothing and avoiding the risks of the stem cell transplant might have been attractive. Since I have a family, however, being with them for as long as possible and for more of my kids' milestones took priority.

Being / Thinking

Partially influenced by Eckhart Tolle, I was struck by simple awareness as distinct from thinking and analyzing. My natural personality is analytical, which has served me well professionally, but has led to struggles at the emotional and psychological levels. Being required to reflect on something like my mortality, which in many ways defies analysis, was salutary and helped me come to greater awareness. In many cases, 'being' was as simple as going for walks and trying to be more observant of and attentive to natural beauty, whether the flowers, trees, birdsong, the way the light played with the leaves, or the spectacularly vibrant fall colours. It was ensuring that I was truly there when talking with my family (the Blackberry was off both literally and figuratively – and it felt good when I finally gave it up!). When I was particularly weak, I found comfort in listening to classical music and just letting the music wash over and through me. My Paris getaway with my wife between treatments gave both of us a much-needed break from the rock and a hard place options before me (and before us). I did not meditate, but made a more conscious effort to find moments when I could simply to be, rather than analyze.

I also found outlets for my analytical tendencies: being on top of my file for when I met with my specialists, doing extensive reading, and writing this blog and my daily journal all helped me analyze what I was going through and helped me feel more in control.

Overall attitude

Finding the right balance between acceptance/anger, surrender/control, individual/group and being/thinking helped me develop the attitude necessary to not only 'carry on,' but also appreciate the good days and moments.

Much of the literature and folk wisdom stresses the importance of attitude. I am not sure this has been empirically demonstrated to affect overall lymphoma success rates (i.e., through control groups – see How positive thinking affects patients with serious illnesses). However, it clearly made the journey easier on me and the people who care about me. It also helped me enjoy and appreciate what I have – especially the people in my life, and time spent with them and doing things I enjoy. Many people commented on my positive attitude, and their comments in turn reinforced this attitude.

I am not referring to the delusional positive thinking that Barbara Ehrenreich rightly criticizes in Bright Sided. After all, cancer, particularly an aggressive form like mantle cell lymphoma, is not just a 'learning opportunity.' Nor can any measure of positive thinking wish it away.

However, given the alternative, having a positive attitude in dealing with cancer, and sharing that attitude with family and friends, makes an enormous difference. When I was suffering from side effects, 'this too must pass' was my way of getting through. When I felt better, I usually made a conscious effort to take advantage of that time, by being with family and friends, going for walks, reading, and doing a number of small projects (organizing family photos and videos, writing this blog).

After relapse, facing a stem cell transplant and attendant risks, having a positive attitude was much harder. The odds were poor (only 2 of 5 people make it) and there was the risk of a seriously compromised quality of life from chronic Graft versus Host Disease (GvHD). For me, this last possibility was a greater fear than death.

Fortunately, I made it to the one-year mark with only mild GvHD, and only a few bumps in the road after the first few rough months.

Living / Dying

The ultimate duality.

While the other dualities came early and easily to me, it was only later on, well after the immediate danger zone of my allo SCT, that I realized that I had missed the obvious duality between living and dying. Perhaps it was already embedded in the decisions I took, my wish to be as active as possible, and my 'this too shall pass' attitude when times were rough.

I think that, for most of us who have cancer or face death for other reasons, the living/dying duality makes us more appreciative of the present moment, not taking time for granted, and shifting our focus to the short-term – when we can do things – from the more uncertain longer-term.

Chapter 7

Faith

We all come from different backgrounds, perspectives and religions. Being in a near-death situation sharpens our internal questions – 'Why me?' We each find our own answers as we become more reflective about our place in the world and how we should live our lives.

As I go through this journey, questions of mortality and of 'why me' are always in the background, no matter how much I try to focus on the here and now.

That this journey has heightened my sense of awe and wonder seems important to me, a feeling that I share with many others who have cancer, heart attacks, or other life threatening conditions. What strikes me are the little things: the interplay of light and shadow; the effervescence of spring and the flameout of autumn; the variety and beauty of cloud formations and colours at sunset; the rhythms of the ocean; a starry sky, and any image from the Hubble; the spirituality of music, whether Bach or Cohen; art, whether classical or modern; babies, and watching and helping my own 'babies' grow up; good design (Apple, not Dell). Others will have their own list, but wondering, rather than taking for granted, is an important change and reflection point.

The combination of wonder and 'why me' questions raises further questions about faith and belief. I am always touched when I hear that family members and friends from a variety of faiths were praying – and continue to pray – for me. I was struck by one remark from close friends, strong believers. They observed, with a combination of surprise and comfort, just how similar our overall perspectives were, irrespective of our individual religious views and practices.

Although I have strong personal connections with all three Abrahamic religions, I am non-practicing and my perspective is, overall, secular. To better understand my thoughts on faith and religion, I did what I always do: I started to read more and more about the subject. My readings ranged from the explicative (Karen Armstrong, Robert Wright) to the more prescriptive (C.S. Lewis), to books that express a sense of wonder at life and the universe (Richard Dawkins, Stephen Hawking, Carlos Eire).

The explicative books resonated strongly for me, as they highlighted the common patterns and universal elements in many world religions, as well as how historical context shaped each religion without disrupting core beliefs.

The combination of friends and family and readings also heightened my appreciation for and understanding of the sense of purpose and community provided by faith and religion, and the comfort and meaning that come from ritual and ceremony. However, this did not speak to me as much as the more universal messages (like the 'Golden Rule': treat others as you would like to be treated), and how these universal messages have evolved and continue to evolve over time (like human rights arguably being an extension of these core messages).

The more science-based readings (*The Greatest Show on Earth*, *A Brief History of Time* and *A Brief History of Eternity*) have all sharpened my sense of wonder at the universe and at the phenomenon of life, reminding me not to take things for granted. Given the sophistication and almost magical quality of nature and scientific laws, these books also gave me an appreciation for how faith might operate at the highest level while being consistent with a scientific understanding of how the world works.

In many ways, this complements the heightened sense of awe at nature that I have developed post-cancer. From a macro perspective, the workings of the universe, relativity, evolution and the scientific laws that underpin them, are all wondrous and impressive. The Eternity book ends with an interesting parallel between modern cosmology and theology, suggesting that these two may be, in a broad sense, complementary and convergent.

I cannot believe in a power that takes personal interest in my fate or the fates of others. Elie Wiesel's denunciation in *Night* rings all too true:

> What are You, my God? I thought angrily. How do You compare to this
> stricken mass gathered to affirm to You their faith, their anger, their
> defiance? What does Your grandeur mean, Master of the Universe, in the
> face of all this cowardice, this decay, and this misery? Why do you go on
> troubling these poor people's wounded minds, their ailing bodies?

Unfortunately, human history is rife with examples other than the Holocaust of when God appears to have been missing, beyond the individual trials and tribulations that we all face during our lifetimes.

Of course, Elie Wiesel's thinking evolved from his immediate anger at God after the Holocaust to a more nuanced and richer view of his faith later on in his life, as described in his book *Coeur ouvert*.

For me, the existence of a less personal power behind the universe (or universes) is more of an open question. Natural and scientific laws, as far as we understand them, do not preclude such a power. I do not mean this in the mechanical sense of intelligent design, but in respect to more general questions: Why a universe? Why life?

I do not mean to be critical of those who do believe in a more personal power or God. I am not opposed to whatever helps people interpret and understand our complex world and our place in it, and provides comfort and a sense of not being alone – as long as faith and its expression allows, recognizes, and respects the universal qualities that unite all of us. Not just tolerating, but welcoming. One example can be found in the film *Of Gods and Men*: the trust and caring between the monks (Catholic) and the local village people (Muslim) and the closing remarks by the lead monk, whose last thoughts are about how much he wants to see the 'Children of Islam' in his next life. There are many more examples of coexistence in our day-to-day lives.

Faith is very much part of the human condition, and thus sterile debates over whether God exists or not appear meaningless to me (hear that, Richard Dawkins!).

So, to answer the questions that I started with: Why me? Why mortality? Luck of the draw, randomness, no great or modest design. It just is, and is where I end up. This may not necessarily be satisfying, but it is something that I accept and live with.

I am only left with the more fundamental question: given the lot we have, how should we live our lives? Whether we arrive at the answer through faith or through a secular approach is secondary.

Chapter 8

Lessons

Some lessons emerge from the experience of having cancer, all of which contribute to our overall attitude towards life and living.

In contrast to my dualities, which helped me understand what I was going through and how I was reacting – and should react – to my lymphoma treatment, a number of themes or general lessons were important to me over the longer term. These first occurred to me about a month or so into my diagnosis, and I kept coming back to them, during good days and bad, as reminders of what I wanted to take away for the future. Thinking about these lessons during treatment, and having them to refer to in the future, is my way of ensuring that I continue to reflect on what matters as I return to 'normal' life.

While my relapse threw into question whether my life would ever be 'normal' again, my perspective on these lessons has remained, at least so far, remarkably consistent with my first thoughts on the subject two years ago.

Time changes

After a cancer diagnosis, one's mortality becomes more imminent, no matter how good – or bad – the prognosis. The question of how to best use one's time in the short, medium, and long term becomes more important. Work-life balance is not just a daily, weekly or monthly matter, but is also crucial in terms of years. What one does in all spheres of life becomes crucial and requires reflection.

After my diagnosis, I was struck by how my focus shifted from questions of short- and medium-term work-life balance to longer-term, almost existential questions. Facing my own mortality made me reflect on the fact that, unlike my parents, I will not live into my eighties – even making it to my sixties is a stretch. I then wondered what this shorter-than-expected lifespan would mean for my retirement plans (the sooner the better) and how I wanted to spend my time in general. I continue to reflect one these questions, coming back to them on a regular basis. My relapse answered the question about my retirement plans – I went on long-term disability, where I will likely stay until shortly before my retirement, marking the end of my professional career.

People are the focus

I learned to appreciate who really cares, who is important, and which relationships will become stronger and which will fade. Some of my friendships became much closer, others withered away. Aside from friendships, I have also become much more conscious of the need to focus on people in general – what drives them, what motivates them – to ensure that I relate to others on a deeper, personal basis.

I stopped taking people for granted. I consciously organized my time to have more 'being there' time with family and friends. Walks are my favourite way of doing this, as I find that I am more engaged when walking than sitting. My daily walks with my wife were particularly important, providing an opportunity for us to talk things through and just enjoy being together.

Of course, I am also more aware of what other people may be going through, and recognize my responsibility to provide them with support when they need it. Looking back, I am not sure that I always fulfilled this responsibility. Now, knowing how important this kind of support is, I will be all the more conscious of the need to make an effort.

To help people help me, I started sharing articles that helped other people have a better sense of what to say or do to a person in my situation. What to Say to Someone who is Sick and A Doctor's Letter to a Patient with Newly Diagnosed Cancer were particularly powerful articles that people commented and reflected upon.

Sharing

Part of putting the emphasis on people is sharing – sharing what you are going through and creating space for others to share. This is an important point whether or not cancer is in the mix. It transforms discussions from mere content and transactions to opportunities for a deeper connection, a connection that helps on both the personal and professional levels.

I made a deliberate effort to increase the depth of my e-mails to friends and coworkers, and later my blog. Many people responded more sincerely in turn, strengthening our relationships. After my relapse, the tone of my blog entries became even more personal, and about twice as long, on average, as they had been before – a reflection of the fact that I was exploring and sharing more.

Count your blessings

My Aunt Myrra, who had a hard life, often told me, 'count your blessings.' I found the saying irritating at the time, but now that I am older and (I hope) wiser, it resonates with me. Materially, I had a very supportive employer with generous sick leave provisions, a good medical plan, and a good long-term disability plan, which allowed me to take time off work without worrying about finances.

Other blessings include the strong emotional support of my family, friends and colleagues, a very comfortable lifestyle compared to most people, and the insights that have come from my journey with cancer. Good days – and most days were good – were also blessings, to be valued and to be made good use of.

Be in the moment

My lessons about Time, People, and Sharing all require that I be in the moment. At the same time, planning moments and making the space for them gives them meaning. When you have ups and downs in your treatment, you will quickly identify whether the present moment is a 'this too shall pass' one, or whether you are in a moment when your health and mental state will allow you to enjoy and be enthusiastic about life.

Given that my first part of the journey could be compared to boxing rounds (knocked down only to get up again) or a roller coaster (choose your metaphor), planning for the moments when I would feel better helped me take advantage of those moments. My plans usually revolved around people: timing my son's visits from Toronto, seeing friends and colleagues, going out to movies and restaurants when my immunity allowed. This really helped put the 'this too shall pass' moments into perspective.

Taking advantage of the break between the 'salvage' chemo and the stem cell transplant for a Paris getaway was another example. Of course, this break was different in character; less 'this too shall pass' and more 'enjoy while you can' in light of what lay ahead.

Do something meaningful, to the extent that your condition and feelings allow. As I mentioned earlier, my focus was on daily walks with my wife, often for two to three hours in a day. The physical activity was secondary to the emotional connection that these walks fostered. To my surprise, I spent relatively little time watching TV or movies, choosing instead to read. I also shared my reading list with friends and colleagues, who appreciated the suggestions, though not without some jealousy about my 'chemo sabbatical.' I also used my time to do some of the things that I had rarely found time for in the past: organizing family photos, videos, the family tree and the like, which was another expression of my focus on family.

My updates and blog engaged me in reflection about what I was going through, gave me a sense of how people reacted to my thoughts, and were also an opportunity for me to learn about blogging. In addition, though I was away from the office (at first temporarily, then permanently), I tried to provide some coaching and mentoring to my replacements, while ensuring that they had the space to grow and develop on their own.

Attitude

All of these lessons – along with my 'dualities' framework – helped me maintain the positive attitude required to get through lymphoma treatment the first time around, and then face the much harder challenge of relapse and an allogeneic stem cell transplant. While there are always 'dark thoughts' in the background (these were darkest at relapse), they are normal and manageable and do not overwhelm me or plunge me into depression. Being open about these also helps my family members deal with their own 'dark thoughts' rather than ignore them.

Following my first round of treatment, I faced the challenge of reintegrating into the workplace and my normal busy life. While I largely 'plunged back in,' these lessons, along with background anxiety about whether or not my treatment was effective, were never far from my thoughts – my experience was too close to me in the short-term.

I never really made it to the medium-term challenge of ensuring that these lessons continued to be lived in my day-to-day existence, since my remission was so short. I was, however, able to come back to the lessons periodically, as I had written them down and shared them through my blog. I also had help from many of the readers who know me (starting with my family), who occasionally reminded me of the lessons when I appeared to stray!

In the longer-term, the lessons I have identified here helped ground me after my relapse, and helped me get through the allogenic stem cell transplant and accompanying period of high risk. As the painful memories continue to recede, these lessons will remain important to remember as I go on with my 'new normal.'

Chapter 9

Relapse

My world is turned upside down when I relapse after only one year's reprieve. I am depressed and despondent. I start salvage chemotherapy and am faced with a difficult choice: certain death if I eschew treatment, or the uncertain odds of an allogeneic stem cell transplant.

ROLLERCOASTER

February 27, 2011

It has been a roller coaster of a month. On the positive side, I have been outside and enjoying the winter weather, cross-country skiing and skating.

On the less good side, I have been having vision and headache issues which came to a head a few weeks ago when I had to go to Emergency. I felt dizzy and had trouble walking, classic stroke symptoms. They ran the usual tests – blood, ECG, movement, brain CT scan – which showed nothing abnormal. These were followed a few days later by ultrasounds of my heart and arteries. Everything was done very quickly, with minimal wait times. As a high-risk patient, I get quicker attention!

Then the neurologist this week. I took the usual motion, coordination and strength tests, plus a lifestyle questionnaire. A stroke was ruled out, but given my history, we will do a MRI brain scan and EEG to ensure that nothing else is going on. I was taken off aspirin, given no restrictions on activity, and we all breathed a real sigh of relief.

A day later, I was in the comical situation of conducting a conference call when the symptoms came back, just as they had before. I soldiered through the call (no one the wiser according to a colleague) and then called 911 to get an ambulance. A bit disruptive to leave the office that way!

There was the usual wait at the hospital, and a repeat of the stroke tests – all negative. Their assessment was that my symptoms were likely just due to a severe migraine. No major restrictions on my activities. Late that night, a severe headache, accompanied by some weakness and dizziness, woke me up. I did the usual stroke tests (which I can now self-administer) and found no issues.

I then went to my regular lymphoma clinic to see my hematologist who said that to have migraines following chemo, while rare, is not unheard of in patients of my age. He put me back on monthly recall pending the results of the remaining tests.

I felt a real fear and sense of despair while waiting in emergency the first time, feeling that just as I was back to being active, things were falling apart. A Doors song, '*The End*,' played over and over in my mind, as I felt that I was letting my family down again. While the routine of hospital tests helped wash the waves of emotion away, this was a sharp reminder of my vulnerability and of how my treatment has aged me. The second time, my reaction was more mixed: the bizarre sensation of conducting a meeting with such thoughts in the background, followed by a more mundane irritation with the whole hospital routine, and then the question of whether I really have the heart for the roller coaster of emotions that these events bring.

I am also part of a study on the psychological effects of lymphoma treatment in terms of memory, concentration and attitude. While I know that I am not as sharp or as focussed before, and that my short-term memory is weaker, the questionnaire reassured me by providing me with the context to see that I am not doing so bad after all.

A few interesting movies of note: *The Kids are All Right*, a well-crafted family drama with a twist; *Blue Valentine*, a claustrophobic tale of romance gone sour; *Biutiful*, an almost unrelievedly depressing, although wonderfully acted by Javier Bardem, life story of death and despair in the slums of Barcelona (these are not the neighbourhoods of *Vicky Christina Barcelona*); and *Winter's Bone*, a depressing tale of Ozark society held together by the strength of a young girl trying to keep her siblings and mother together. I will have to watch some more cheery movies in the future.

NOT OUT OF THE WOODS

March 6, 2011

A busy week. I had an EEG on Monday to rule out seizures, and a MRI Tuesday to get a finer view. It was my first time with both tests. Each have elements of Chinese water torture (EEG features intense flashing light at varying frequency, and an MRI is like being inside a jack hammer with all the vibration and noise). Ironically, these tests took place during the same week as my daughter's school play on brain disorders, *Night Sky*, her videos for which included MRI brain scans.

The results of the tests were mixed. The EEG was clear, but the MRI showed advanced arthritis in my neck, which explains my neck pain and stiffness. More significantly, however, it also showed inflammation of the leptomeninges, two of the membranes surrounding the brain. This could simply be due to post-chemo irritation of a pre-existing condition, or more seriously, it could signal the return of lymphoma. The end result is another test – a lumbar puncture for a sample of my brain/spinal cord fluid, to examine the blood cells and, hopefully, rule out lymphoma.

Not great news, but I am not yet sure to what extent. I will know about a week after the lumbar puncture, which is this coming Friday.

In the meantime, the headaches and vision blurring episodes have been minor and manageable. I am also adapting to my hearing aids, and finding that they sometimes trigger an episode. Finding the right balance between hearing better and not getting headaches is a bit of a challenge. Trade-offs!

I have started letting people at work know about what I am going through. It is never easy, but going through this the second time is more matter of fact than, as before, existential. Family and friends are harder to tell, as none of us expected this possibility so soon. It's not over until it's over, however. While my normal optimism and glass-half-full perspective are being severely tested, I am still trying to focus on living rather than dwell on what might be. Still, I feel frustration, irritation and anger at having to go through this so soon after my last series of treatment – it's hard to be zen.

I was, however, able to schedule the lumbar puncture without impacting our family March break plans, which will help keep my focus on the positive and on those special family moments.

NOT GOOD

March 16, 2011

The nice, relaxed attitude of the doctor and staff during my lumbar puncture Friday – they said the results could wait until after our planned March break week – didn't last. I knew something was up when I received a call late Monday afternoon to come into the lymphoma clinic on Tuesday. Just what my wife and daughter needed before they flew off ahead of me!

Going to the clinic, I felt a real sense of foreboding, which reminded me of earlier times.

My regular hematologist started off the discussion by saying that the results were 'not good' – semi-joking that calls from the hospital are rarely 'good.' Essentially, the lymphoma is back. The test on my spinal cord fluid showed the presence of white blood cells, meaning that the lymphoma has crossed my brain membrane. Final cell-level pathology will likely confirm that in a few days.

All of this took place with the backdrop of the unfolding disaster in Japan, an ongoing reminder of the fragility of life that put my situation into perspective.

As always, there is a plan. Short-term, a bout of chemo targeted to address lymphoma in the nervous system, which should stabilize things and provide immediate relief – this is important given the instability of mantle cell lymphoma. A 'cocktail' with relatively minor side effects. This needs to be done quickly, so there will be no March break for me (sigh…). This initial treatment will be followed, after a month or so, by another MRI or lumbar puncture to see how I have responded. Then it will be time to look at longer-term options, including allogeneic stem cell transplants.

All in all, not much fun ahead. I asked the awkward but necessary question about quality of life trade-offs involved in the longer-term treatment options. My hematologist said that we are not there yet, given my age and that some of the treatments have reasonably good prospects, but we will have more such discussions in the future.

The usual mixed emotions: mainly down, swirl around, everything from the minor (missed March break and interesting business trips) to the major (longer-term mortality worries and the realization that I may need to retire earlier or have a less demanding and less interesting job).

Then came the harder part. Talking to my wife in Europe, letting her know. Letting some of my staff know. Talking to my son. To my brother. Letting my bosses know. As I noted in the last entry, I am getting better at this, but it's not a skill that I pride myself on.

I am back to this feeling of being in limbo. Focussing on work and the daily routine helps. Today, the chemo was scheduled for Sunday/Monday, and I have started arranging everything around that.

I am more resigned than depressed, knowing that I need to go through with this. Again, thoughts about my family. A wonderful exchange with my son when I tell him, 'This sounds stupid, but I don't want you to worry,' and he says, 'Dad, it is stupid.' And so it is.

TRANSITIONING

March 21, 2011

Over the past few days, I have been mulling over how to 'will myself' into the neutral zone, that space between the past and the future, between letting go and embracing (or at least accepting!), as described in William Bridges classic, *The Way Of Transition: Embracing Life's Most Difficult Moments*. Funny how I have come back to a book that I once read to help me manage much more banal and mundane work-related transitions.

My first strategy was keeping busy, getting more work-related stuff done, as well as a lot of work around the house. Talking to friends and family varied by conversation – while the love and support all helped, some conversations brought me back to the sense of loss. Some music brought me up (Springsteen), some down (Cohen, given his emotional power); even some 60s bouncy music, given associations of loss; but mostly all brought out the emotional side, and again the sense of loss. Yesterday, the pretense dropped, and all the normal apprehension about going back to chemo surfaced. The chores around the house were left undone. This was all, of course, aggravated by the fact that my whole family was away. While texting, phoning and Skype do help, they are not the same as physical presence.

However, getting back into the hospital routine, with its familiarity and matter-of-factness, helped me move towards the neutral zone and focus on the present. There, I found a number of familiar faces, the same wonderful attitude on the part of the staff (and the same awful food). There were also some improvements, like the addition of bike machines to distract me and keep me in shape.

I had a good discussion about the chemo with the hematologist and pharmacist today. Essentially, it will involve getting a high dose of methotrexate ('juicing' me with a higher dose in a shorter period of time than previously) to help clear out the presence of lymphoma in the brain and spinal fluid and tissue, followed by complementary medication to reduce side effects and help clear the from my body. The side effects are expected to be manageable (I reacted well to this drug last time), but of course I will need to be careful given the normal drop in immunity that will occur about a week after treatment. I am getting myself into the 'neutral zone' before we start discussing longer-term treatment options. Although, funnily enough, the options came out in dribs and drabs through this last discussion and one with the head nurse: another stem cell transplant, but this time with a donor. More details to come, but this will not be an easy process to go through.

More movies than reading so far: *Carlos*, a fictional biopic on the world's most famous terrorist of the 70s, brought back memories of that time; Terry Gilliam's *Twelve Monkeys*, which was not as good as *Brazil* but still a well-done sci-fi dystopia that plays around with time and reality (I also watched *La Jetée*, the French film it was based on); and *A Matter of Life and Death*, an old movie that also plays with the reality/imagination theme.

One book that I have finished, however, is *The Central Liberal Truth* by Lawrence Harrison. It discusses and illustrates, through case studies, the importance of culture to history and development. While some of the case studies (at least of countries that I have experience with) are somewhat superficial in terms of the interplay between culture, economic and social factors, and while the tone appears triumphalist to post-2008 crash eyes, it nevertheless provides a good basis for reflection and discussion.

Throughout, I have benefitted tremendously from the support of my colleagues, at all levels, who have seen me go through this once before, as well as a from working in an organizational culture that is very supportive of employees under circumstances such as mine. This has been a reminder, behind all the debates, discussions, and sometimes absurdities of the workplace, of our fundamental humanity. Although I would not recommend such extreme measures, my bad news has increased readership of my blog!

About a year after returning to work at the end of my last treatment, I am back in my familiar hospital ward, looking out the window and reflecting. It's the first day of spring, but since this is Ottawa, we had a blizzard outside!

'SALVAGE' CHEMOTHERAPY

In contrast to my previous treatment in 2009, where I followed a standard protocol with standard sequencing and fairly rigid timing, this time I received more custom or 'bespoke' treatment to stabilize my lymphoma in my central nervous system (CNS). The following table, written after the fact, summarizes the approach taken.

Round	Dates	Treatment	Purpose/Comments
1	Mar 21-24	Methotrexate	Address lymphoma in CNS – methotrexate is preferred chemo to get behind the blood/brain membrane
2	Apr 12-14	Methotrexate Cytarabine (Ara-C)	Ara-C injected into spinal fluid directly following lumbar puncture No change in white blood cell counts in spinal fluid
3	Apr 26-28	Cytarabine	Shifted to Cytarabine given Methotrexate is too hard on my kidneys (creatine level high) Ara-C injected into spinal fluid directly following lumbar puncture White blood cell counts in spinal fluid have dropped – chemo is working
4	May 25-27	Cytarabine	Ara-C injected into spinal fluid directly following lumbar puncture After this round, my condition stabilized with no white blood cells in spinal fluid

GETTING BACK INTO THE ROUTINE

March 27, 2011

I had forgotten how crummy chemo makes me feel once it starts to kick in three to four days after the fact. I am calling it the chemo hangover: a mix of headache, mild heartburn, a bad taste in the mouth, fatigue and the return of the chemo pale and wan 'tan.' And this is an easier cycle! However, I seem to be through the worst of this particular round, so hopefully the bounce back is starting although I really feel tired this time.

I have to drink lots to help my kidneys recover from the chemo. This week, I will enter the (low immunity) phase, where I will have to be hyper-careful to avoid infection.

I am strong enough to get back into my routine of walks, even if the weather is still too cold to really think of spring and renewal.

Part of being in the neutral transition zone is getting back to the rhythm of the chemo cycle: feel OK, get chemo, feel sick, feel weak, build up strength and repeat!

I have started to review websites and the like for information on allogeneic stem cell transplants (SCT), the likely longer-term treatment option (e.g., National Marrow Donor Program, Blood and Marrow Transplant Information Network). This treatment will be intense and rough; I will get more details during my clinic visit on Tuesday. As always, with the web, the challenge is finding the balance between enough information to be realistic about what lies ahead, and too much, which tends to push one towards worry and depression.

While I was able to approach the first round of chemo somewhat tongue-in-cheek, as a 'learning experience,' I am not yet in that space this time. The second round feels very different from the first. I am more realistic, more apprehensive, and more resigned – but still determined (stubborn?) to give it my best shot.

Having my family back from their trip keeps my focus. While emotions continue to wash over me, the 'in front of my eyes' reminder of why I need to go through this gives me strength.

Music, rather than bring me down as it did last week, brings me up – whether it be Mercedes Sosa or some classics from the Beatles and Dylan.

Similarly, I have been having fun with movies. I am currently watching a series of Elizabeth Taylor classics (*Who's Afraid of Virginia Woolf?*; *Suddenly, Last Summer*; and *Cat on a Hot Tin Roof*), which feature great casts and great writing. Other films I have seen recently include *Get Low*, a charming piece starring Robert Duvall and Bill Murray, with a theme of reconciliation and putting things right; and *The Fountain*, a somewhat odd film by Darren Aronofsky (Director of *Black Swan*) on immortality and love.

I finally got around to reading *The Sentimentalists* by Johanna Skibsrud. While well crafted, neither the story nor the observations particularly moved me – though that may just reflect the space I am in now.

Getting back into the weekly blogging routine, and my daily journal routine, is helping me work through and reflect on this second journey. The warmth and support of my family, friends and colleagues, sometimes in the context of the blog, sometimes not, keeps me going.

Bouncing Back

April 3, 2011

I have largely bounced back from the chemo. The side effects are gone, my energy levels are back up, and no sickness has resulted from my current low immunity. I feel the contrast in conference calls comparing Monday to Friday; I also feel my lower haemoglobin count during my regular – and increasingly long – walks. Every time I go through the bounce-back phase, I feel a sense of wonder at both the body's ability to recover and the knowledge of my medical team, who calibrate so finely how much my body can take without crossing the line.

Emotionally, the bounce back also helps. While the worries remain, feeling well enough to be able to go for walks, work part-time remotely and putter around the house make a big difference. In addition, I am coming to terms with the implications for my professional life – getting to the neutral zone instead of dwelling on the transition from a leadership position, with the profile and satisfaction that this entails, to some yet undefined, but more low-key, role.

I had a somewhat funny, if frustrating, clinic visit on Friday. As part of the Surrender/ Control duality, I try to control what I can and surrender to what I cannot. Part of having control is knowledge, and I had dutifully, following chats with the hematologist during my stay at the hospital, reviewed some of the web sites he suggested on allogeneic stem cell transplants. The result was that I was prepared with a question list and a table to help me understand the various steps, risks, outcomes (the polite term for survival rates!), and side effects.

However, the clinician said that this is premature – they will walk me through everything once they find a donor. A fair amount of bobbing and weaving was required as I continued to try to get more clarity (with the backdrop of a Canadian politicians doing their own bobbing and weaving during a national election, it seemed kind of funny to be playing this game with a doctor and not a politician). Ultimately, however, did get a fair amount of clarity on the following:

- The treatment aims at providing me with a new immune system that is less susceptible to mantle cell lymphoma, rather than at completely wiping out any traces of my existing lymphoma (a nuance which I need to understand better).

- I will only have a reduced intensity conditioning regimes (in contrast to the high intensity regime). While everything is relative – and I need to get a better sense of how this compares to my conditioning regime last time – lower intensity sounds a lot better than high intensity.

- In order for the transplant to work, my lymphoma needs to be stable. This may require some 'salvage' chemo, given that the original chemo was not as effective as it should have been. I will get all the requisite scans, etc., over the next few weeks to decide what kind of chemo may be necessary.

I also pressed the clinician on timelines – for my family and I to plan around, as well as for the sake of my colleagues at work. Essentially, should one of my brothers be a match, the transplant could take place in as few as six to eight weeks; if not, it could take an additional four to eight weeks to arrange. We did not discuss the 'if there is no donor' scenario – again, a 'layers of an onion' approach to imparting information.

All in all, there is still a fair amount of uncertainty, but enough general clarification that I can help ensure as smooth a transition as possible at work, and also find a week off to sneak away with my wife before this next stage begins.

As I have been working part time this week, there has been less time for fun reading. Amazing how work gets in the way! I am halfway through *Atonement* by Ian McEwan, a wonderfully written and crafted novel (the movie adaptation is also good).

We have watched fewer movies as we are back into the school routine. However, we have seen one more Elizabeth Taylor movie (*Butterfield 8*, overly 'Hollywood' and conventional); *Made in Dagenham*, a formulaic feel-good movie, but based on a true story of the struggle in England for equal pay for equal work; and *Inside Job*, a documentary on the 2008 economic meltdown and the banking sector.

Inside Job complements an earlier reading, *How Markets Fail: The Logic of Economic Calamities* by John Cassidy. His book provides a good overview of the history of economic thought and the development of the range of financial instruments and deregulation decisions and their consequences.

GETTING ON WITH IT

April 10, 2011

> *Do not go gentle into that good night,*
> *Old age should burn and rage at close of day;*
> *Rage, rage against the dying of the light. Though wise men at their end know dark is*
> *right,*
> *Because their words had forked no lightning they*
> *Do not go gentle into that good night.*
>
> *Good men, the last wave by, crying how bright*
> *Their frail deeds might have danced in a green bay,*
> *Rage, rage against the dying of the light.*
>
> *Wild men who caught and sang the sun in flight,*
> *And learn, too late, they grieved it on its way,*
> *Do not go gentle into that good night.*
>
> *Grave men, near death, who see with blinding sight*
> *Blind eyes could blaze like meteors and be gay,*
> *Rage, rage against the dying of the light.*
>
> *And you, my father, there on the sad height,*
> *Curse, bless me now with your fierce tears, I pray.*
> *Do not go gentle into that good night.*
> *Rage, rage against the dying of the light.*

Dylan Thomas

This was an intense week, helping me move forward and firming up plans and approach for future treatment.

My hematologist laid out a general plan, but like last week, she stressed that there is no regular protocol or sequence for me to organize my life around. The treatment will vary based on how my body responds, with a fair amount of uncertainty/flexibility where timing is concerned; it will, however, likely include two to three more rounds of chemo ('salvage chemo') to address the lymphoma in my nervous system. The transplant will likely take place this summer, and I should know in a week whether one of my brothers is a match. My kids rather sweetly asked whether they could be donors so we inquired with the medical team but apparently the odds are no better than in the general donor bank. As to the inevitable question – will we find a donor? –

my hematologist was categoric: with my background and seven million potential donors, a match will be found.

I probed a bit on the subject of the transplant procedure itself. Again noting that we should not get ahead of ourselves, she told us that the conditioning regime will likely be closer to high intensity than low (in contrast with last week), and will involve radiation not only for conditioning, but possibly for treatment as well. This makes the treatment harder, but also more effective. The usual balance and risk management.

She told me not to drive in the meantime, given the remote chance of a seizure, and said that I should not plan to return to work, but instead explore early retirement options.

Clear, brutal, but delivered in a wonderfully compassionate and thoughtful manner.

We then had a good session with the counsellor. Again, going back to the individual/group duality, a lot of my worry revolves around my wife and kids – both our son, who is at university, and our daughter, who is still at home. It was a good and helpful discussion, with follow-up sessions for us and/or the kids as needed, given the pressure on my family. She then turned to me and asked the inevitable 'what about you?' in light of the fact that I seemed to be more concerned about my family and work team than myself.

It was helpful to articulate the real sense of loss I felt at the premature end of my professional career, the sense that this second time was so much harder, and that I was finding it difficult to get into the zen space that I was able to access the first time. I also seem to be more emotionally fragile, more sensitive to both minor professional issues and to new health information (I never sleep well after a clinic visit!). The counsellor reassuringly said that this is normal, and noted that I was processing a lot of information – implications on health, profession, family and place in society – all of which takes time, and for which there are no real shortcuts.

However, she noted that my journalling and blogging, given the self-awareness that it fosters, are both good techniques to help me through this. Equally reassuring was her doing a signal check with my wife, who confirmed that none of this was new, which means that I have been sharing my emotions with her.

Given all this, I have let people at work know that I will not be coming back – although I will be engaged remotely (love the technology) over the next few months to help my group transition and to transfer my knowledge and experience. All of my colleagues were very supportive. It is never easy to have these discussions and there is no way to sugarcoat this. While I cannot control what is happening, I can at least manage how I exit, and try to do so in a manner that is as supportive of the team as possible.

I have also been getting some great comments from readers of my blog and via other on-line fora, all of which help to broaden my support network.

My metaphor seems to be changing; I had earlier cited an article that spoke to me, In Search of a Better Metaphor, which challenged the notion of 'fighting' cancer. Now I seem to be coming back to the fight metaphor, as best expressed in the Dylan Thomas poem above. Maybe getting back into the zen space will change this; we shall see. Ironically, *The Ottawa Citizen* seems to have deleted this article from their archives, a reminder of how transitory the electronic world we live in can be.

I watched just two movies this week. First, *Precious Life*, a documentary about a Palestinian baby who received a stem cell transplant in Israel, and the hopes, politics, and realities that this entailed on all sides. A bit too close for comfort for me on the medical front, but it made for some good additional information on what I am about to go through, less the charged environment. The second film was *Four Lions*, a black comedy on suicide bombers that works devastatingly well.

I have started a twitter feed (predictably called @LymphomaJourney) to allow for short updates when appropriate while I continue with my weekly posts.

Other than that, I have been feeling well enough to be walking a lot, doing a fair amount of work, and this weekend, to go out for a few bike rides and savour the first few days of nice weather. As will be going back in the hospital for round 2 on Monday, I am enjoying this weekend with my family, which has been particularly nice since our son came home to spend the time with us.

GOOD NEWS, BAD NEWS

April 17, 2011

I was at the hospital this week for my second round of chemo. The usual routines. Being a human pincushion becomes harder and my veins protest more, but all in all it went well. I had the same kind of chemo as last time, with similar side effects towards the end of the week. All manageable – although as I write this post I am still in the 'feeling crummy' and very tired stage, which should pass in a few days.

I received a mix of good and bad news. The good news is that my CT scan was clear.

As for the bad news, the lumbar puncture and brain/spine MRI showed little to no improvement, which means that I have not been responding to my previous round of chemo. While the current round may be more effective, since some chemo was injected directly into my spinal cord fluid, the medical team is considering other options, including radiation. This is more fodder for discussion at my next clinic session on Tuesday. 'Of concern,' say the doctors; 'worrisome,' says I. This would mean a longer a longer and rockier road to getting me stable enough for a stem cell transplant.

My medical team had warned me that this stage would involve adjusting the treatment based on my response to it, but knowing this theoretically and actually experiencing it are two different things. The normal routine of 'chemo, body responds' is no longer, and we are going into uncharted (for me) territory. Surprisingly, I seem to be more zen about it, at least for the moment, than I would have expected. Perhaps the accumulation of bad news over the past months is making me more resilient – a kind of perverse impact.

Despite all this, I have remained involved at work, working part time on the areas where I can help most and doing the necessary 'letting go' of files that are less important. An e-mail that previously would have irritated me became a 'whatever,' so I have made progress!

On the nice side, I was 'beamed in' via FaceTime to a retirement lunch, which allowed me to reconnect and recognize a colleague's professional and personal contribution over the years. I love the technology when it reconnects and reinforces bonds, rather than do the opposite (see *Keep Your Thumbs Still While I am Talking to You*).

I only watched one movie this week, *The Station Agent*, a low-key off-beat story about lonely characters and how they are brought together by chance and life. I also watched the Canadian election debates, and the commentariat analysis (I much preferred the more engaging and substantive French debate). My son recommended a fun book, which I enjoyed: *Green Grass Running Water* by Thomas King, a playful and inventive aboriginal novel. Finally, at the end of the week, my iPad that I had ordered arrived. It will keep me amused – or at least distracted – over the next number of months.

Next week should be a recovery week. I will be getting back into my walking routine (assuming the weather picks up again), figuring out next steps with my medical team, and getting together with everyone for the Easter weekend.

Made It To the Neutral Zone

April 24, 2011

A good bounce-back and recovery week. My energy returned, the chemo aftertaste dissipated, and my wife and I were able to resume our regular walks together.

I had my regular clinic visit, which gave me a more nuanced view of what may be happening in terms of my response to the chemo. My regular (and favourite) hematologist was not willing to write off chemo yet, given that the medical team did not know the exact baseline of lymphoma in my central nervous system before I had the first round, thus not knowing whether the lymphoma was, in fact, responding to treatment.

Another round of chemo and another analysis of my spinal cord fluid will answer that question – hopefully confirming that treatment is in fact working. My body is recovering well enough that I can be on the regular (and more effective) two-week cycle, so back to the hospital I go next week.

My hematologist was very responsive to my wish for a second opinion. She said that this is very normal in cases like mine, and that they can arrange for me to meet with someone at the Princess Margaret Hospital in Toronto. I do not expect to hear anything radically different (I have not seen many alternatives on the web), but it will give all of us piece of mind.

As the circle of people who are aware of my situation grows, I have been getting some wonderful support from friends and neighbours – and also from readers of my blog, in the form of both reading suggestions and comments. My favourite comes from a colleague, who said that anyone who has read my blog will have 'probably taken some time to live a little more in the now and perhaps hug their wife and kids a little longer.' As always, people have that very human urge of wanting to help; for the moment, expressing support and keeping in touch make all the difference. In future stages of my treatment, the opportunities to help may evolve into something more concrete.

I think I have made the shift, with respect to work, from experiencing a sense of loss to enjoying the process of watching – and coaching – my team. My colleagues are rising to the challenge of going on without me there, all while continuing to do some really good work. No one is indispensable, least of all in large bureaucracies; but I am really focussing on my transition role, which is to provide advice and direction where needed (and hopefully only where needed) and just help the team to continue developing their abilities and delivering on government priorities. A turning point for me.

If I have not quite made it to the 'zen space,' I have at least made progress towards the acceptance side of the acceptance/anger duality.

I did some fun reading this week: *If Nobody Speaks of Remarkable Things* by Jon McGregor, a delightfully written (almost poetic, even) story about day-to-day life on a street in England – although the characters are less engaging than the writing. I also watched a really imaginative visual essay, by Stephen Fry, on Language.

Rabbit Hole, a film about how a young couple tries to overcome their grief after the death of their only child, depicts the tensions and overwhelming emotion involved in such loss. The screenplay captures the intensity in some brilliant scenes, which range from the deep (a mother-daughter scene about whether the pain ever goes away) to the comic (a group therapy session). This was all particularly poignant for me, as I watched – but as a teenager, could not fully understand – as my parents coped with the death of one of my brothers.

On the lighter side, we have been watching some *30 Rock* episodes as a family. The writing, if uneven, is always entertaining. I also saw *Source Code*, which was not a great thriller; it had an interesting *Groundhog Day*-like premise, but lacked originality (unlike *Inception*). Finally, I watched *Tristam Shandy*, featuring British comedians Steve Coogan and Rob Brydon, which had its moments but seemed forced to my taste.

I have been discovering the world of 'Apps' on my iPad, which has almost become my default device now (apart from when I work or write longer pieces).

I am having a wonderful weekend; both our kids and my brother are here, and I received clearance from my hematologist to go to an Easter brunch. It's always nice when the chemo cycle lines up with family events!

Best wishes to all of you this Easter and Passover season.

GOOD NEWS – CHEMO IS WORKING

May 1, 2011

A hospital week, but with good news. The test results from the   show a dramatic decline (90 percent) of white blood cells (WBC) in my spinal fluid. The chemo is working, contrary to our fears after last time. Hopefully this round will get me to 0 percent, which is where I need to be. According to the hematologist, this is of more significance than the MRI results; some of the brain membrane damage may remain, but it should not get worse.

This round involved a slight change in strategy. The previous type of chemo (methotrexate) appears to have been too hard on my kidneys, so the team switched to another drug (cytarabarine) that also addresses lymphoma in the central the nervous system. I have had it before (as part of Cycle B of), so the side effects should be manageable. Ironically, the blood indicator (creatinine) for kidney stress went up when I arrived at the hospital (psychosomatic?) and then fell back again the second day. The hematologist joked that had they known, they might not have changed the strategy.

When I asked him about the next steps should the count reach 0 percent, he just smiled and said, 'We are playing it by ear.' In any case, so far so good – a great relief for all of us.

And on an amusing note, they were testing patients for early signs of dementia, and I fortunately failed (despite one of the side effects of the various rounds being weaker short-term memory).

One piece of bad news: we were shocked to learn that another of the hematologists had been seriously ill and would not be able to come back to work full time. The transition from healer to patient must be a difficult one, and the news touched us more than we would have expected.

I did some great reading this week. On the light side, *The Uncommon Reader* by Alan Bennett, a hilarious story in which the Queen of England becomes such a voracious reader that she starts to neglect her duties. A good complement to the royal wedding, which yes, I did watch – at the hospital, along with most of the nurses. It brought to mind contrasting memories of my own far simpler wedding, and I wondered, without being morbid about it, whether I will be there to witness such a milestone for our kids.

On the serious side, I read *At the Will of the Body* by Arthur Frank, which a reader recommended to me (thank you, Richard!). The book is an account of Frank's experience with, and reflections on, illness, occasioned by his having a heart attack and then cancer. His reflections are very similar to those that I have been exploring in this blog, but more coherent and articulate. A real affirmation and example of fully savouring life. While we cannot choose our illness, we do have some choice in terms of how we respond to it and live it. Interestingly, Frank also picked up on the theme of dualities, though his were not the same as mine (they included struggle vs. fighting, denial vs. affirmation, comforters vs. accusers).

I have been much more fortunate than he was in that most members of my medical team have been more compassionate about my experience than his medical team was when the book was published (1991). One wonderful *bon mot* to share, however: 'one is a patient because one must be patient.' I highly recommended the book for anyone experiencing (or caring for someone with) a serious or chronic illness.

There are a few movies to note. During the last night of the Easter weekend, we all watched *How to Train a Dragon*. While formulaic (an outsider, a father-son conflict and resolution), it was delightfully done, and it was fun to watch an animated film with the kids again. On the more serious side I watched *Vision*, a film about a 12th-century Benedictine nun, Hildegarde von Bingen. It captures the atmosphere – religious, social and political – of the period, and particularly of a cloister, and shows how she applied her more humanistic and compassionate views as she navigated the politics and gender roles of the time.

Lastly, I finally saw *Incendies*, Denis Villeneuve's film about the calamities experienced by one woman during the Lebanese civil war. It is told, in part, through the eyes of her children, who have to discover the truth about a father she had told them was dead and a brother that they never knew existed. A very powerful depiction of the brutality and savagery of the war. Moving between the perspective of the mother, who lived the experience, and that of the daughter, who asks questions to discover the story, works well; the ending, however, is too contrived to be believable.

Should be a quiet week ahead as I am back home to work through the side effects. Fortunately, warmer weather ahead for walking to assist recovery, while work will focus on follow-up to the election results.

Recovery – A Bit Longer This Time

May 8, 2011

A recovery week. The side effects felt deeper this round, which was likely a reflection of the particular chemo used, and perhaps the result of a cumulative effect. Nothing serious, just the usual – the crumminess, chemo aftertaste and dryness, and brain fog from more fatigue – but I not able to brush it off quite as quickly as in previous rounds. By the end of the week, however, the slow bounce back was underway, and my wife and I were back to our regular walking routine. For those of you who are curious, yes, my hair is thinning, but it is still there.

As this phase progresses, I become more and more conscious of the need to prepare myself, emotionally and physically, for what might lie ahead. The physical aspect is easy: exercise, eat and rest, or, as the expression goes, 'fatten myself up' for the transplant procedure. The emotional preparation is more complex. I feel both dread and an eagerness to just get it over with, and am also trying to find a balance between knowing enough and knowing too much about the potential risks and complications. I have seen a range of experiences on other blogs; for some patients the transplant process was hard but on track, whereas others ran into complication after complication. As was the case with my previous stem cell transplant, the medical team and I will only know the outcome once I go through the procedure.

At the weekly clinic visit, I was initially a bit put out to find that my appointment was with an internationally trained resident, and not one of my regular hematologist. However, unlike the 'regulars,' who just refer to scans and medical imaging, she actually physically examined me to make sure no signs of lymph inflammation or swelling – a more human touch. She found nothing. I have yet to find out when I will be getting the second opinion we requested; I will likely have another round of chemo in two weeks, followed by another clinic visit next week to confirm that the treatment is working.

Unfortunately, the DNA swabs for my brothers were not usable, so they are proceeding to getting their blood work done. This has no impact on the timeline, but reminded me of the ongoing need to watch things closely – part of 'owning the file' (i.e., me and my care) and ensuring that nothing slips by me (and the medical team!).

While I still do not have a firm timeline for the transplant, it will take place during the summer. In the meantime, my mind turns to the other things that I need to do to in the next few months. Most of the morbid stuff (my will, etc.) was taken care of during the first round, but I had good discussions with the pay and benefits people at work, who have clarified my options. I realize how fortunate I am to have such a good benefits and retirement package, which takes away most of the financial worries.

Work-wise, I am also in the process of winding things down. The performance reviews of my staff are done, and I had the odd experience of writing a draft performance agreement, setting out work objectives for my successor (and doing it in a responsible way!). I am also letting stakeholders know about my departure, helping with some individual files, and preparing some reflections on how my files have evolved and developed over the past few years. The deeper side effects this round, in addition to some considerations related to my pay and benefit options, are forcing me to reflect on how long it will be before I need to go on medical leave full time and 'cut the cord' with work. Another subject for discussion at the clinic next week.

I had a lot of fun reading *The General and his Labyrinth* by Gabriel Garcia Marquez. The novel is about the last voyage of Bolivar, hero of Latin America's struggle for independence, and his reflections on what he achieved and failed to achieve during his life as 'the Liberator.' It brings me back a bit to my time in Latin America in the 1980s: the richness of life and of the people, and the failed hopes of a continent. As always, Marquez's writing is sublime, his descriptions rich, and his humour at times fiendish. The themes of looking back on a life (the achievements and failures) and of the transitory and ephemeral nature of much in the temporal world, are powerful reminders as I look back on my own modest career with an appropriate perspective.

We watched *The Messenger*, a post-Iraq film about the soldiers who have to notify family members that their child or spouse has been killed in the line of duty. The intense dynamic between the official and the human is well captured by the two contrasting soldiers, superbly played, who deliver the news. Ultimately, the film ends up on the human side, but without being too cloying: 'they're all people,' as the lead character says. For Woody Allen fans: his article on his latest film, Midnight in Paris, is amusing.

It was a big week for news, featuring both the Canadian election results and the death of Osama bin Laden. 9/11 was one of those events where we can all remember where we were and what we were doing when it happened. We were in Los Angeles at the time, and thus lived it more intensely than had we lived in Canada.

Perhaps fittingly, this week ends with Mother's Day – a reaffirmation of life, and a time to appreciate the mothers who made and raised us and the strong women with whom we share our lives and children.

A Frustrating Week

May 15, 2011

This week has been harder than expected.

First, my wife caught a very severe flu, just when time my immunity was lowest and I had to be the most careful. I was consequently pretty useless as a caregiver (role reversal) and painfully aware of my dependence on her, both emotionally and practically. Emotionally, I missed our walks for the connection and support time they entail (and it was odd to be talking over the phone from different parts of the house to avoid catching her flu); practically, having no one to drive me to my appointments became a real issue.

Fortunately, we have a number of really good friends and neighbours who helped us out, whether by bringing food, taking me to the hospital, or letting her know that they cared. Our teenage daughter became more helpful as well. Once again, I really appreciate what we have in terms of support as we go through this.

I had an equally frustrating time at the clinic. The hematologist who had originally put my treatment plan in place (and who had told me that I couldn't travel to Paris for March break) was visibly frustrated at how little the planning for the stem cell transplant had advanced. My assumption that my case was being reviewed regularly at the weekly case meetings appears to have been misplaced. There was little action on the issue of getting my brothers' blood work, and the medical team had not anticipated that the stronger side effects of cytarabine should have made them consider giving me Neupogen (which accelerates the production of blood cells following chemo). As my hematologist noted, my bone marrow was 'pooped out,' and I would need another week of recovery, as well as a dose of platelets to bring up my levels, before undergoing a further round of chemo. Not to mention that there is still no word on the second opinion from Princess Margaret Hospital (and this hematologist appeared less receptive the second opinion than the other hematologist).

I chalked it up to another lesson learned about the Healthcare System and took ownership again. I sent an email to the clinic asking them to get on with things, which will hopefully reinforce the hematologist's intervention. I am also really pushing for an early appointment at the Princess Margaret Hospital next week, when travel will be easiest for me given my schedule. No word yet, so I will keep pushing. Things are starting to fall into place for my brothers' blood work. The process for family members who life out of town has been complicated, which surprises me as we cannot be the only family that is scattered around.

I did, however, get some clarity on my work situation. I was told that I should stop working and begin long-term disability on May 30th, the week after my next round of chemo is expected to take place. Although the date is set, I still have some mixed feelings, but I am also satisfied that I have helped my team with the transition process over the past few months.

I enjoyed *The Greatest Show on Earth* by Richard Dawkins, which helped me learn and re-learn about evolution and the incredible diversity of life (The Guardian review here captures some of the limitations of his book). A real antidote to some of my cancer-related readings! Also, we watched Robert Altman's funny (if not totally successful take on the fashion world), *Prêt-à-Porter*; as well as a classic spaghetti Western, *A Fistful of Dollars*, featuring Clint Eastwood in a classic Clint role, and the usual great pacing, shots and score.

Other than that, it has been a quiet week. My slightly lower energy level has resulted in shorter walks (partly for physical reasons, partly because they are not so much fun on one's own); I have been wrapping up files at work, and above all, ensuring that I don't catch anything during this period of my low immunity. Next week should be easier on all levels, since my wife is now better, and I hope to go into the office to pick up my things and clean up, in addition to touching base with people.

A MUCH BETTER WEEK

May 22, 2011

Things got back on track this week.

First, my wife got better, and we were able to get back into our routine of regular walks, even though weather was mixed.

Secondly, things at the clinic started to move. One brother flew up here to do his blood work, and arrangements for the other to do get his done in the States early next week were confirmed. I finally got an appointment for the second opinion at the Princess Margaret Hospital (PMH), for June 6th. My counts had bounced back at the end of the week, which means that I can undergo another round of chemo next week, rather than wait through a further delay – although my haemoglobin remains low, reducing my energy level.

All of this was a reminded me that the healthcare system is a big bureaucracy, and that I have to use my bureaucratic skills, honed by 30 years of working for the government, to advance my case. For example, the delay in getting the appointment for a second opinion was caused by my hematologist and the clinic, who took 3 weeks to get the requisition to the PMH. The PMH only took about a week to respond. I need to keep track of what is going on, follow-up and be persistent.

I have asked for a full copy of my file and a CD of my images (requested by the PMH) to ensure that I have all the necessary information on hand, and to make things easier should we decide to seek a third opinion.

I also had a good appointment with the clinician, who is more generous with her time than some of the hematologists. I asked about whether I am still banned from driving given that I no longer appear to have the headache and vision symptoms as before. The ban remains, although there is some flexibility for short distances in the city; but no driving on the highway or during rush hour. No biking, either. As the clinician told me with a smile, I need to consider the level of risk and how I would feel if something happened, like 'breaking open [my] skull,' that would delay my treatment plans! I also pressed her to make sure that I am prescribed Neupogen (fortunately covered by my drug plan) for the next round of chemo to reduce the period of low immunity.

It has also been a good week on a personal level. Our daughter turned 17, so we had a nice family celebration, and were joined by our son who was visiting for the Victoria Day weekend. The weather has shifted from a cold rain to nice and spring-like, the flowers are in bloom and the trees are green. The sight of this wonderful renewal and growth has been making our walks more enjoyable.

With our son the film buff at home, we have watched some interesting movies as a family. *Repulsion*, an early Roman Polanski film starring Catherine Deneuve, captures one woman's descent into madness and paranoia. It was an uncomfortable film to watch, but one that demonstrates Polanski's skill as a director. We also saw *Limitless*, which despite starting with an interesting concept was not a successful thriller; it follows what happens to a man who takes a miracle drug to make himself smarter (a bit too Hollywood – he makes a lot of money, gets his girl back, and then becomes a politician to save the world!).

I did not go into the office this week as my counts were initially still a bit low, but I will do so Tuesday. It will be time to hand in my laptop and Blackberry, marking a further transition, although I will still have access to my corporate email through my desktop computer (and eventually my iPad).

I am currently reading *Bloodlands: Europe Between Hitler and Stalin*, by Timothy Snyder. It is a powerful book that captures the atrocities committed by both Stalin, in the name of collectivization and 'revolution,' and Hitler, in the name of ethnic purity and cleansing. Snyder explores the links between the two, without diminishing the centrality of the Holocaust and the unprecedented industrialized cruelty involved in the 'final solution.' There is a fair amount of controversy on this point, to which Snyder replies in his article, The Fatal Fact of the Nazi-Soviet Pact. Given my work with the various communities affected by Stalism and Nazism, it was helpful to broaden my understanding. Highly recommended, but not an easy read. *Bloodlands* was also my first e-book. While I miss the tactile sense involved in turning pages, the electronic format is so much more convenient!

I have started adding some health or life-related articles that I find interesting to my blog; I will try to be judicious in my selection.

Next week will be another hospital week, and I will be undergoing the same kind of chemo as before: Ara C (another name for Cytarabine), since it is easier on my kidneys, even though it is harsher in other respects. The usual triage decisions we have to make!

ANOTHER ROUND DONE

May 29, 2011

Another round is done and I am back home to recover.

I have the perception, however, that things are not clicking together as smoothly as they should. Some things are easy to judge; when I went to the hospital on Tuesday afternoon, I found out that the staff had forgotten to order my chemo! On the bright side, I was able to go home that evening for dinner and a walk (seize and savour the opportunity), but the error wasted time and caused a delay in treatment.

Given my new 'take charge' approach, I arrived at the hospital with a list of specific treatment questions: about the use of Neulasta or Neupogen to accelerate my blood count recovery; whether to have a lumbar puncture to see how well the chemo is working; whether to reschedule the Princess Margaret Hospital visit given that I will have low immunity on June 6; what the next steps pre-stem cell transplant are; and finally, I asked about when we might know whether either of my brothers is a potential donor.

Perhaps it was the style and demeanor of the intern to whom I spoke, but nothing is so frustrating as to ask questions and then be told that she would need to check with the doctor on each and every one. This was compounded by the impression that she had not reviewed my file, as the answers were already – or should have been – on file. Our meeting was in strong contrast to my last three sessions, at which I dealt directly with the doctor (and unlike government, where detailed expertise is often at relatively junior levels, in the medical world, experience and knowledge happen at more senior levels).

Part of the exchange was comic: the intern wanted to know why I was curious about my brothers' potential compatibility at this stage. After some toing and froing, I said that the issue is worry and that this knowledge will remove one potential layer of uncertainty, which is important to all of us. Duh!

The lumbar puncture was more complicated and painful this time. A great learning opportunity for another intern – and don't get me wrong, I know that is part of the bargain for the next generation – but I did miss being on my previous doctor's shift. Maybe I had just become too comfortable with the procedure and needed a reminder (sharp!) that it is somewhat complicated.

In the end, I did get clarity on most of the points I raised, and the doctor came in just prior to my release (yes to Neulasta, the PMH has been rescheduled to June 20, and I was told that this was likely my last round of salvage chemo if the test results are good and I have no more symptoms). I got a blood transfusion to bring up my haemoglobin, but they forgot to prescribe anti-nausea meds. Fortunately, I had some remaining at home.

My medical file and CD were given to me in person at the hospital, giving me the opportunity to meet the clinic assistant. I often speak to her on the phone and was glad to finally have a chance to thank her in person. The nurses were as helpful as always; some of the really outstanding ones were there this week. Still, I had more negative feedback to pass on to the clinic; maybe I am just grumpier the second time round. I will need to watch the grumpiness factor and balance it with graciousness and thankfulness!

I cleaned up my office this week, just before my hospital check in. I brought back three boxes of career-related stuff to sift through later at home, plus the usual family pictures and art. I did a walk-around to thank people. At this stage, it was less emotionally draining than I had expected; having worked through the issues over the past few months has made a difference. Of course, I miss the people and the discussions. I was lucky to have worked with a fun and proficient team.

I have been watching some fun stuff. First, *Summer Heights High*, an Australian sitcom about eccentric characters at a high school (delinquent, spoiled rich girl, egotistical drama teacher). It was very funny and our kids love it – they are closer to the high school life than my wife and I are, but it brought back some memories for us, too. I then started going through some Sergio Leone movies: *Once Upon a Time in the West*, arguably his best and certainly my favourite for its tight and sparse plot and the fact that it is so well written, filmed, scored and paced; and *Once Upon a Time in America*, his gangster movie, which has a more epic but slower pace than *The Godfather*. I prefer his westerns; *Once Upon a Time in America* was a mixed bag. Though powerful in places, it ultimately drags on and is not successful.

I finished *Bloodlands*. It is a long book, but as its subject matter involves some 14 million mass killings over 15 years by two major totalitarian regimes, there was lot of ground to cover. Three particular points resonated with me:

- First, the importance of recognizing the humanity of the individuals involved, and that each number has a name, an identity, and a family history behind it. It is not 14 million, but 14 million 'ones,' as Snyder puts it;

- Secondly, I gained a greater appreciation of Eastern European histories, particularly those of Poland and Ukraine, and the particular challenges of capturing their national stories, their collaboration, and the distinctions between Stalinist repression and the Holocaust (rather than blurring them together); and

- Thirdly, the question of what I or others would do in similar moral and ethical situations, either as individuals or as government officials. Joy Kogawa's *Obasan*, a novel recounting of the internment of Japanese-Canadians in Canada during WWII, which featured savage and biting commentary on the actions of government officials, prompted similar reflections. Snyder, without excusing the actions of collaborators, provides an explanation and context for their choices, thus making those who resisted appear all the more remarkable as individuals. For me, in the context of government service, it really boils down to being confident that one has provided the thorough analysis and fearless advice that inform better decision-making, but of course I had the luxury of working in a context where I was not really tested.

Since I turned in my laptop and blackberry, I have been using the iPad exclusively (including to write the draft of this post). The iPad is not as efficient as a regular laptop since it lacks a keyboard and a full browser, but is nonetheless more than adequate – and there is only one device to keep charged, to consult and to worry about.

Next week should be a normal recovery week, when I will get to 'enjoy' the bulk of the side effects of chemo. The Neulasta should at least help reduce the length of my low immunity period.

'SALVAGED' – ONE MILESTONE ACHIEVED

June 2, 2011

Overall, this has been a recovery week. The side effects were more mild than those that accompanied the last round. Be thankful for small mercies! The only major effects were low blood counts, in terms of both immunity and haemoglobin; the latter means anemia and consequently low energy levels. Short walks, not long walks, this week.

I also had a good, long discussion with the senior hematologist this week. The lumbar puncture found no white blood cells in my spinal fluid, meaning that the 'salvage' chemo has worked as it should and that this particular stage is complete. It was clear from our discussion that there was some 'hit or miss' uncertainty about whether my disease, stubborn as it is, would respond to treatment; that it has done so is encouraging and means that we can continue to 'plan for success'.

The discussion then turned to preparations for and the timing of the stem cell transplant (SCT). The search for an unrelated donor has begun in parallel with the process of my brothers' blood typing (although this hematologist had promised me that we will know whether either one is a match by this past Friday – and I had been given similar assurances last week during my hospital stay – the procedure was still marked as 'in progress' in the system despite efforts by my brothers and I to get a clear response. This is frustrating, and my own personal take is that this likely means that there was no match and that we will likely have to go the route of an unrelated donor. Just in case, however, I have e-mailed the senior hematologist to remind him to look into my brothers' results.

Without going into the (horrific?) details, the hematologist reiterated that the SCT conditioning regime will involve a mix of radiation and chemo (cyclosphosphamide), and that he will be setting up a meeting with the radiation oncologist. I have already had cyclophosphamide before (for my previous auto SCT), in both 'moderate' and high doses, so I know that taking it in combination with radiation is really going to be fun!

He then said, looking me in the eye, that they would not go ahead unless I was fully committed to the allogeneic SCT despite what I had read and learned about the risks, both short- and long-term. One of those serious and intense doctor-patient moments.

In response, I went back to our discussion in March, when I had asked the 'quality of life' and prognosis questions and he had replied in the positive. I told him that I had to rely on the expertise of he and his colleagues (including the those who will provide the upcoming consultation at Princess Margaret), and that if this treatment offered the best chance of remission, and could take place before any symptoms came back, I was committed. My answer highlighted the awkward realization that if my symptoms were to come back quickly, the SCT would no longer be an option, and we would be in a very different world.

To reduce this risk, given that there is only a temporary window of opportunity before my spinal fluid lymphoma returns, the SCT will be scheduled to take place as soon as possible (in early July if one of my brothers is a match, or later July if an unrelated donor is needed). The timing is an issue, because my wife and I are trying to ensure that we can have a quick getaway together before what will be a very difficult year. Not having an answer about my brothers makes it harder to book tickets! Doctors do understand. It is all based on risk calculation: the risk of symptoms returning versus the risk of missing an important chance to spend time together.

I downloaded a special software (which is fortunately free and open source – OsiriX), I was finally able to view the CD of my CTs and MRIs. I have spared you the 'home movies' version, but this shot should give you an idea of what the scans look like. The images are quite impressive, but from the point of view of interpretation and meaning, the dry radiologist reports are more useful.

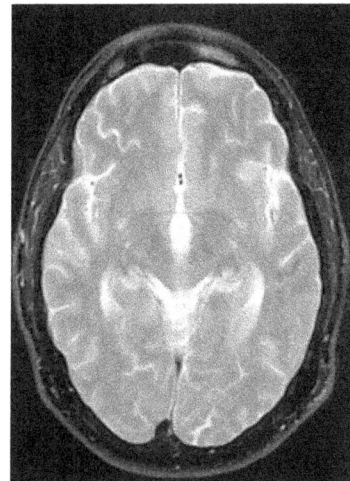

My inner mug shot

I have not done any reading this week, but have instead worked on the more personal administrative clean-up of household files and the like. I went through everything, chucked out a lot, and am keeping (and neatly organizing) just the essentials.

I also went through the boxes of stuff from my office. It was fairly easy to be ruthless. Interestingly, I had kept every one of my performance review since joining the government some 30 years ago. The reviews capture a decent record of my career in terms of the major files and issues and where they occurred. Of course, these reports were a bit self-serving, with a stronger focus on my achievements and less emphasis on my screw-ups (fortunately, I don't think there were too many of those!). Worth keeping, at least for now.

I am finding that keeping up with the various websites, twitter pages and other online platforms that I follow takes a fair amount of time. I have been using *Reeder*, *Zite* and *Flipboard* to compile articles of interest (and sharing the most interesting ones), and have also been corralling interesting feeds, which range from heartbreaking to hucksterism and everything in between, on my Twitter account. It is easy to drown in all the information, particularly given the richness of some of the experiences being shared. I have been trying to manage my time and focus better. After all, it is better to do some in-depth and more outward-focussed reading and go for more walks than to get caught up in the vortex of the internet.

In addition, I finally completed and circulated my 'reflections /lessons-learned' presentation on my work on Canadian citizenship and multiculturalism issues over the past four years. Thinking it through and putting it together was a good process. I will be presenting this presentation to our Department's senior management team in a few weeks, which will be a nice way to share and also connect on a personal level.

I watched a couple of Woody Allen movies this week. One new: *Cassandra's Dream*, rather mixed, on the themes of murder, remorse and consequences; one old: *Crimes and Misdemeanors*, one of his stronger films, which develops much the same themes much better (*Matchpoint* is another Allen film that addresses the same themes better). I am also waiting for *Midnight in Paris* to arrive in theaters here.

I am looking forward to what should be a good week, and to building up my strength. The Neulasta should have done its work by then and I should be past the period of low immunity, and thus more free of the risk of infection. I may need a blood transfusion to help bring up my haemoglobin levels and my energy, and I will certainly be doing what I can to nail the SCT donor question.

GETTING READY

June 12, 2011

The week started off slowly, as my anemia shortened the length and slowed the pace of our regular walks. I remember my mother, who also had lymphoma, telling me that she could judge her blood counts by the effort needed to walk up a very gentle hill, and I am now in the same situation – albeit in my 50s, not in my 80s!

However, I soon received a blood transfusion 'booster,' which made all the difference, and I was back to my regular walks by midweek. On top of that, the Neulasta worked, so my period of low immunity was over quickly.

The process of arranging my SCT has started to move forward. Unfortunately, neither of my brothers is a suitable donor, but other potential donors have been identified, and their suitability is being confirmed. While this route takes more time, the rate of success from the siblings and unrelated donors is virtually identical.

Since my opportunity to get a stem cell transplant is dependent on the kindness of strangers, my public service message is to encourage those who can to join a bone marrow registry: in Canada, OneMatch, or in the USA: Be the Match (those of you in other countries can Google 'bone marrow registry' or 'stem cell donation' in the local language). I hope some of you will check it out.

My health baseline is being established pre-transplant through more tests (a heart ultrasound and a test of my pulmonary capacity). I have 'negotiated' the dates of my end-of-June getaway with the medical team, and have had good discussions with the clinical doctor and the advanced practice nurse regarding what lies ahead. As always, different members of the medical team take a range of approaches, some more reassuring and some more frightening.

On the reassuring side, if confirming a donor goes according to plan, the transplant should take place in four to six weeks. The actual allo transplant process will be similar to, though more intense than, the auto transplant I had over a year and a half ago; it too will require a mixture of in- and out-patient treatment. The risk of infection and side effects (particularly on the liver and kidneys) resulting from the immunosuppressant drugs required this time is something that they will be paying close attention to. While the conditioning regime, a mix of chemo and radiation, will be harder on me, there are a number of medications that can alleviate treatment side effects.

On the frightening side are the numerous risks associated with any transplant. The clinical doctor noted that we would have another conversation with key doctors about these risks, the main one being Graft versus Host Disease (GvHD). GvHD can cause problems in the short-term as well as in the longer-term, in the form of chronic and ongoing GvHD.

The aim of these discussions is be to make us aware (the polite term; 'frightened' would more accurate) of all the bad things that could happen. These include death, diarrhea, skin problems, the perpetual need to be on oxygen, and other unpleasant chronic problems. Of course, some people also sail through the treatment. The problem is that while doctors know the overall odds, they cannot predict with certainty what will happen at the individual level. I mentioned to the clinical doctor having had similar discussions with one of the hematologists, and she noted that he tends to be 'overly soft.' I will thus be exposed to the 'scare' approach from now on to make sure that we fully understand the risks.

This information was delivered with compassion, but was still fairly brutal. Then again, so is my situation, and having a range of approaches is actually helpful. It prepares us for the inevitable decision about whether to go ahead, aware of the risks; hoping for the best, but preparing for the worst, as the cliché goes. The information from the medical team dovetails with a lot of the commentary from survivors and others on the web, though that discussion is naturally biased towards the survivors since they alone can continue to write.

All this helps us sharpen our questions before our consultation at the Princess Margaret Hospital on June 20th. We plan to inquire about options, alternatives, risks and implications. The main issue for my family and I (and the focus of my fear) with respect to my options and alternatives is the potential impact on my quality of life.

There was strong and practical support on the part of medical staff for my planned getaway, which I have been encouraged to take it sooner rather than later. They scheduled tests around our plans, providing me with medication (and accompanying instructions) in case it is needed, and even tentatively scheduled another blood transfusion just before we leave to ensure that I have enough energy to enjoy the trip. Life-affirming.

With our son being home this weekend, we have had some good family discussions about what I am going through and the seriousness of and risks involved in what I and the family as a whole are facing. Finding a balance between honesty and despair in sharing my vulnerabilities and fears is a challenge. One never knows how to get this exactly right, but given our shared need for support, I prefer to err on the side of being more open. I certainly I felt better after our discussion.

On a more prosaic level, I also had a very good exchange with the quality control person at the leukemia and lymphoma ward regarding the issues I identified during my last visit (at the end of May) and had captured in a detailed e-mail (not anonymously). Her response was positive; she took my points in the spirit of improvement that I intended, shared key elements with the medical team, and provided me with a concrete list of follow-up actions. I guess I can no longer pretend to be a 'mystery shopper,' and I did note that feedback on me as a patient was fair game!

My staff and colleagues sent me a wonderful book of memories, filled with their messages and photos. The messages – whether funny or serious, personal or less so, longer or shorter, general or particular – were a wonderful reflection of their diverse personalities, as well as the common humanity that we share. My eyes welled up a number of times!

I have been getting back into my reading, but started with something light. *What am I Doing Here*, by Bruce Chatwin, is a collection of short, interesting essays, most of which reflect his travel writing interests. While not necessarily deep, they were all engaging and thoughtful reminders of the rich variety of societies and cultures on the planet.

Movie-wise, the big screen movies that I want to see (*Midnight in Paris, The Tree of Life*) have yet to open in Ottawa, so we watched a few light movies at home instead. First was *Wild Target*, a British comedy-thriller, which doesn't quite come together but has its entertaining moments; then our kids did a *Back to the Future* marathon, so I watched the first movie in the trilogy with them – a bit dated, but fun.

Next week will be a further recovery week, building up my strength before the visit to Toronto and our getaway.

A Good Recovery Week

June 19, 2011

This week's post is shorter, as I have no intense clinic discussions to report on. In that sense, I have been enjoying a break from treatment and difficult discussions, and am just savouring life. I have been out and about, doing lots of walking (including some nice walks with friends) and enjoying the warm weather.

I enjoyed going into work to present my 'reflections' piece on the files that have consumed and interested me over the past four years. It took more preparation than my other presentations (I am not used to writing speaking notes anymore, and of course I could not delegate this one!). It was good to see the senior management team again. The presentation appeared to be well received (it is rare for employees to hear these kinds of reflection pieces), and it generated some good discussion. Of course, at the end of the day, files and issues will evolve, and how people handle them will vary depending on the current context. It was nevertheless satisfying to share my observations and increase awareness of certain issues. A nice way to close on both personal and professional levels.

As a 'regular' visitor for blood work (from frequent flyer to this!), I noticed that hospital has changed from standard needles, which worked well, to retractable ones, which seem to cause more problems for the nurses (and for me). I began to ask the nurse, each time I went in, whether or not they liked the new needles. The response was overwhelmingly negative. I also provided my own negative feedback to the clinic (part of my role as a non-mystery shopper!) and we will see if there is any change over the next few weeks.

I am becoming more interested in the 'metrics' of, or hits on, my blog. This week, I reached the milestone of 10,000 hits – not a lot when averaged over the number of posts I have made over the months, but it still feels significant. What is more interesting is seeing which articles, posts and links, apart from my weekly updates, resonate most with readers (in terms of active clicks). The top 5, over the past quarter, were:

1. What to Say to Someone Who's Sick
2. Fact Sheet on Mantle Cell Lymphoma
3. A Doctor's Letter to a Patient with Newly Diagnosed Cancer
4. Managing Mantle Cell Lymphoma
5. The Expert Patient

An interesting mix of more general interest articles and specific information about mantle cell lymphoma. I am not surprised that 'What to Say to Someone Who's Sick' was at the 'top of the charts;' it covers an issue that everyone can relate to and find helpful.

No reading this week – that time was devoted to a combination of preparing for the presentation and working through other stuff that needed to get done. I did, however, see some good movies: Mike Leigh's *Another Year*, a strong ensemble piece on intimacy and loneliness that beautifully captures family and friend dynamics; Kubrick's *Full Metal Jacket*, his Vietnam film, the first half of which was particularly powerful in its scenes of Marine basic training; and lastly, *Midnight in Paris*, which finally came out in Ottawa. I thoroughly enjoyed it. While it covers many of Woody Allen's favourite themes (creativity, relationships, meaning and compromise), it is all set in a wonderfully nostalgic Paris, and features some great character sketches (Hemingway and Dali were my favourites) and asides (the pedantic character Paul, Inez's parents' politics). Fun!

As noted in *A doctor's letter to a patient*, being at family events is part of what keeps patients going. This weekend included what was a good Father's Day for me. I attended our daughter's high school closing ceremony. While not as major a milestone as graduation, she still made herself and us proud by getting recognition for her achievements. As always, being at one milestone makes me reflect on the other milestones that I want to be around for, and gives me all the more reason to go press on. Later today, we are all off to Toronto to spend time with my son before the Princess Margaret consultation on Monday.

Overall, I had a relaxing recovery week, and appreciated that my medical team kindly organized the timing of the required 'booster' blood transfusion to fit between our daughter's school closing ceremony and our getaway, which will optimize my energy levels. And so, with more colour in my cheeks, and more spring in my step, I am ready to go!

I expect Monday's session at the Princess Margaret to be intense as we continue to come to grips with the next phase before getting on the plane for our getaway. However, the opinion will provide us with greater certainty with which to go ahead, or will open up some more options for consideration; either way, we will be better informed as we move forward and make the necessary decisions.

It should be a quiet week for the blog, but I will stick with the weekly updates.

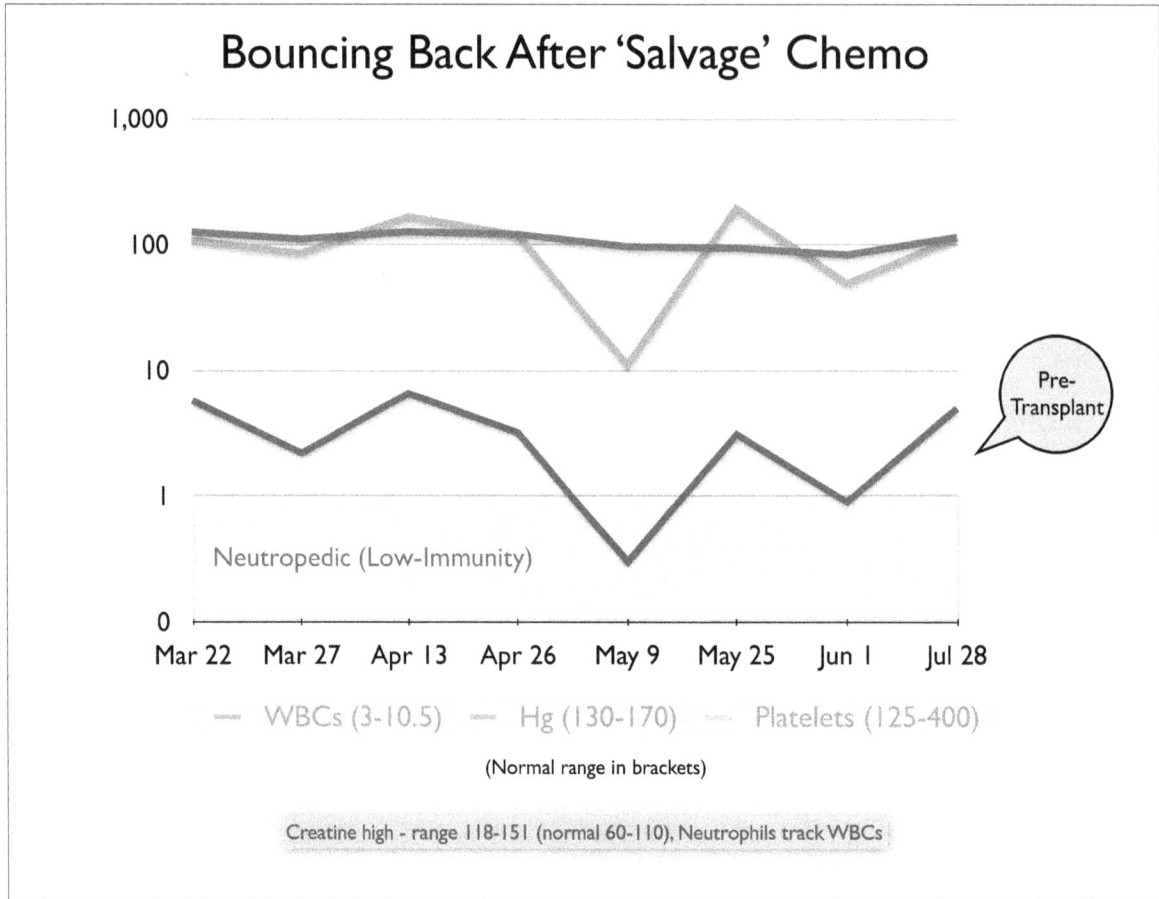

Bouncing Back After 'Salvage' Chemo

SECOND OPINION – GRIM BUT HELPFUL

June 21, 2011

I had a good and thorough session at the Princess Margaret Hospital (PMH) first with a resident, later joined by one of the hematologists. Both were knowledgeable and generous with their time – we spent close to an hour with them. Our son came with us, providing strong support and a third pair of ears to hear and absorb what was being said.

With respect to my previous treatment, the PMH uses different protocols: R-CHOP followed by maintenance Rituximab treatment, as the evidence base is more sound than that for R Hyper CVAD. However, the evidence to date suggests that the latter option is also an acceptable treatment regime. The PMH staff were surprised, however, that no bone marrow biopsy had been performed at any stage in my treatment to assess how systemic my MCL is.

In terms of going forward, the hematologist noted that mortality rates were often deceptive. For example, Seattle, which has the best (that is, lowest) mortality rates, benefits from its selection of patients (they must be healthy and wealthy enough to travel there); public systems like those in the UK and

Certainty or Hope - The Choice

- Do nothing - 1 year max
- Allo SCT - high risk
- Health, age improve odds
- Many discussions
- Philosophical choice
- Family driving force

20%

40%

40%

- Death within 3 Months
- Death within 2 years
- 3-5 year survival

Canada, in contrast, do not filter or select patients in the same manner, and consequently have higher mortality rates. These rates are pretty brutal: 20 percent mortality in the initial treatment phase (the first three months), and an additional 40 percent or so in the first two years. The overall success rates are in the order of 35-40 percent, where success is defined as living for three to five years with no remission.

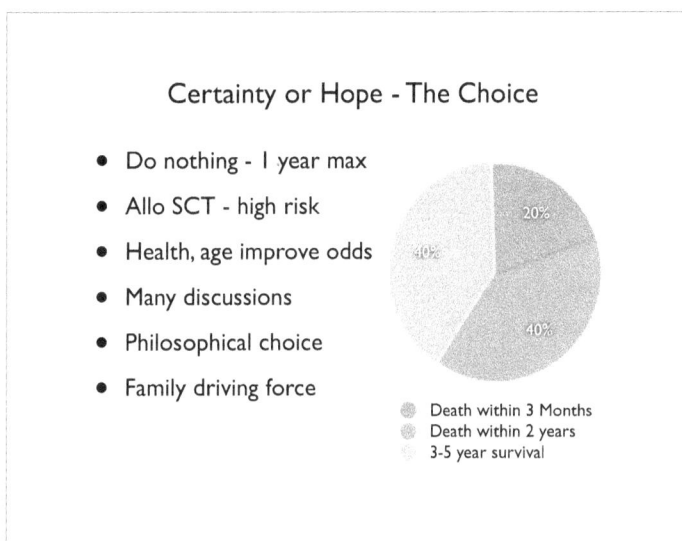

On the other hand, doing nothing would mean that my lymphoma will return. Typically, the period of remission becomes shorter following each round of treatment. After the first round, I got fourteen months; after the second round of salvage chemo that I have undergone over the past few months, the hematologist said I may get nine months. A third round would likely give me even less time in remission. This is all based on averages, of course, but the pattern is clear and fairly certain.

He phrased the choice between doing nothing and an allo stem cell transplant almost philosophically: either the certainty of succumbing to MCL in less than two years, or the risk and hope involved in getting an allo SCT for longer-term results. My relapse has shown me the limits of chemo. An allo SCT provides the alternative of an immunity-based approach, though with all the high risks that such an approach entails.

While the risk of Graft versus Host Disease is most acute during the first three months, it really takes two years before one can know whether one is all clear. Typically, reactions will diminish during that period as one's body and new immune system come to terms with one another, but the process is still definitely a long haul.

Assuming that the bone marrow biopsy confirms that I am in remission, my age and general health make me a candidate that the hematologist would, like my medical team in Ottawa, recommend for an allo SCT. The physical exam confirmed what my CT scan showed: my lymph nodes are normal. I am a bit of an oddity in that the lymphoma in my central nervous system (CNS) is not present elsewhere. This means a combination of aggressive and indolent lymphoma, although the hematologist suspects that a bone marrow biopsy earlier on would have shown lymphoma there as well (making it systemic). Fortunately the treatment I received to address the lymphoma in my central nervous system is also effective in the bone marrow, and should have cleared that up too.

He did, however, recommend a low-intensity conditioning regime of chemo given the amount of chemo my body has already endured and that the chemo has not had a long lasting effect. At least the chemo part of the treatment would be easier than what I undergone during my auto SCT over a year and a half ago; in other words, I will 'just' have to worry about radiation treatment, and particularly, about GvHD.

Some practical suggestions that he made regarding the next phase:

- do a bone marrow biopsy to confirm remission – he would not proceed to SCT without it

- consider some immunotherapy (Rituximab) in the interim

- review recent Canada health study on some new GvHD drugs that are proving to be effective

While he will make his formal report to the Ottawa team, whom he clearly knows, later, I have already flagged the need for a bone marrow biopsy and will share these notes with my medical team to ensure that we heard and absorbed the information correctly.

I did receive some compliments from both the resident and the hematologist – I looked better than expected, and I am a very knowledgable patient. Filing everything on my iPad allowed me to call things up quickly. Small stuff, but a nice counterpoint to the serious medical information and good for the ego!

All-in-all, a really helpful visit to clarify my options, though the choices are not easy ones and the situation feels surreal.

Away From it All

June 26, 2011

My wife and I had a wonderful Paris getaway, just what we needed after the discussion on options at the Princess Margaret Hospital.

To get a European perspective on my options, we also chatted with the father of one of my son's friends, who confirmed the general approach, signaled some possible complementary treatment options (immunotherapy) and highlighted that we might eventually consider participating in clinical trials – but noted that the SCT is the best option for now.

With that out of the way, we are enjoying our vacation. This is not a 'bucket list' trip, but rather a return to one of our favourite cities and one that each of us has visited frequently – both together and separately. Paris is a great walking city, with many neighborhoods to explore and revisit. We went to our preferred museums and saw some special exhibits, savoured the food, and enjoyed the street life, seeing friends and just being and enjoying. Hard to beat!

I have certainly been making use of the 'booster shot' blood transfusions – we are walking for three to four hours per day, and my energy levels are still good.

I have been reading *The Best Laid Plans* by Terry Fallis, a delightfully light and funny political satire. It captures the Ottawa milieu all too well.

While we do come back to discussing my options from time-to-time – I seem to be between a known hard rock and a less known hard place – our focus is on being in the here and now. The decisions can await our next series of discussions in Ottawa.

WAITING FOR THE NEXT STEP

July 3, 2011

Our break in Paris has come to an end, not without reflection on how good a break it was, and how necessary to get away from hospital visits and consultations. My wife and I were both re-energized and recharged by our time there, and have largely been able to put aside what lies ahead. I am curious, of course, to see what impact if any the trip had on my blood counts; ideally, we could schedule such a break every three to four months as part of my treatment plan!

During the plane trip back, I worked on refreshing the background pages on my blog (Dualities, Lessons Learned, Healthcare System) post-relapse. I posted the updated versions yesterday. The Dualities piece struck a chord with readers through StumbleUpon, judging by the spike in blog stats; of the three pieces, that one helped me most of all – and continues to help me – work through the issues.

Writing these on the plane reminded me of old times, when I would business trip and meeting reports while flying. I always find airplane time to be incredibly productive. I also started writing some reflections on faith, which, not surprisingly, are taking some time to work through.

This was my first trip using the iPad as a laptop substitute. It is very workable in a travel context, although the virtual keyboard is not as precise as a regular keyboard. In addition to its lightness, another advantage of the iPad is it can remain in my bag through airport security – one less hassle.

Of course, coming back home means coming back to reality. I have to visit the hospital for blood work, and next week, the clinic to discuss next steps. I have been having some discussions with the kids (our son is making a concerted effort to come home whenever possible) on the rock and hard place options.

As I felt a bit guilty to be leaving our son so soon after the brutal discussion at Princess Margaret, it was good to have a follow-up chat with him in person this weekend. He expressed incredible support, both practical and more importantly, emotional, for both my wife and I, as well as a real openness and willingness to engage in these difficult discussions. This makes a big difference. I have also had some equally supportive discussions with my brothers as we proceed to the big decision.

Disappointingly, there has been no news from the hospital about scheduling the bone marrow biopsy, so I am working through a list of topics to bring up at the clinic on Tuesday. These will include my notes from the Princess Margaret Hospital (I will likely just give them a copy of my blog entry to suggest gently that their responsiveness, or lack thereof, will also be noted in the blog!). Of course, I am also equally interested in knowing the results of any testing for the compatibility of potential donors.

We had a great Canada Day, which was kicked off with one of my last work-related activities – we were able to attend the Canada Day citizenship ceremony, witnessed by the Duke and Duchess of Cambridge, Will and Kate, and presided over by our Governor General. While this ceremony was unique given the presence of the Royal couple, I find all of our citizenship ceremonies moving; it is powerful to see people who have chosen Canada formalize their decision by becoming new Canadian citizens.

It was impressive to see just how good Will and Kate are at working the crowd, engaging in conversations, and communicating interest in the people they were talking to. Our daughter was lucky enough to have a short conversation with Will, and she was really impressed with how engaged (and engaging) he was. Naturally, she updated her Facebook page to share the news, and her friends were impressed – especially when a number of them saw her in the TV coverage of Will and Kate interacting with the crowd.

While we let our kids disappear to enjoy the Canada Day concert and other events, my wife and I did catch the fireworks. These are always enjoyable and were a cut above the usual this year given the presence of the Royals. I made use of the 45-minute walk to and from our viewing spot to confirm that my blood counts were OK.

Next week's focus will be on the clinic visit and related discussions on my options. While I am leaning towards going ahead with the stem cell transplant, a key factor will be the results of the bone marrow biopsy (the PMH doctor was particularly adamant on that point) to ensure that I am in full remission and thus completely ready for the transplant.

A FEW MORE WEEKS

July 10, 2011

Paris was good for me – I now have the data to prove it. All my blood counts have improved, particularly my haemoglobin and creatinine (which signals kidney stress, or lack thereof). Getaways are good for the body as well as the soul.

I had a good clinic visit with the senior hematologist, walking through what we heard from the PMH and related questions and issues. I summarized what I learned from the medical team there, noting their agreement that a stem cell transplant (SCT) was the recommended option and their emphasis on my getting a bone marrow biopsy beforehand.

I also provided the hematologist with a copy of my blog entry.

While he was pleased that the overall recommendations were the same at the PMH as in Ottawa, he suggested that the bone marrow biopsy was not necessary as it would not tell us anything new. The presence of lymphoma in my central nervous system already showed that the lymphoma was systemic (the PMH doctors had also noted this), and the absence or presence of a few more cells in my bone marrow would not change the recommended course of treatment. The hematologist agreed, however, to schedule a biopsy as part of the normal pre-transplant re-staging (assessing how advanced my lymphoma is) process. His explanation about the biopsy was reasonable to my lay ears, but I was pleased that he agreed to have the biopsy done in any case.

No word on donor status yet, but I will get an update next week. The hematologist referred again to the three to six weeks required to arrange the transplant, which means that it will now more likely take place in August than July. I expressed surprise and concern at this new timeline, as I had imagined that some of those three to six weeks had already elapsed. He replied that he understood that the transplant may seem like a 'mirage,' ever receding, to me. However, the delay reflected the need for my firm confirmation that I wanted to proceed in light of the PMH second opinion before setting everything in motion.

A few more weeks of comfort have I. Half-jokingly, I said that I would like to go back to Paris if I must wait! He took this seriously – the medical staff is very supportive of things that help us get through the waiting period. Something else to consider once the time frame is confirmed.

There was no real discussion of the protocol and treatment plan at this meeting; the hematologist merely noted (again) that it will involve Total Body Irradiatio – TBI). An August transplant date would likely mean that I will not need any more chemo to keep my condition stable. I asked about immunotherapy (Rituximab), and he replied that any effect would be marginal and not needed.

I challenged him a bit on the different communication styles of doctors, and how some prefer a 'shock and awe' approach while he, in contrast, was much more reassuring. He laughed and acknowledged the point, but placed it in the context of the seriousness of mantle cell lymphoma

146

(i.e., there are no great options). While the transplant was serious and risky, he responded effectively with the following points:

- he had nothing else to offer that would get me to next summer;

- the normal tendency was to dramatize side effects and risks (citing the detailed description of risks that accompanies Aspirin);

- I got through the auto SCT relatively easily;

- I have read and am well-informed enough to make a decision (there can never be 100% certainty); and,

- overall, given the alternative, the risks are worth taking.

He ended with the compliment that I had worked through the issues in a very timely manner. I noted that not having much time helped, but clearly he has other patients who find it harder – for their own valid reasons – to make this decision.

He ended by turning to my wife to make sure that she was OK (she is a bit overwhelmed, as we all are), noting that while there was little support during the waiting stage, there would be more help available to accompany the transplant process.

I also had a good meeting with the social worker, during which I worked through my impressions and reactions to the different approaches of doctors towards communications (noting that personally, these different approaches help me sift through information, but that others may react differently), and my feelings about some of our family dynamics as I undergo the transplant. I suggested that having another session with the whole family before the transplant could be helpful. She also gave some practical advice: worry about the transplant first, as any effects would occur subsequent to the transplant phase – a 'chewable chunk' approach.

On the life and living side, I have had many of long walks and am enjoying the summer weather. Our son is back again this weekend and we have been experimenting with new barbecue recipes; a quintessential Canadian summer activity, and an opportunity for father-son bonding!

I saw some interesting movies this week. In the ambitious but failed category, Terrence Mallick's *The Tree of Life* (pretentious, incoherent and silly) – although we also watched his *Thin Red Line*, which is much more focused and effective, if still meandering. I also watched *Of Gods and Men*, a French movie about monks who decided to remain with their village during the period of violence between the government and Islamic groups in Algeria. A very powerful depiction of the positive power of faith, and the courage that can accompany it.

I read *And Then They Came for Me*, Maziar Bahari's recounting, from the perspective of a Newsweek journalist, of Iran's Green Revolution and of his subsequent imprisonment. It was not as sophisticated as Haleh Esfandiari's *My Prison My Home*, but included many insights into Iran, the interrogation process, being courageous and keeping one's sanity, and finally, the important role played by international pressure in getting Bahari and his fellow hostages released. The book featured some wonderful asides on Leonard Cohen (Bahari's strongest Canadian connection), which reveal both his cynical side (Bahari mentions the song 'Everybody Knows' as he realizes the election results will be fixed) and his romantic or hopeful side ('Sisters of Mercy' comes to him during his time in prison). Another powerful and depressing account of Iran today.

This week, we also visited the Caravaggio exhibit at the National Art Gallery. The exhibit was a manageable size, and contrasted his style of painting with that of other Renaissance artists, showing that he was one of the key painters involved in creating a more naturalistic style.

I hope to get a few more details on treatment plans and timelines this week, which would help me figure out how best to use the waiting period. As I understand it, things can move quickly once a donor is confirmed. While I am enjoying the current break, my normal inclination, once I make a decision, is to get on with it. Hopefully the wait will not be too long.

Chapter 10

Transplant

Day 0 to 30

I receive new stem cells from my donor. The first month brings the risk of these failing to 'engraft' onto my own blood marrow. I have a high risk for infection, given my low immunity. I am weak and feeling extremely crummy.

WE HAVE A DONOR

July 17, 2011

Good news: I have a 'perfect' donor lined up and the medical team is now working out dates. My team has proposed that the transplant take place during the first week of August, and pre-transplant planning is proceeding with that date in mind even though things could change if the time is not convenient for the donor.

This has taken a major load off our minds; we were concerned despite having been assured repeatedly that finding a match would not be a problem. The machine is now in motion, which means new scans, more exhaustive blood work and other tests are being scheduled, along with a few pre-treatment planning sessions. The heart test ('perfect' – all that walking must help) and lung test ('normal') are complete, and show that and I am fit enough to handle the transplant.

Of course, after the emotional relief of knowing that a donor has been secured, my worries about the transplant and GvHD have re-emerged. Funny how the mind can compartmentalize. Though the planning sessions will help us deal with our worries, some of the 'what if' discussions of potential side effects will not exactly be cheery.

The restrictions on my driving and biking have largely been lifted (though I must still be extra careful) which will help me enjoy the next few weeks. While driving is a major help for convenience and autonomy, biking makes a big difference on the emotional and spiritual levels – there is a wonderful 45-minute bike ride that I like to take, and which allows me to appreciate nature. It will be part of my new daily routine.

I am getting through some of the stuff that needs to get done before I re-enter the world of weakness and low immunity, ranging from the mundane (visiting the dentist) to the enjoyable (seeing friends).

I have had a good cultural program these days. My thoughts on one film, *Beginners*, were mixed; the story is about a father (played by Christopher Plummer) who comes out in his mid-70s, following his relationship with his son and the parallels and differences in the romantic relationships that each develops. It was not fully successful, but had a good feel for the discovery and intensity involved in falling in love. It did include some great cancer-related black humour: when the son is trying to get the father to tell his friends that he has cancer, he dramatizes the point by noting, 'You have stage IV cancer; there is no stage V.' The father calmly replies, 'Stage IV just comes after Stage III; it is just a number' – he is focussed on life and living.

I got permission to go to Stratford and see some plays (one last getaway), so my wife and I took our daughter to see the *Merry Wives of Windsor* and *Twelfth Night*. Our choice of plays was determined by the timing of my treatment, but I really enjoyed being back in Stratford with my wife and daughter. It reminded me of going there regularly with my parents when my brothers and I were teenagers. And at one of the plays, we saw Christopher Plummer in the audience!

I have been re-reading the two plays we saw to help me enjoy (and follow!) the performances better. Reading Shakespeare again has brought back the richness of his language, the quickness of his wit, and the degree to which his work is engrained in our consciousness. It also reminds me of the need, when reading the work of Shakespeare and other great writers, to slow down and savour the words. The usual scanning-type reading that we do on a daily basis does not cut it.

We reached another milestone this week, as we wrapped up the process of coaching our daughter for her driver's test, which she passed. As is the case for all parents, this transition caused new worries to emerge, but that is just another part of the cycle of life.

The next few weeks will be a mix of seeing people, savouring my remaining time pre-transplant, getting scans and tests done, having planning sessions with the medical team, and continuing to build up my strength so that I will be as prepared as possible for the transplant and aftermath.

WE HAVE A DATE – THE COUNTDOWN BEGINS

July 24, 2011

It has been a good but split week: my 'honeymoon' from treatment ended Wednesday with another lumbar puncture and the accompanying top up of chemo (methotrexate) for my spinal fluid. This meant that I was unable to bike and felt really tired for a few days, but today (Sunday) I got back into my biking routine.

My transplant is set for August 12th, and the conditioning process will begin about a week earlier. In contrast to my previous stem cell transplant, I am going into this feeling strong and relatively 'normal,' so I expect that the negative effects will feel even more like hitting a brick wall than they did last time.

We had an excellent discussion at the clinic with the new head of the Blood and Marrow Transplant (BMT) team – so I have more detailed information in this week's post.

I will be getting what is known as the full myeloblative treatment, which involves high intensity chemo (my old favourite, cyclophosphomide) and Total Body Irradiation (TBI). The radiation is used to get at the parts of my body that chemo has difficulty reaching (it gets across the blood-brain barrier better than methotrexate and Ara C, which are in turn most effective in the Central Nervous System – CNS).

This high intensity functions both as treatment (to get at any remaining lymphoma cells) and as the all-important conditioning for my stem cell transplant; its purpose in that regard is essentially to 'kill' my existing immune system. The radiation, in particular, provides a few months before the new immune system is active, reduces risk of rejection of my new stem cells, and is able to either kill or suppress any remaining bad cells.

I asked about the possibility of lower intensity regimes, as per the suggestion of Princess Margaret Hospital medical team. The head of the BMT team noted that the pendulum of evidence tends to shift between low and high intensity regimes, and that it currently appears to be shifting back towards high intensity, which of the two (with comparable toxicity) seems to get at the CNS more effectively.

After the transplant, the engraftment of the new stem cells onto my bone marrow takes between two and three weeks, after which point we should start having a sense of whether Graft versus Host Disease will develop. Most of the treatment will occur on an out-patient basis, although I requested that it in-patient when I am administered cyclophosphomide (given my past experience with a mega dose, after which I had severe nausea and vomiting and had to go back to the hospital).

The Allogeneic Transplant Process

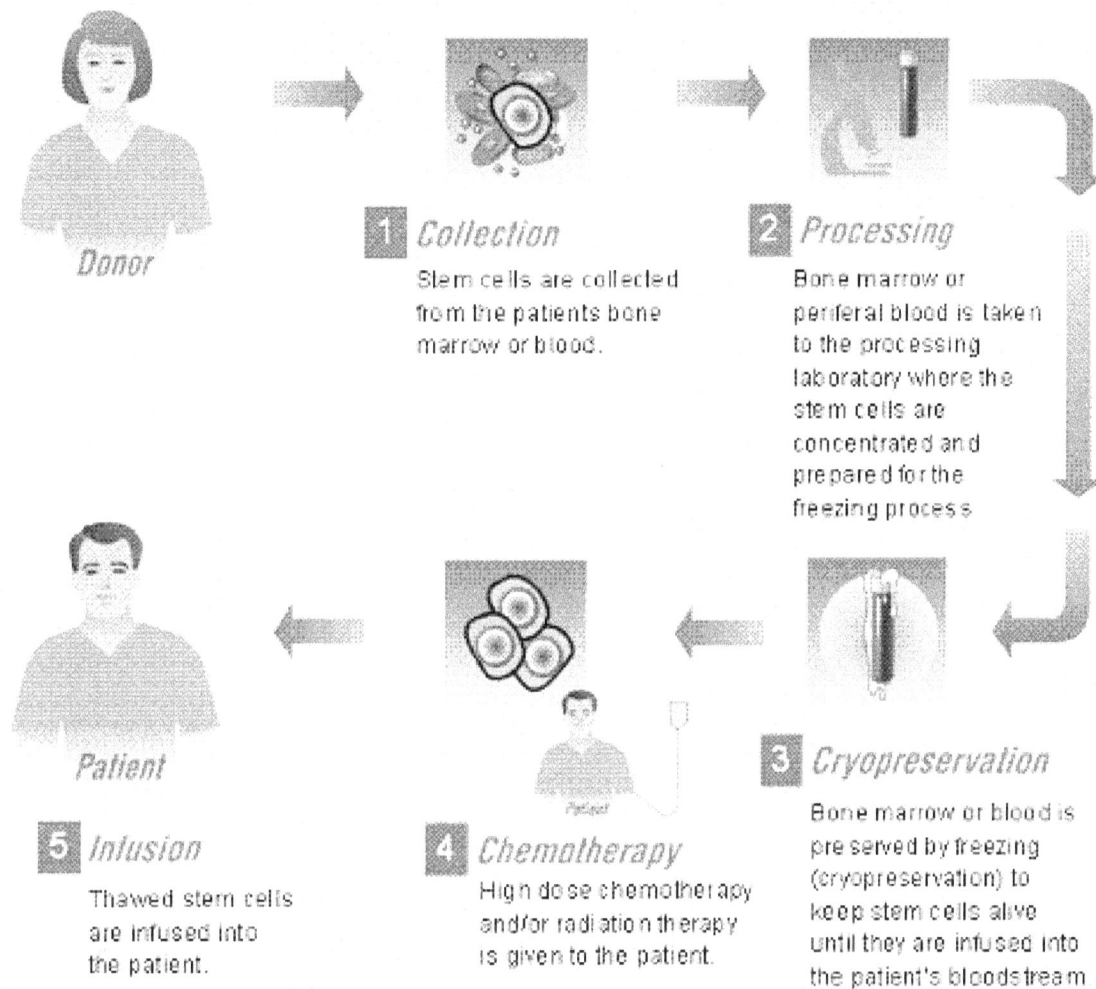

Donor

1 *Collection*

Stem cells are collected from the patients bone marrow or blood.

2 *Processing*

Bone marrow or periferal blood is taken to the processing laboratory where the stem cells are concentrated and prepared for the freezing process

Patient

5 *Infusion*

Thawed stem cells are infused into the patient.

4 *Chemotherapy*

High dose chemotherapy and/or radiation therapy is given to the patient.

3 *Cryopreservation*

Bone marrow or blood is preserved by freezing (cryopreservation) to keep stem cells alive until they are infused into the patient's bloodstream

Biomed.brown.edu

We covered – again – the potential risks. The risk of acute (possibly fatal) GvHD is about 10 percent. The main consequences would be rashes, diarrhea and damage to the liver. Overall, exposure to GvHD is managed by a combination of 'little squirts' of methotrexate and pills over the short term, which would range from between three to twelve months depending on my response. The long-term effects of GvHD affect a broader range of organs (e.g., lungs, kidneys, eyes, mouth).

We must strike a fine balance between keeping GvHD under control and eliminating it completely; after all, some GvHD is necessary to keep my under control. I will be on a knife's edge, and consequently will be closely monitored. About 50 percent of patients experience some form of chronic GvHD.

As usual, the risk decreases with time. Making it through each stage further reduces risk, with the first three to six months being the most critical. The BMT team head noted, with a smile, that despite my relapse I am still alive and have made it through the last few months of chemo without any major issues. While there are no guarantees, these are encouraging signs from his perspective.

The recovery period is about a year, and will be followed by monitoring for an additional two years. In addition, I will need to redo my vaccinations (again!) for my new immune system after a bit more than a year.

There was some further discussion about my lung test, since my oxygen diffusion was apparently low. As this may have been related to my low haemoglobin count at the time (85 compared to the normal range of 130-170, it does not seem to be an issue.

I also raised the question of whether any other immunotherapy would be used in parallel with the chemo and radiation. With respect to Velcade, he noted that there was no real data and that it would bring an additional risk of neural toxicity; similarly, with respect to Rituxan ('prescribed like water in the US'), there is no real data on its effectiveness for someone in my situation.

The results from my lumbar puncture are excellent: 0 white blood cells. The head of the BMT team confirmed the opinion of his colleague, who had suggested that a bone marrow test would not show anything new or change the treatment approach (apparently these are largely done for research reasons to ensure comparability of results between different patients). His view in a nutshell: why undergo the additional discomfort? I agreed, as I would rather have more time to spend bike riding and being with the family.

Ironically, although I had been warned that this particular hematologist tends to deliver the message of risks in a pretty brutal fashion, that was not the case at all (or maybe I have been 'conditioned' to no longer find this kind of news brutal!).

All-in-all, it was a helpful and even encouraging session. I had adequate time to go through the issues, and I have a high degree of confidence in their approach, which I believe has been well thought through. How I respond, of course, is still up to the luck of the draw, but as the doctor noted, the most serious threat at this point remains mantle cell lymphoma.

I did finally break down and get *The Emperor of Maladies: A Biography of Cancer*. I should have read it earlier, as it provides great historical and scientific context for everything I have learned, and continue to learn, through my journey − all in a very readable form. The book is not necessarily cheery, and some of the history of early clinical trials is particularly gruesome, but I am surprised at how much I am enjoying the read. It has aroused my intellectual curiosity, and I have gained a deep appreciation of how much I have benefitted from earlier research and trials (and a particular appreciation for many of the patients involved, who were little more than guinea pigs at that time). Highly recommended for those interested.

While our kids saw the last Harry Potter film on opening night, my wife and I went to see it this week. Like so many others, our kids grew up with the books and the films (I remember them disappearing for a few days after each book came out). We saw the early films together before they became older and started going with their friends, and so the end of the films symbolizes in many ways the end of their childhood. And yes, I enjoyed the movie!

Everything else is falling into place. I have a meeting with the radiation oncologist, a related scan, and a detailed planning session scheduled for next week, and the MRI has been scheduled for the beginning of the following week. My blood work (5 vials!) was done this week.

As I gather all of this information, much of it familiar, some of it new or more detailed, the imminence of what I am about to go through strikes me anew. Theoretical worries remain theoretical for now, but I feel a bit more jumpy and worried. I am still, however, still comfortable with going ahead. I am far from relaxed about it all, but at least in a space where I am ready to go for it and give it my best shot. As good as it can get!

ALLOGENEIC STEM CELL TRANSPLANT TIMELINE

At a high level, this graphic captures the overall transplant process and timeline from conditioning regime to recovery. The clinic had been meaning to develop such a graphic and was really happy with my handiwork – an opportunity for me to give back.

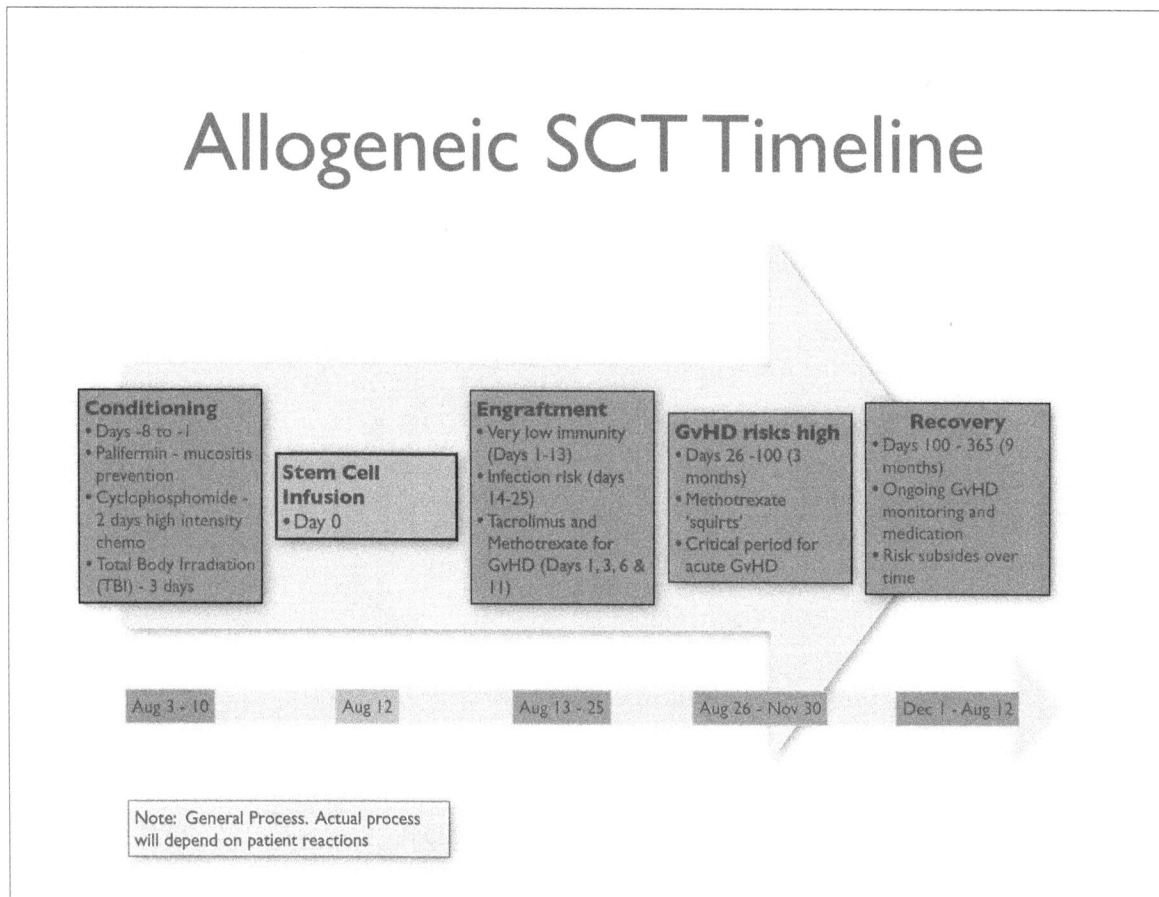

LAST FEW DAYS BEFORE IT STARTS

July 31, 2011

> *Because I know that time is always time*
>
> *And place is always and only place*
>
> *And what is actual is actual only for one time*
>
> *And only for one place*
>
> *I rejoice that things are as they are and*
>
> *I renounce the blessèd face*
>
> *And renounce the voice*
>
> *Because I cannot hope to turn again*
>
> *Consequently I rejoice, having to construct something*
>
> *Upon which to rejoice*

From T.S. Elliot, *Ash Wednesday*

It has been a good week, spent making the last preparations before things really get moving next week. I had with sessions with both the radiation oncologist and the Blood and Marrow Transplant (BMT) liaison nurse. There may be more details than necessary below, so be forewarned.

The week started with a hiccup. My donor's wife contracted Hepatitis C a few weeks ago. The donor assured the team that they had had no intimate relations since then (the things we learn!). From my medical team's perspective, the overall risk of transmission is low, even if he did catch it from his wife.

The alternative – checking out the other potential donor – would mean a six week delay (and confirming whether or not my current donor had or had not contracted Hep C would mean a six *month* delay because of the incubation period). The risks involved in waiting would be high for me, since I am currently at the optimum point for a transplant. The kicker for me: on the off-chance that I become infected, the negative effects would be 10 years out. This is a risk I can live with given my much more immediate concerns. Relatively speaking, this is a minor worry in relation to my overall worries – though one that I did not need, of course. I have put the need to get tested for Hep C on my b/f (bring forward) list six to nine months post-transplant if, as I hope, my other worries and risks have passed by then.

The BMT liaison nurse, my wife and I walked through the detailed transplant regime. The process was familiar because of my previous transplant, but tougher. The chemo used (cyclosphosphomide) will be at a much higher dose than ever before. It will be administered on an in-patient basis given my extreme nausea last time (the benefit of experience!). This treatment, in combination with Total Body Irradiation (TBI), means that the normal post-chemo side effects (nausea, mucositis, diarrhea, low immunity, risk of infection, need for transfusions, etc.) will be more severe. The latter half of August will not be an easy time for me.

The donor cells will be collected on August 10th and 11th, and will then miraculously arrive in Ottawa for the 'infusion' on the 12th (fresh, not frozen!).

I asked about taking probiotics to help alleviate bowel problems and reduce the risk of C. difficile (which I caught after my last transplant). The BMT liaison nurse said to check with the pharmacists before my chemo starts. She also reminded me that hand sanitizer does not kill the C. difficile bacteria, and that a good, rubbing hand washing is the best way to reduce my risk.

She also gave me the usual reminders about Graft versus Host Disease (GvHD), ranging from dreary to cheery, that I covered in earlier posts. As I have been told a number of times, it is important that I manage my expectations. The transplant process is a one-year marathon and it is normal to need two to three readmissions within that year.

The post-transplant medication program is a mix of Tacrolimus and Methotrexate, which serve to reduce the likelihood of GvHD. I mentioned the previous issues that Methotrexate has caused me in terms of kidney stress; the BMT liaison nurse responded that the medical team will be monitoring me very closely and will adjust the dose – or take me off the drug completely – as needed. While the Methotrexate dose alone is low, the cumulative impact of Cyclophosphomide, TBI and the transplant increase the potential stress on my body, making the treatment a real balancing act.

Overall, though she gave me the necessary reminders of side effects and risks, the BMT liaison nurse did so in an encouraging manner. It also helps that I have enough knowledge and experience to ask the right questions (as the Dutch soccer player and coach Johan Cruijiff put it, 'There is an advantage to every disadvantage').

After our discussion (and a lengthy wait), I was joined by an intern, who was an annoying waste of time. He knew nothing about my medical history. How many times do I have to tell people about my previous treatment? After reading my file, he proceeded to reiterate, in a more confusing and depressing manner, all of the risks that I had just been told about. Why not just come in and say:

> You have had a number of sessions with the medical team on the
> treatment plan, potential risks and complications. Are there any remaining
> issues that you have or would like to discuss?

Clean, simple, and provides a final opportunity to raise concerns. Sigh. I will need to provide some feedback. Overall, however, the process – while sometimes frustrating and lengthy – has helped my family and I work out the issues as best we can.

I also had a session with the radiation oncologists. While the short-term effects are as noted earlier, the longer-term effects could be as follows:

- Medium-term (six months to a year): thyroid impairment, lung impairment (i.e., shortness of breath); and,

- Long-term (ten or more years): brain cancer, bowel cancer, cataracts; in fifteen to twenty years, kidney impairment.

These are manageable, and some are so far off in the future as to not be an issue in my case. Regardless, all pale in significance to the more immediate risks related to the transplant itself and GvHD. As a result, I am definitely 'living in the now' (the Keynesian formulation, "in the long run, we are dead," has a particular resonance!). It is kind of funny to have this kind of briefing, my response to which has a 'whatever' aspect to it – i.e., I should be so lucky as to have some of these complications, since they will only occur if my treatment works and prolongs my life by ten years or more!

On a more interesting note, I really enjoyed reading Karen Armstrong's *The Spiral Staircase*, which recounts the author's spiritual journey from a cloistered novice to a crusading rejectionist of religion and spirituality, and then finally to the discovery of a more universal belief in faith and spirituality.

It is not surprising that her conclusion emerged from visiting Jerusalem, where she was confronted with the three Abrahamic religions operating literally within blocks of each other. This prompted her to learn about Judaism and Islam, and thus the similarities and differences between these and Christianity. Well worth reading. In retrospect, I should have read this before writing my Reflections on Faith page, but better late than never. Armstrong repeatedly cites a poem by T.S. Elliot, *Ash Wednesday*, that resonates particularly with her journey. It spoke to me, too, though from a more secular perspective; hence the excerpt above.

My wife and I have been watching a number of older movies with our daughter, ranging from *My Fair Lady* to *Groundhog Day* to *Scarface*. We also rented *Winter in Wartime*, a Dutch film about a boy's coming of age and his involvement in the resistance during World War II. A good and interesting film.

I have been savouring the summer weather and continuing my bike rides, which I can now do in 40 minutes compared to my earlier 45 minutes. I now have an additional pre-transplant baseline as reference. On top of that, my son and I will be going for a long bike ride this weekend, on one of my favourite routes through parks and by the water – just to enjoy, not to prove anything.

My son is home for the long weekend, and I am enjoying the time with my family during these last few days of feeling healthy, engaged and alert before I start the next phase of the journey – my 'marathon' – on Saturday. I feel as strong and prepared as possible, am hopeful within reason, and am ready to get on with it.

Until then, I am enjoying myself while and when I can!

IT HAS STARTED

August 7, 2011

A few pictorial metaphors for what I have started to go through.

The first, naturally, is a brick wall. Over the past few months, I really built my strength up. I am stronger now than I was during my last stem cell transplant, at which point I had just finished a heavy series of chemo. Consequently, I expect that this round, with its blast of high intensity chemo and total body irradiation, will hit me even more like a brick wall since I am used to feeling healthy. We shall see – the full effects of yesterday's chemo have yet to set in.

The second image is that of a roller coaster, which represents the ups and downs, the 'thrills' and (hopefully few) spills of the next few months and beyond. The other relevant aspect of this metaphor, which struck me just this week, is the anticipation (dread?) that one feels when waiting in line and going up that first hill – knowing that the ride has started, and that there are no off-ramps!

I will know which metaphor works best in about a month or so.

This week, we moved from discussing to doing. I spent most of the week preparing: a MRI of my brain and spine to provide baseline information (a charming hour or so inside the 'jackhammer,' as I refer to it), some pre-radiation meds (no real side effects), the installation of my Hickman line (which I will likely need for three to six months), and the unfortunate end of my bike rides. Once the line is in, one's tolerance of risk (e.g., less able to handle a bike crash) decreases rapidly.

As a result of my worries shifting from theoretical to real, I slept less well, and was much more nervous than I expected during the minor operation to install the Hickman line. I expect that this reflected my overall worries, which happened to crystalize in that moment; fortunately, some 'happy juice' (Ativan, a drug to treat anxiety) helped relax me.

I had a good session with the pharmacist, who walked me through some of my meds (those to control nausea, etc.). She was was fairly upbeat as she walked me through the stages: nausea in week one; crumminess, low immunity and possible mucositis in weeks two and three; and recovery in week four (at least, that's the plan).

All in all, this past week has been a hybrid between enjoying the last few days with family and friends, lots of biking and walking, and savouring good food while I could taste it, and on the other hand, getting ready for my treatment. In many ways, there is a 'last supper' element to many of these activities. This is not so much due to a sense of finality (I remain cautiously optimistic), but rather to the realization that I am beginning a long process and it will be a long time before I am back to normal (and my normal activities). Hence the imperative to have really enjoyed this break.

A number of you have noticed that in July, I broadened my blog beyond the weekly updates, posting links to articles of interest. It was interesting to see the direct correlation between the increased number of posts (over 70) and increased number of hits (almost 6,000). StumbleUpon was the best vehicle (better than Twitter) for attracting readers. The five posts (apart from the Home page) that received the most hits were:

1. David Servan-Schreiber (French obituaries, NYT obit) – by an overwhelming margin, which is surprising given the lack of English-language coverage

2. Some reflections on faith

3. Learning from Insect Swarms: Smart Cancer Targeting

4. Cancer Sucks – Synovate Insights Blog

5. Handwashing alone won't stop C. difficile, experts warn

Needless to say, I expect to be less prolific – and possibly less coherent – in these coming weeks, perhaps to the relief of some of you!

No week of preparation would have been complete without more paperwork. While my long-term disability insurance was approved, I also had to apply for the Canada Pension Plan – Disability as part of the terms of my insurance. The forms remain as cumbersome as they were when I was working on making government service more citizen-friendly over five years ago. In addition, there was duplication between the form for the private insurer and for CPP-Disability, which was a total waste of time – the medical information should be the same for both applications, and one should just have to fill out the relevant consent forms. Sigh...

No reading this week, but I expect to have time next week. I did get a chance to watch some light, fun movies; first, *Singing in the Rain*, and then *An American in Paris* – and now, to distract me during chemo, some real shlock: *Terminator* (incredibly bad) and *Die Hard*.

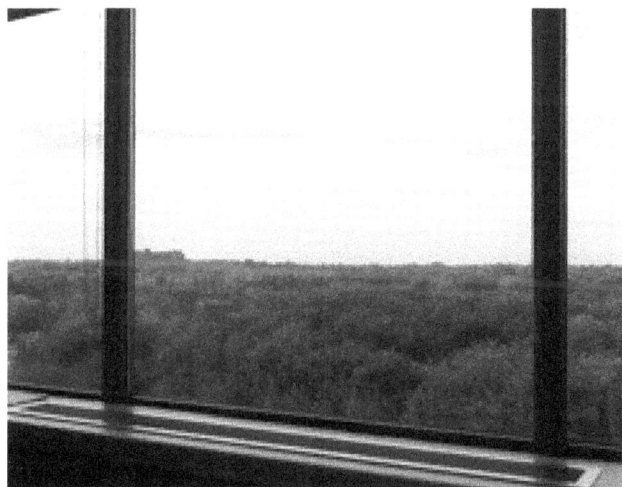

The chemo, in-patient (the photo at left is of the view from my 'suite' – lucky to have this room) this Saturday and Sunday requires a lot of fluid to flush out the system, and consequently, washroom breaks every hour. There is a similar requirement for today and tonight as well, which means 48 hours of sleep deprivation. A form of torture; no rest for the wicked.

The other effects to date (chemo generally has a delayed effect) have been manageable, but I certainly had a 'stuffed up head' feeling and some nausea within the first hour. The brick wall metaphor is just. We will see how next week goes, as the effect is cumulative.

In sum, this week is largely about getting through the chemo and Total Body Irradiation (TBI), hopefully as an out-patient as of Monday; the stem cell transplant itself will take place on Friday. The next stage will involve a few weeks with a high risk of infection due to low immunity before the new stem cells do their magic and start to rebuild my blood counts.

I am not quite sure how soon I will get back into my walking routine, but I do not expect to be up to it before next week.

WEEK 0 – I HAVE MY NEW STEM CELLS

August 14, 2011

'This too shall pass.'

This has been the foundation week for the marathon that lies ahead.

In the process of getting through this week, I recalled one thought that I often idly, in retrospect, used during my first round of treatment: 'this too shall pass.' I came back to it this week during the difficult days, and to help me get through the following:

- two days of intensive chemo (cyclophosphomide, a derivative of mustard gas from WWI!), which was a great time to listen to the Glenn Gould recording of Bach's *Goldberg Variations*;

- three days of Total Body Irradiation (TBI) in the morning and afternoon; I felt marked and 'trussed' like a chicken, 'toasted' for six minutes per side; counting and focussing on my breathing helped me get through it;

- two days (one of which overlapped with TBI) of treatment with ATG (antithymocite globulin), another drug used to kill off part of my immune system (specifically my T-cells) – I just felt a flush and some finger tingling;

- the start of taking Tacrolimus, my new friend for the next three to six months, which will ensure that any remaining lymphoma cells are suppressed until my new system kicks in; and,

- the infusion of the donor stem cells Friday, accompanied by having no immunity (being neutropedic), which marked the beginning of the next phase.

The first part was rough. Forewarned is forearmed, but living it is harder. In the end, the weekend with the chemo and the first day of TBI were the hardest on me. I experienced a fair amount of nausea, with a few 'aggressive' vomiting sessions. My worry and fear that this would continue for a while were thankfully misplaced, and the rest of the week had me weak but generally OK. I am very thankful for small mercies!

The actual stem cell infusion was almost anticlimactic. I walked in, followed the same procedure as with a normal transfusion (which took about an hour), was carefully observed for immediate reactions (of which there were none), spent another on hydration, and then walked out again.

To my surprise, I was quite emotional about it all, and got choked up at the wonder and the power of what was happening to me. It was humbling to be given this second chance, and I felt something very deep that went beyond my previous thoughts, hopes, and fears.

Last week, I talked about the brick wall being the metaphor for having to slow down so quickly. In line with that theme, and this being a foundation week, I was drawn to the adjacent image from Sacsayhuaman, the ancient Inca fortress above Cuzco. It reflects just how interlocking the various pieces of treatment – the protocols, drugs and procedures – must be in order to create the best possible foundation for success of my transplant. There is real craftsmanship and design in the work, built up over time and through the contributions of many people. The modern scientific process, with its standardization, protocols, checklists, and so on has made these foundations look more bland, but also means that they can be applied more broadly. Overall, as I think back to what I could

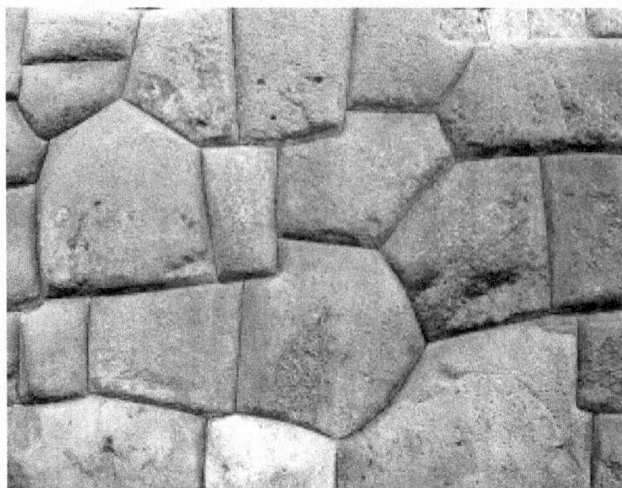

Sacsayhuaman, Cuzco, Peru

do just ten days ago, the feeling of having stopped suddenly, my normal life suspended, remains – but so does my wonder at the original artistry involved in designing treatments, and how it has been refined and broadened.

Next Steps

Now, of course, the long process of rebuilding begins: first, two to three weeks with absolutely no immunity, and then the gradual building up of my new immune and blood systems (my blood type will gradually become the same as my donor's).

In contrast to my previous autologous SCT, during which Neupogen was used to stimulate production of white blood cells, Tacrolimus is the drug of choice for allo SCTs. Its purpose is to delay the possible return of lymphoma or of my own white blood cells (it is likely that a few still remain) until the new immune system is up and running and (hopefully) able to deal with either.

It is a fine balancing act. My blood counts are taken daily. On three days per week, I do not take Tacrolimus unless my blood counts indicate that I need it. Another example of the knife's-edge scenario we will be living over the next months, and the delicate balance between my body and my new blood. Scary, but fascinating at the same time.

I lucked out in one respect: the hospital is doing a comparability study of whether to administer transfusions when haemoglobin levels are below 90 or below 80 (the current standard). I 'won the lottery' and am in the 90 group, which means that I should be more energetic and consequently, more active if I so choose. All other things being equal, of course.

One of the nice things about the Ottawa medical team is that they do their best to ensure that as much of my treatment as possible take place on an out-patient basis. We live close enough to the hospital to make this very practical, and the emotional and practical benefits are enormous.

Another great benefit is the staff. At this moment of vulnerability, I am particularly touched by the empathy and support expressed by everyone from the 'newbies' to the old timers. They seem to genuinely care about patients, rather than just trudge through their work. They even arranged to get a bike in my room during one long day-visit, and I was able to use it a bit!

I had some good discussions, first with one of the nurses, about whether I want to know who the donor is. My initial reaction was hesitant; while I am tremendously grateful for his life-saving gift (as long as I don't get Hepatitis C!), I am not sure how much I really wish to know, though I am curious about him in a general way. What if I don't like him? What if we are from completely different religious, political or other backgrounds? As usual, my wife brought me back to reality: he is a good person who has done something incredibly kind and generous, and that is all we need to know. Once again, my overly analytical character is tempered by her common sense. I still have a few months to make a final decision, however.

I have been experimenting with a meditation app on my iPad to help me relieve some emotional and psychological pressure (Simply Being is the one I use) and I am finding it helpful. I am also, strength permitting, trying some yoga. Both of these will be interrupted occasionally due to medical ups and downs, but help give me more of the emotional strength I need.

I finally got around to reading the Susan Sontag classic, *Illness as Metaphor*. I was much less impressed than I expected. It read very dated, likely reflecting views on cancer in the late 70s, when it was written. The literary and political references are impressive and the comparison between TB and cancer well drawn, but it somehow left me cold – too distant and too intellectual.

Our son is back for a week, so we had one of our regular 'family conferences' to chat on how things are going. I covered the medical side, of course, but more importantly also addressed my need for assistance from everyone in the family over the coming weeks. I also noted, given the amount of pressure on all of us, the importance of being generous and understanding with each other. It was quite an emotional discussion; not easy for me or, I imagine, anyone else. Again, I noticed a big difference between our earlier, theoretical discussions and actually living the experience.

Taking inspiration from managing transitions at work, I developed written 'talking points' to make sure that I say what I need to at the system (family) level, working with my wife to ensure that the messages were consistent and helpful in her efforts as primary caregiver (and in so many other critical aspects). Helpful, I think, for all of us.

There were many supportive emails and phone calls, and a few visits, to encourage me over the past week; these make a big difference to all of us.

Since the effects of chemo and radiation really kick in after about a week, this coming week will be a difficult one. Some of the side effects are already making themselves known, to varying degrees: mucositis, gut irritation and diarrhea, and yesterday, extreme fatigue. I have already shaved my head in anticipation of the inevitable hair loss, which gives me one less thing to worry about.

We will see whether I can get away with staying at home or will need to be in the hospital due to possible complications.

WEEK 1 – BETTER THAN EXPECTED

August 21, 2011

Last week's post ended on the note that the side effects were beginning to kick in, and that these would likely not be fun to experience.

Looking back on the week, there were far fewer 'this too shall pass' moments than I had expected, and the week was easier than I would have anticipated. A less intense post than last week's, both physically and emotionally!

Apart from the fatigue, thanks to which I am always either sleeping or listless (with a perpetual state of chemo/radiation brain fog), the main effects of the treatment have been on my gut, resulting in ongoing diarrhea. However, I have experienced no major nausea and little mucositis to date, and do not have any other major side effects to report. I consider myself very lucky indeed (sometimes expecting the worst pays off!).

Food-wise, I am eating a very bland diet to make things easier on my stomach, plus some protein supplements. Since my taste buds are currently dead, this is not a real sacrifice, but I am so glad that I took advantage of flavourful food while I could. I have been somewhat frustrated given that our son is home and continues to experiment with the BBQ quite successfully, but I can look forward to better meals in the future.

My need to stay close to a washroom has affected our walks, since I am only willing to risk a block or so. This has become one of my bigger 'this too shall pass' issues, as walking makes such a difference physically and emotionally. While my mental fatigue is significant, I would be physically able to go for good walks were it not for the washroom issue. My metaphor for how I feel, given the sensitivity of my stomach and the related constraints, is that I am walking on eggshells.

I have settled into the daily routine of spending a few hours at the hospital starting at 8 am for the following elements of treatment:

- blood counts;
- Hydration;
- transfusions when needed (I have had both blood and platelets to date; blood is about once a week, platelets more frequently);
- ongoing antibiotics;
- other medication as required (e.g., when called for by the protocol – Days 1, 3, 6 and 11 – and a magnesium booster); and,
- regular checkup and vital signs.

The medical team is pleased with my progress, and particularly the fact that my liver and kidneys are holding up well. This means that I can get the occasional 'squirts' of methotrexate that make up part of the contra-GvHD regime. No plan B required so far.

I was amused to live out a cliché moment. Monday morning, the senior hematologist and the transplant coordinator came into my room with big smiles of congratulations. A classic post-successful-operation scene, but it reminded me of just how human and caring the medical team is, that they also feel the pressure of the risks involved in treatment, and that they are rooting for me as much as anyone. Sweet.

They are all impressed at how I am tracking everything on the iPad, and by some of the apps that I am using for monitoring purposes. It is a bit of a Rube Goldberg approach as I use a fair number of separate applications to track my temperature, weight, blood pressure, counts, narrative log/journal and treatment schedule, but it works for me and keeps me in focus.

Given my low energy levels, it has been easier to read short news and other articles than start a book. To my surprise, I have been able to absorb some articles and maintain a (reduced) posting schedule, which is more than I had expected. Hopefully next week will bring a bit more energy in that regard, and my gut will settle down to allow for longer walks.

I have been watching a number of light films with the family: *Ratatouille* (the food and kitchen scenes are fun), *Everything You Always Wanted to Know About Sex* (very dated, but it was one Woody Allen movie our son had not not yet seen), a few French comedies – *Trois hommes et un couffin (Three Men and a Cradle*, a very French comedy, somewhat successful) and *Potiche* (or *Trophy Wife*, in which Catherine Deneuve emerges as an empowered woman; dated but entertaining) – and the classic Jack Nicholson film *Five Easy Pieces*. I also watched *Land without Bread*, not a light film, the classic 1930s documentary by Luis Buñuel on the abject poverty in Hurdos, Spain. A reminder of just how poor parts of Europe once were (and of the fact that Buñuel could do a straight documentary before he became a well-known surrealist).

I continue to get many emails and phone calls of support, all of which help, and have taken advantage of feeling 'reasonable' to get some overdue thank you's to a number of people who have been particularly helpful. In addition, the 'family conference' and some subsequent discussion has really helped me in getting the support I need from everyone as I go through this.

I have started to up the frequency of my short walks, as too much inactivity increases the risk of pneumonia, and it does feel very good to get out of the house.

I expect the next week to be much of the same, and hope for gradual improvement despite the possible ups and downs. Only when the engraftment takes place in about a week, and new blood cells are produced, should I expect to notice a more significant improvement.

I attained my objective for this week, which was to remaining an out-patient, with all the advantages that entails. That will remain my objective for the coming week. Whether I reach it or not is another matter, but it is always good to have short-term goals!

WEEK 2 – BACK TO THE BRICK WALL

August 28, 2011

Well, Week 2 recalled both my metaphors: the roller coaster, in reminding me that things can change quickly, and the brick wall, which I hit hard after the comparative easiness of Week 1.

Essentially, mucositis caught up with me early in the week. It caused a lot of mouth pain, but also more critical, sharper swallowing pain. While it is a normal side effect of the chemo/radiation combo, I had hoped (out of hubris?) that I might avoid it. There is nothing much to be done about , apart from rinsing one's mouth every hour or so (with salt or soda water), gratefully accepting the painkillers offered by the hospital, and making a few other changes to ease the pain for the week or so that this lasts.

The mucositis has given me a case of the Godfather jowls, and my hoarse voice contributes to the effect – but the Godfather look is dissipated by my having lost what little hair I had left! Speaking is also painful, so I have not been very talkative these days.

Mid week, the inevitable happened: a high fever. I made it to Day 12 (the medical team was impressed that I had made it that far, or they just were being nice!) before checking into the hospital on Wednesday. I will be here for about a week to ten days for more antibiotics and greater control over my health. My blood culture tests revealed a blood infection (bacteria from the gut, a side effect of mucositis), but a type of infection that is fortunately treated by the antibiotics that I am already taking. Once my counts are up (by Day 21), I should be able to return home.

Eating is more of a challenge. My medical team's dietician is a strict taskmaster, trying to convince me to develop a 'taste' for the various supplements. Her approach is a bit much sometimes. However, by eating soft foods (soups, purees and yoghurt, with some neutral protein supplement mixed in), I have been able to stay on a 'normal' (under the circumstances) diet. Eating is a slow process, as a break between each swallow helps things go down.

Fortunately, I am not dependent on hospital food (if the chemo doesn't kill you, the food will!) and am forever grateful to my wife for bringing me food from home.

While I was thankful when my diarrhea seemed to go away, by the end of the week it had returned (a side effect of the heavy antibiotics). Oh well, this too shall pass!

At the same time, I have been blocked up with a dry cough. It has slowly been dissipating over the past day or so, but contributes to the general feeling of crumminess. The combination of drug-induced fatigue and a sore throat makes me a poor conversation partner; this really is a good time to veg out. I had a chest x-ray to make sure that the cough was not serious. It wasn't, but my body let me know it had not forgotten my last bout of radiation by having me promptly throw up. Next time they suggest an x-ray...

In sum, I am back to the hospital routine, where I am well looked-after, under close supervision, and hoping to keep things stable until my counts come back up. Since I am in isolation, I do get a bit stir crazy, but (fortunately? unfortunately?) I am not feeling good enough for that to become a real issue.

I was going through my medication list the other day, which continues to get refined as my doctors adjust the dosages. I have never taken so many pills in my life:

- Tacrolimus (immunosuppressant): two pills (1 mg and 0.5 mg) twice per day, adjusted occasionally depending on its level in my blood

- Famvir (anti-viral, helps with): one pill three times per day

- Pantaloc (heartburn): one pill once per day

- Fluconazole (anti-fungal): four pills once per day, in the morning

- Delaudid (for pain): one to two pills every 4 hours plus patch, or as needed

I had a chance to ask about the procedure should we wish to know the identity of the donor. In Canada, the waiting period is one year (by that time, the success of the treatment is reasonably well established). The only other details I have is that the donor was a healthy young male and by inference, that he must be Canadian (other countries have different waiting periods).

I have not had the energy level to read books or watch movies given my general and drug-induced drowsiness. Somebody commented on my last post that I was a bit unfair to dismiss *Potiche* as dated, arguing that it was more significant for the époque than I let on (and one could argue that the Dominique Strauss-Kahn affair shows that things in today's France remain far from ideal!). I do still scan a lot of newspapers and websites (*Zite*, *Flipboard*, Twitter, etc.), which are perfect for my attention span these days.

On the good news side, I have gotten the first sign that the transplant is working and that engraftment is taking place. My white blood cell (WBC) count moved from 'not countable' to 0.1, which signals the start of the process. As my counts increase, all of my current side effects should decrease, and the worst – for this stage – may be over. I am not sure how soon this will happen, as Neupogen is only prescribed to accelerate white blood cell production for auto stem cell transplants (like I had a few years ago), not the allo stem cell transplant I have just had. The reason is to maintain the delicate balance between any remainder of my existing immune system and my new incoming system.

With any luck I should start to feel better in Week 3 and return to out-patient status, feeling strong enough to start walking again. Then I can start worrying about GvHD.

As always, just taking it day-by-day and week-by-week, appreciating every small bit of progress.

WEEK 3 – ON THE MEND

September 4, 2011

What a difference a week makes! Coming back to my metaphors, the roller coaster took an easy turn and I have been in full (albeit slow) recovery mode, and I have broken through the first of the brick walls of this marathon.

The transplant is working. My bone marrow has come back to life and is producing blood cells again. I am no longer neutropedic and my white blood cells (WBCs) and neutrophils have increased, the result of which is that my new immune system is starting to address all the side effects that were making my life miserable last week. My platelets are also up, and Saturday, my haemoglobin was up as well – all good signs.

At this point, it is worth stepping back a bit and reflecting on just what has been happening. Essentially, the conditioning regime killed off my blood marrow and left me unable to produce blood cells. The new stem cells from my donor successfully 'engrafted' into my dead bone marrow, made themselves at home, and brought the marrow back from the dead. Again, I feel a sense of awe and wonder at all of this. Seeing and feeling my new bone marrow working and making me feel better feels miraculous, even though I more or less understand the science behind it. Not to be taken for granted, that's for sure.

While I am still feeling far from great, the main irritants of last week (and pain eating and swallowing, cold and sore throat) are largely gone and I am beginning to feel more human again. So many of my 'this too shall pass' moments have indeed passed!

I still have a number of side effects that preclude my feeling fully human:

- extreme fatigue (I tend to sleep on and off for about 14-16 hours per day, and have too little energy to read anything serious);

- a disgusting, post-chemo leathery and metallic taste in my mouth;

- diarrhea, partly the tail end of my mucositis, partly due to the heavy antibiotics I am on (I finish the antibiotics Sunday so hopefully that will make a difference);

- bland eating since my stomach is sensitive and rejects anything with flavour – quickly (although interestingly, liquids that are too bland – i.e., water – are hard for transplant patients to drink, so diluted juice it is); and,

- general crumminess, about 5 out of 10 on the 'crumminess index,' from the combination of of fatigue, the taste in my mouth, and mental fog in general

On a more positive note, I started walking the hospital corridors and got up to 10 laps or 1 km – at a very slow pace, but moving nevertheless. The hospital also gave me day 'parole' passes that allowed me to spend a few hours at home a on few days this week, in preparation for my return on Friday (when I will be back to being an out-patient, again with daily check-ups). At home, I have been able to start going for short walks (one block). These walks are slow, too, but it is good to be outside and moving.

All in all, the medical team is very happy with my progress to date and commented that my own personal conditioning likely helped me get through better than most.

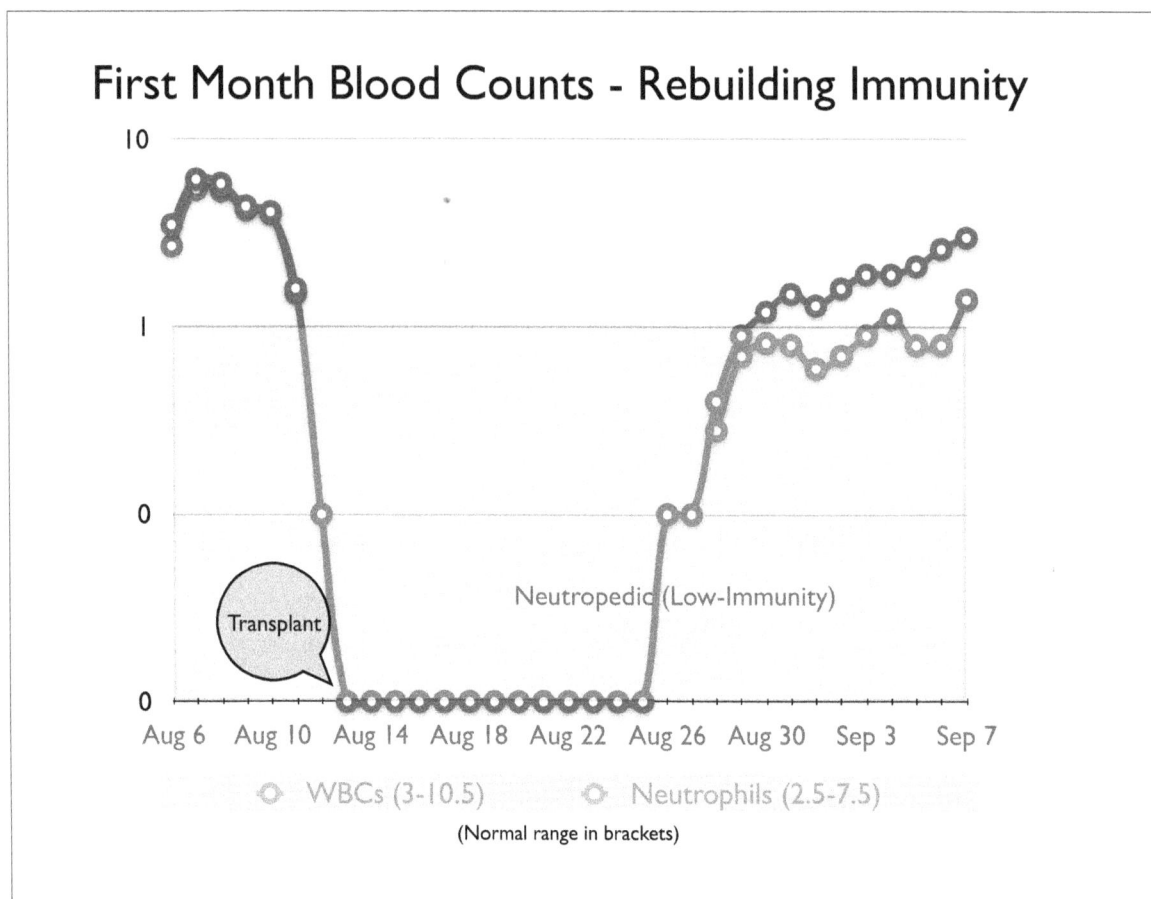

First Month Blood Counts - Rebuilding Immunity

I have had the 'privilege' of undergoing both an auto SCT (my stem cells) in 2009 and the allo SCT (external donor's) this past month. No matter how much the medical team warned me that the two are like night and day, it took going through it myself for me to realize how true this is. The fatigue is probably the biggest difference (I was reading by week two after my auto SCT), although the side effects (e.g., mucositis) were also more severe. Looking back over my notes and posts from after the auto SCT, and experiencing the last few weeks, makes the risks and the need for time and patience all the more evident.

Of course, with this stage almost over, worries about Graft versus Host Disease arise. The main short-term risks are skin rashes, which develop gradually, or stronger diarrhea, which would come on much more quickly. As always, if anything happens, I need to call in to and likely go back to the hospital. I really hope, of course, that I avoid most of this, but as a minimum, I want to have a few quiet weeks to recover from this stage and start feeling more like myself. Of course, I have no choice in the matter!

I have surprised myself by maintaining a decent pace when it comes to blog posts (over 60) and page views (over 5,000) this past month, despite what I have been going through. The articles and my comments may have been less insightful than usual, but the blog is still something that keeps me going. The five pages with the most views this month – apart from the Home page – were:

1. Health Plans Much Costlier for Docs in U.S.

2. Cultural competency improves patient care and patient satisfaction

3. David Servan-Schreiber – various (Death of David Servan-Schreiber, Le combat contre la mort, Exponent of cancer treatments). I am somewhat surprised that this continues to be of such interest

4. Learning From Insect Swarms: Smart Cancer Targeting

5. Jack Layton – various (Jack Layton in his own words, Layton Funeral: Some Reflections, Jack Layton's courageous, gracious fight)

If all goes well, my slow recovery should continue next week, with the remaining side effects becoming less and less intense. I will transition from coming into the BMT clinic every day for blood work and hydration to coming into the clinic a few days per week. The less time spent in the hospital, the better.

I have largely completed the first phase (the transplant phase) of month 1, with months 2 and 3 involving the highest risk for acute GvHD. We will see what happens, but so far so good.

WEEK 4 – DISCHARGED, ONE MAJOR MILESTONE

September 11, 2011

Well, if last week signalled my technical 'return from the dead' with the reactivation of my bone marrow and the production of new cells, this week signalled my coming back from the dead psychologically. I have a bit more energy, experienced a small but significant decrease in side effects, and am starting to feel a bit bored (funny how boredom can be a good sign!).

All my counts – white blood cells, , haemoglobin, platelets – are close to the normal range now. Other indicators, like creatinine (a barometer of kidney stress), have also shown similar improvements, as have the side effects of last week (fatigue, leathery and metallic taste in mouth, and general crumminess).

Type	Count
WBCs	5.0
Neutrophils	3.1
Haemoglobin	107
Platelets	167

However, in contrast to last week's plan for my early discharge, I have continued to visit the hospital every morning, where I am being given additional antibiotics, a stronger anti-viral IV to help address my remaining mouth and throat issues, and hydration to ease the strain on my kidneys. It is reassuring to be doing this for one more week.

Just in time for the weekend, 28 days after my transplant, I was formally discharged and 'graduated' to the clinic. This is a significant milestone, as it marks the successful end of the transplant phase, and while I am not up to champagne, it is a champagne moment along the marathon. I received many congratulations from the medical team; they really do acknowledge and celebrate these milestones with their patients.

My doctor, rather amusingly, noted that in addition to the medical requirements for release (e.g., no infections, functioning and maturing bone marrow, no serious GvHD), the other requirements include being able to walk and talk, neither of which are issues for me!

Keeping out of the hospital, my new objective, requires me to stay hydrated by drinking between two to three litres of liquid per day, and avoid infection and fever.

While my counts have improved vastly, they are only good relative to being and in a post-transplant context – my overall immunity remains fairly weak. I have to practice the usual post-chemo precautions, staying away from crowds, washing my hands frequently, and taking it easy.

This is essential if one's body is to rebuild and recover from all the 'toxicities,' so my lifestyle has to remain fairly monastic for the next month or two.

The only thing that has not improved is my diarrhea, which has not been helped by the continuation of antibiotics. The medical team is not worried – their usual refrain of this being a marathon rings true (the extended version of 'this too shall pass'!) – but hopefully next week, when I stop taking antibiotics, I will start to see a slow but steady improvement.

A downside of being out of the hospital is that I am now financially responsible for my meds. At these times, I am grateful to have a good drug plan. One of my meds costs $1,500 for a two-week supply, so 80-percent coverage makes a big difference.

I am going for more regular walks (albeit still only as far as a block or so at a time) in addition to pottering around the house more. I do want to take advantage of the fall weather, so I will continue to push myself gently.

Food-wise, I am still in the bland zone but am eating more and progressing to solid foods. This is a move in the right direction, and I will hopefully be able to start eating more interesting fare again next week.

An equally important improvement, this one on the emotional level, is that I am starting to have enough energy for more phone calls with family and friends. These still take some effort (my throat is not completely normal yet) but they also, through the connections they bring, give me energy. Hopefully my ability to interact with others will also continue to improve, with visits becoming possible once my immunity strengthens further.

All-in-all, while I would still place myself at about a 4 on the crumminess scale (down 1), the trend line is good. To date, there are no significant signs of Graft versus Host Disease. Of course, as my medical team reminded me, they want to see some GvHD, which is evidence that my new immune system will also work against any remaining mantle cell lymphoma.

No real 'cultural program' yet; I am not quite there. I have been watching more TV news, and the occasional light movie or TV series with my kids (*Robin Hood: Men in Tights*, *Black Adder*), but find surfing channels the least taxing these days.

Now that school has started, both kids are busy and the rhythm of the house changes. Our son is less able to come home each weekend, due to both school and other activities (including volunteering for TIFF, the Toronto International Film Festival). However, it is really good to see both kids engaged and interested, and always fun to see them building up their lives.

This post happens to fall on the 10th anniversary of 9/11. I am not going to offer any analysis of what it meant and continues to mean – there is enough out there for people to sift through and reflect upon. However, when I look back at some of the key moments in history that have taken place during my lifetime – the moonwalk, the fall of the Iron Curtain and 9/11 being the major ones – it is clear that 9/11 had the biggest direct impact on North American daily life. The impacts range from the annoying (the circus or theatre-like security at airports) to the broad (forcing us to question what kind of society and what kind of world we want to live in).

As if often the case with traumatic events, we all remember where we were when the towers fell. As mentioned earlier, my family and I were in LA when I received a call from a colleague who told me to turn on the TV. When I started watching, it was six in the morning, LA time. I remember driving downtown to my office, one of the few cars on the road. Being in charge of the team, as my boss was stuck in Canada. The surreal nature of driving around LA without encountering any traffic during the first week. My family huddled at home watching the TV. Dealing with Canadians stuck in California trying to leave, and advising them the safest thing to do was to stay put. Watching and contrasting the Canadian memorial on Parliament Hill with the U.S. memorial at the National Cathedral. Seeing the first planes in the sky over downtown LA a few days later and having the inevitable worries flash through my mind. Then the stranger sensation, a few weeks later, of getting on a plane myself, wondering – what if...? And finally, gradually getting back to the normal routines at work and at home. I, like many others, will be watching the coverage that will flood the media at this ten-year mark, looking back and reflecting on how our lives have changed, and how the world has changed, over the past decade.

Next week, I will continue my slow recovery, GvHD permitting. Slow and steady is fine with me, even if I am naturally impatient. Not having to visit the hospital daily gives me more time; that, and my increasing level of boredom, will hopefully motivate me to get back to reading and other activities (though at a reasonable pace).

Chapter 11

Graft versus Host Disease

Day 31 to 100

My new stem cells are working and the main threat to my health becomes Graft vs Host Disease (GvHD). I continue to live like a hermit because of my low immunity, and still feel crummy.

WEEK 5 – SLOW AND STEADY

September 18, 2011

My ongoing recovery continues, albeit slowly (the marathon metaphor still holds).

It is refreshing and nice not to have to go into the hospital every day; the weekly Tuesday clinic visits and Friday home care visits (to change my dressing) leave me that much more time to relax and recover without being stuck in the hospital environment.

The head of the Blood and Marrow Transplant (BMT) team was very pleased with my progress this week, in terms of my charts, my general appearance, and his examination. He had pride in his voice as he noted the benefits of the out-patient program for accelerating recovery times, telling my wife and I that other cancer centres might still have me in hospital. Nice to know that I lucked out!

He gave me some good information about eating, saying that I should just eat what I can, and if it works, stick with it until I get sick of it; I shouldn't feel the need to experiment too much or too early. So I am still on my rather bland and mainly liquid diet, which seems to be working for me, and my weight loss has largely bottomed out. He also reiterated that it will take time to for me to recover my strength and energy, and that I should just take things day by day.

Where I am now:

- The leathery and sticky feelings in my throat and tongue are slowly (*very* slowly) diminishing;

- My drippy nose and cough are largely gone, although I will have to be careful with the change of seasons as I am more sensitive to the cold;

- The diarrhea and unsettled stomach are mostly over with, since I am no longer on antibiotics;

- I have very mild – my skin is slightly sensitive but there is no major rash; and,

- My hair is starting to come back.

Despite having made major progress, I would still place myself at about a 4 on the 'crumminess' index because of my overall fatigue and the tongue/throat issues. However, the trend is one of improvement, and I just have to let the recovery process run its course and take the time it takes.

I have been walking much more this week. Nothing too long – about 15-20 minutes, and at a slow pace – but at least I can get out and start building up my strength. At this point, I feel it in my legs, and am usually a bit short of breath when I get home.

I have started reading again, starting Arthur Frank's *The Wounded Storyteller* (I enjoyed his earlier book that recounted his experience with cancer, *At the Will of the Body*). It is a fairly heavy book (in retrospect, I should have started with something lighter!), that explores some interesting frameworks (he uses Control, Body-Relatedness, Other-Relationships, and Desire), so he and I share some of these). Frank also reinforces the importance of storytelling, as storytelling allows the ill person to assert his or her identity as he or she goes through the healthcare system, whether the stories fall under the category of restitution (getting better), chaotic (chronic) or quest (transformation). The concepts in Frank's book ring true to me, although it is bit too heavy at times.

We watched Suzanne Bier's *In A Better World*, a film that examines choices between violence and non-violence The story alternates between Sudan and Denmark, focussing on two young boys and their complicated family situations. Beautifully filmed, with outstanding acting.

A friend of mine sent me Bach's Chaconne in D (the Busoni arrangement) as powerful music for facing obstacles and dealing with them with strength, confidence and energy – very inspiring:

One nice thing is that my slowly increasing energy means that I am more talkative and more engaged, whether during phone calls or when our son came back this weekend, recounting his celebrity sightings at TIFF. Two weeks ago, I was sleeping most of the time!

For the week ahead, I expect – and hope for – more of the same slow, steady recovery, gradually building up my strength and waiting for the side effects to dissipate. Hopefully, as the weeks go on, these posts will become more 'boring' – boring is good under the circumstances.

WEEK 6 – CONTINUING ON THE SAME TRACK

September 25, 2011

Another slow and steady recovery week. Boring is good!

The two issues I have been dealing with this week are a rash and kidney stress.

The former had me back at the clinic (after Tuesday's visit) this Friday to ensure that it was not getting worse. It was not, and they gave me some cream to alleviate the itchiness. The rash is more of an irritation than anything else, and the medical team thinks that it is more chronic than acute. This is a good signal that my body and my donor are coming to terms with each other in the desired manner. While that could change at any time, so far so good.

As for the kidney stress, it is normal after what I have been through, but the medical staff were worried about the fact that my levels of creatinine remained high. They 'threatened' me with the possibility of having to come back into the hospital for dehydration, and admonished me to drink more (I am already at more than two litres per day), but fortunately my count showed an improvement by Friday. This means that I get a free weekend and no time at the hospital. A gift!

I had two separate and funny discussions on nutrition. The doctor I met with on Tuesday encouraged me to branch out a bit, so I did – but I must have gone a bit too far (although having new tastes was wonderful), as my stomach quickly told me to back off (great feedback mechanism). The doctor I talked to on Friday emphasized that calories and fluids are important than protein these days, so I have my marching orders. I am increasing the amount of both in my diet, being a bit – but not too –adventurous. When I try 'new' foods, the intensity of the taste is refreshing after six or more weeks of blandness. Even carrots have more flavour than I remembered!

My other side effects continue to dissipate and are a bit less aggravating. Again, I am doing very well overall according to the team, and just need to keep going in the same direction.

I asked the team about the extent to which I can push myself in lengthening my walks, recalling their earlier admonitions. They answered with good, practical advice. Essentially, if I can't get out of bed the next day, I have pushed myself too far! But given that I have been taking three 20-minute walks per day, I am free to try some longer walks. Given the wonderful fall weather this year, that is another gift that makes a difference. though pacing remains important.

Emotionally, I have been feeling, if not depressed, lacking in my usual bounce and enthusiasm – a bit world-weary and listless. I take a questionnaire on a regular basis that poses attitude- and emotion-related questions, and it confirmed my thoughts. This is not to say that I am not optimistic about getting through this – I am. Rather, I have noticed a sense that I am dragging my feet and having to make myself do things, rather than just enjoying my life. This transplant has been harder than the last on an emotional level.

I asked the BMT liaison nurse (who is wonderful) whether this was normal and what the cause might be – the transplant, the drugs, or a combination? She said that three factors are at play:

- the transplant itself, including my body's accommodation with my donor's stem cells and immune system, which takes a lot out of me;

- one of my drugs, Tacrolimus, which combined with some of my other drugs, decreases my testosterone level; and,

- the stress on my kidneys, which adds to both effects.

In sum, this dip in my emotional state is not unexpected, and should correct itself once I come off Tacrolimus and some of my other drugs, hopefully around the three-month mark. In the broader scheme of things, it is not that big a deal, and though it may stick around longer than I would like, I can contextualize my negative emotions as a 'this too shall pass' moment.

Psychologically, my frame of reference is starting to shift from a focus on reaching six weeks post-transplant to making it past the three-month mark. Every week on the way is another mini-milestone.

The medical team through the BMT liaison nurse has asked me for some feedback on the care I have received and the overall process that I have experienced. I focussed on three points:

- I am impressed by and appreciative of the quality and warmth of the nursing staff. The nurses have a wide range of personal styles, as is normal (and which makes life interesting), but I felt well cared-for, not just as a patient but as a person.

- Rather than giving oral instructions alone when patients are discharged, a short written summary would help. In my experience, there was a large amount of information to absorb, and on top of that, my ability to focus was often below normal. I do not think I personally missed anything important, but other patients may have similar issues. She noted that the possibility of changing the current practice is under consideration for these reasons.

- While the overall process of 'conditioning' me psychologically and emotionally for the transplant worked well, in particular the final long sessions with the head of the clinic and with the BMT liaison nurse, the clumsy intervention by the intern following my discussion (where he essentially went over the basic risks for yet another time, just when I was ready and psyched up to go ahead, making my wife and I feel like lead balloons) needs to be rethought. Both the head of the clinic and the liaison nurse understood my point exactly. The nurse noted that they do not usually let interns intervene at that stage, since interns do things by the book and lack the knowledge of how best to deal with people that comes with time.

I have been reading S.C. Gwynne's *Empire of the Summer Moon*, the history of the Indian settler wars in Texas, which mainly involved the Comanche tribe. It has been a reminder just how brutal (on both sides) life was back then. The pressure of the settlers was so relentless, and nomadic groups like the Comanches were so dependent on Buffalo herds, that in in the end, despite the success of their early resistance, the Plains Indians had no chance. The extent of the violence from the Comanche side – they were raiders by nature, and outstanding warriors who often killed and tortured enemies – was of course matched by the Texas Rangers, and the Comanches were pushed off their land. There are likely some echoes of this in Texan culture today.

We have been watching some old Paul Newman movies: *Cool Hand Luke*, the story of life on a Southern U.S. chain gang; and *Sweet Bird of Youth*, A Tennessee Williams' play which involves separate plots about a corrupt governor on the one hand and an aging Hollywood actress on the other. Paul Newman serves as the link between these two. He is the actress' driver, handler and more, and comes back to his old home town to see the governor's daughter, his old sweetheart. Both movies worth seeing.

I am still living a relatively hermit-like existence. My counts are getting stronger, so I might be able to relax this restriction a bit, but I prefer to err on the side of caution for the moment. Phone calls and emails will have to do the trick for now.

Hopefully next week will be another 'stay the course' week, and I will be able to continue trying longer walks and also work more on building up my strength.

WEEK 7 – ON TRACK

October 2, 2011

It has been another good recovery week. My remaining side effects continue to dissipate, my rash is very stable, and the stress on my kidneys has declined. I have been walking for longer and more frequently to build up my strength (again, a slow but steady process), my weight is stable (I have lost about 6 kg in total, but had some padding beforehand so that is not an issue), and I have been needing less sleep.

Last Friday, I was prescribed some medication to move my digestion along. It was too effective, and caused diarrhea on the weekend. My diagnostic skills are getting better, so I called the BMT liaison nurse and asked whether I could suppress the meds. She gave me the green light, and sure enough, problem solved. It is nice that my analysis skills seem to be transferable and practical! However, I still have to be careful with what I eat as my stomach remains, as they say, 'fragile.'

The only other issue was that I sounded congested. However, this has been the case for the past number of weeks and my lungs were 'clear as a bell' then. The congestion is likely an ongoing side effect; if I get away with this and the mild rash, I will be doing very well.

I asked the hematologist how long I will have to remain in the 'bubble,' and when I might be able to go, if not go to malls and movies, to the occasional coffee shop. The answer: around Thanksgiving, when my neutrophils have been strong for a solid month or so. Of course, while my neutrophils are strong, their efficacy is weakened by the immunosuppressant (Tacrolimus) that I am taking. Another reminder of the fine balance in my body and that I am far from being 'normal' again. I will have to be careful for a number of months yet.

On the bright side, I am spared from having to do yard work this fall!

A good friend, who calls me on a regular basis, passed on the regards and concerns of a number of mutual colleagues that we both know well. After I thanked him, some of my usual feistiness came back, and I said, 'Why don't they e-mail me? I'm not on my deathbed!' This recalled some of the difficult discussions I had with one of my brothers. During one of these, I got the sense that people thought I was already dead! I quickly disabused everyone of that notion, at one time telling them, 'I'm not dead yet and don't intend to go!'

I was a bit surprised by the strength of my reaction. I know intellectually that people mean well when they pass on their concerns, and I appreciate the thought and intent behind the act. I also know that in my previous life, I would have done the same.

In addition, I have noticed that while a number of colleagues e-mail me on a regular basis (thank you!), others are either unsure of whether it is safe to contact me or are too busy with their lives, but are nevertheless following my weekly updates (for those interested in methodology, I can infer that from the 200 hits or so that occur regularly on Sunday and Monday, when the lead post is always and only the weekly update).

I find it amusing that I am triggered this way. In one sense this is good as it means that I am not in a deep funk but alive. I had hoped that some of the tools and guidance in my blog (e.g., What to Say to Someone Who's Sick, one of the all-time most popular posts), combined with the fact that I answer the awkward question of how I am doing in my weekly updates, would help people communicate better (and be more comfortable) when faced with situations like mine. I guess the lack of contact is just part of the blogosphere and the busy lives people lead – and again, I can recognize my previous self. However, e-mails, comments or even clicks on the 'like' button are always welcome (WordPress does not, unfortunately, have a 'dislike' button for those inclined!).

I hope this did not sound like whining!

Time for my monthly update on top articles and click-throughs. The top 5 posts (apart from the Home page and weekly updates) were:

1. How to Make Medical Decisions – WSJ.com

2. Flesh and Stone – Piercing the Veil, More Drug Companies Reveal Payments to Doctors

3. Monday's medical myth: a diet high in antioxidants slows the aging process

4. Dignity Therapy: For The Dying, A Chance To Rewrite Life : NPR

5. Social gaming to engage patients and improve wellness

I finished *The Empire of the Sun*, and its inevitably brutal dénouement. It gave me a bit more detail than was likely necessary, but was compelling and tragic at the same time, and the transformation of the last great Comanche warrior chief, Quanah, into his new role as leader and advocate for his people after their surrender, was impressive.

With our son home, I have watched more interesting movies. First was *Hanna*, an innovative and captivating, if somewhat strange, thriller. The protagonist is a 13-year-old girl, raised far from civilization by her assassin father. The movie follows her and her father as they are chased by an organization going after rogue agents.

Last night, we watched the classic James Dean movie *Rebel Without a Cause*. I still find that it does a good job of capturing teenagers and family dynamics during the period when it was filmed, though it takes this portrait to the extreme.

Next week will hopefully be more of the same, steady recovery; five weeks to go to the three-month milestone.

WEEK 8 – LARGELY ON THE RIGHT TRACK

October 9, 2011

While overall it has been another slow but steady recovery week, with lots of walks, my experiments with increasing the variety of my diet have been less successful. I have had nausea around dinner time for the last few days, which is new. I hope it is merely an after-effect of some of the new foods I have tried, and will dissipate. It makes it hard to eat as much as I need to, but hopefully 'this too shall pass.' The medical team did warn me that there would be a few ups and downs, and I was overdue for a down; fortunately, this is a mild one.

On the good news side, my regular clinic visit went well and both the BMT liaison nurse and hematologist are pleased with my overall progress; in particular, my blood counts are 'perfect' (for someone post-transplant). My rash is stable (although there was an interesting difference of opinion between the nurse, who was relaxed about it, and the hematologist, who is starting to look for signs that it is diminishing and wants me to continue using the cream I was prescribed).

Some other points we discussed:

- I have noticed some brown spots on my face and asked whether they were of concern. They potentially are, so I need to watch for any change in colour, size or shape. I will also need to use sunscreen all the time, even in winter, 'for the rest of my life.' No more beach holidays!

- I asked whether we could travel to Toronto in mid-November for my son's birthday. The liaison nurse urged caution, whereas the hematologist said that it should be fine as long as we don't stay in a Super 8 and eat at Harvey's! We will go with the more cautious approach and not risk a visit at this time.

- Once again, all of my family members need to get flu shots to 'cocoon' me (it would not make a difference for me to get one this year given where I am in the post-transplant process).

- I also asked about when I will be taken off my immunosuppressant (Tacrolimus) and when the Hickman line can be removed (it has not been used for a month and is largely an insurance policy in case I need to be hospitalized). The hematologist said that we will start having this discussion at the three-month mark, and the decision will depend on how I am doing at that time. Getting off the immunosuppressant will be another milestone as it will allow me to build up to normal immunity.

- Lastly, I have started using e-mail to flag any changes that I am concerned about for the liaison nurse. I asked her whether this made her life easier and she said yes; she can print these e-mails and stick them on the file, and said that she will reply by e-mail when hospital policies allow (some things can only be done in person or over the phone).

I am following some issues at work a bit more, trying to find the balance between getting involved and just letting the team run with things. Only they know whether I am achieving this!

I have not watched many movies. since my brothers (not only the one from Toronto, who comes up regularly, but also my other brother, who flew in from Mexico) and my son are in Ottawa for the Thanksgiving weekend. It is really nice for all of us to be together and for me to be well enough to enjoy it, even if I cannot fully partake of the food. We did re-watch *Amélie*, a wonderfully quirky and clever French movie – well worth seeing.

I am slowly wading through David Landes' The Wealth and Poverty of Nations, which explores why some societies are rich and others are not. An enjoyable and interesting book, but a bit heavy going – the link connects to a review that lists some of the weaknesses of his arguments but not deny the value of the book.

One of my faithful readers pointed out to me, in light of my surprise that I have not been getting more messages from colleagues, that it was hard to figure out how to send private messages (for those not comfortable with using the public comments function). To give people another option, I have added a 'Contact me' button to my blog.

This week, I also received confirmation that my Canada Pension Plan - Disability application has been approved, as this works alongside my private long-term disability insurance. I managed my expectations well; the normal period of adjudication is listed as three months, but mine came through in a single month.

Hopefully my nausea will clear up, allowing me to eat more and start to put on some weight over the next week.

WEEK 9 – A BUMP IN THE ROAD

October 16, 2011

It has been a rather mixed week. While it was nice to have my brothers and son with us for Thanksgiving weekend, the holiday was marred by my nausea, inability to eat much food, and a fever. I consequently felt very weak and lacked my usual energy.

I had more blood work done during my clinic visit on Tuesday. My counts were good with the exception of those for my kidneys (the level of creatinine is still too high). On the other hand, my blood cultures test was negative, ruling out some kinds of infection. The clinical doctor gave me some practical suggestions on how to get my food consumption and energy levels up (salty beef broth is the miracle drug; I was also prescribed Entocort, a steroid that helps the stomach deal with GvHD, of which I seem to have a mild case).

Other things that she is watching out is for a liver reaction to the transplant, which is common around the two-month mark – so far there is no evidence of this happening. They also hope that I can get away with only taking Entocort rather than Prednisone, a steroid that affects parts of the body other than the stomach.

Less than 24 hours after visiting the clinic, I bounced back (thanks to the miracle broth). I was able to eat better and more, and my energy picked up enough for walks. Quite remarkable and quite a relief.

I have also started drinking energy drinks (by which I mean Boost, not the Red Bull variety) to get an extra 700 calories a day, which brings me up to my normal intake.

On Friday, I was back at the clinic where the medical staff, too, marvelled at my recovery. The nurse gave me some further advice on how to increase my protein and calorie intake, and also told me which starches digest quickly for immediate energy (e.g., pasta and potatoes) and which have more lasting power (bread). I have been incorporating more foods – tabouleh, tofu pudding, more meat, more pasta, etc. – into my diet, and my stomach seems to be able to handle it. Progress.

Since the side effects of Tacrolimus include shaking hands and the reaction in my stomach, the doctor slightly lowered my evening dose (down to 0.5 mg from the previous 1 mg; but it stays at 1 mg in the mornings). Later that evening, my rash got worse and the itching came back so we will see if this settles in a few days, or whether I need to go back to my previous does (it seems to be settling down). Amazing how quick the reaction was. Similarly, on Saturday I forgot to take my mid-day dose of Entocort and immediately developed heartburn and shivers. I learned my lesson!

I have been cleared to start driving, albeit only for short distances. Another bit of progress.

A roller coaster of a week. I had been having it too easy lately, and I expect that the next few weeks will bring, if not a brick wall, more ups and downs as doses are tweaked and my body adjusts accordingly. Part of the journey.

In terms of movies, we watched *When We Leave*, a film about a Turkish woman who takes her son and leaves her abusive husband in Turkey to go back to her family in Germany. Her family's code of honour means that they cannot accept her separation from her husband. Although she makes repeated efforts to make amends (her attempts are excessive and futile), her family's emphasis on 'honour' is too strong for her to succeed. An insightful movie, and while some elements are a bit unbelievable (the wedding scene is over the top), it is worth seeing.

We also watched *L'Amour fou*, a film about Yves Saint-Laurent, his long-term lover and business partner Pierre Bergé, their incredible collection of art and objets d'art, and the life and times during which Saint-Laurent worked. It was captivating, as a 'bio-pic,' a film about the Époque, and as a story in itself.

I installed iOS 5, the latest Apple update to iPhones and iPads this week (once I could get through to Apple's servers), which includes a new feature, iCloud. Now all our calendars, to-do lists, contacts and so on are synchronized across devices, so I will no longer need to shift this kind of information from one device to another. As the ad says, 'it just works,' eliminating one of the little hassles of modern life.

All the ups and downs this week make it harder to predict the days ahead, but I hope things will stabilize more (just like my appetite and digestion did), and that the improvements will follow a more linear path. However, I always knew – and the team reminded me – that there would be some ups and downs. I have no choice but to plow through, happy that I am only three weeks away from the three-month milestone.

WEEK 10 – BOUNCE BACK

October 23, 2011

What a difference a week makes – this has been a real bounce-back week, though it started with a few bumps.

The combination of Entocort and salty broth settled my stomach and brought back my normal appetite, allowed me to increase my food intake and include greater variety of foods, and made a marked difference in my energy level. It also eased the stress on my kidneys, which had been of concern to my medical team.

I am back to feeling human. While it is still taking longer than after the auto transplant for me to gain weight, at least I am no longer losing weight (I have lost a total of 20 lbs since the beginning of treatment, only some of which was 'surplus'!) and am eating mostly normally. This past weekend was a breakthrough in that respect, and it makes a big difference physically and psychologically (real food with real taste!).

The bumps in the road included reacting to the reduction of my evening dose of Tacrolimus a week ago Friday. My rash flared up almost immediately and remained worse for about 24 hours. While I debated whether or not to call the hospital, in the end I decided to wait for a bit. Sure enough, it went away on its own, showing that my body and my donor are learning to get along. Now I have virtually no rash left, which so far does not seem to be an issue either (it is always hard to know how much of a rash the medical team wants to see and when – more questions for my next clinic visit).

Ironically, I am back on the original dose as my level wound up being too low, but it was an experience! Interestingly, the protocol on how long one takes Tacro for has changed. The previous head of the clinic favoured a relatively short period, but the current head recommends six months, so six months it is (he believes that this controls for longer and we have to trust his judgement). This means that the next milestone after month three will likely be month six – a landmark every quarter.

I also had a quick scare because of some some vision issues (blurring) similar to those that I experienced when my MCL relapsed. All the old fears came back, but the doctors were not worried about it. They assured me that it could just be a fluke, but obviously I need to tell them if it comes back again. I have to trust that my new immune system will wipe out any remaining MCL cells.

While my blood counts are strong, another aspect of my immune system is doing less well, so I will get monthly boosters of intravenous immunoglobulin (IVIG, a blood product) to help out in that regard. Not a big deal, just another thing to have to deal with. The only benefit is that I get to see the nice staff at the Medical Day Care Unit again!

I have witnessed a few vignettes recently that gave me perspective and reminded me of what I have:

- At clinic this week, my wife and I had our usual neutral, glum and (I guess) worried expressions on our faces when another couple came up to us. The woman – the caregiver – spontaneously embraced my wife, and then started a warm conversation about how they understood what we were going through, having gone through it themselves five years ago. It was a rare moment of humanity in what is a fairly sombre waiting area, and it was so nice to see how they both rolled with the punches involved in treatment with such a positive attitude. Touching.

- In contrast, I found myself admiring the cut of an executive's suit. He was obviously impatient, waiting to get on with it, which reminded me of how I felt after I made it through the first round of treatment – I was completely back at work, and focussed on the day-to-day aspects of my job. I could not help thinking, 'please give him more time than I had to enjoy that life, and make him careful not to take it for granted.'

- I got great news from one of my readers, Avi, who discovered my blog when he was diagnosed with MCL, and with whom I started to have a back and forth conversation that helped both of us get through our various treatments and complications. He informed me that he has finally made it through his Hyper CVAD successfully and is now in recovery mode.

- I got less great news from Brian, another reader. He stumbled across my blog while looking for a photo of a roller coaster to describe what he was going through with his son's AML (a form of leukemia; see his blog Walking with the Waltons), and we started a thoughtful and caring discussion on faith and religion. No child or parent should have to undergo what the Waltons are. Their faith is a great comfort to them, and my thoughts are with them.

- Closer to home, some colleagues were involved in biking accidents, which reminded me again of the fragility of life. One young woman, by all accounts well-liked and respected, was, to everyone's shock, killed. Another, with whom I worked closely for about four years, and who had wonderful spark, energy and drive, has been off for the past few months recovering from a concussion. Sad and sobering.

These vignettes are a mixture of good and bad news, but regardless they are reminders to treasure what we have, savour life, not take things for granted, and, as one of my favourite quotes from another colleague goes, 'Give an extra hug to your kids, spouse or significant other as you go out the door each day.'

On a more mundane level, I am having fun with some work-related files (it is nice, however, to be free of the day-to-day worries and responsibilities!). I have been working with litigators on an affidavit for a court case that not only brings back some of the work that I did previously, but more interestingly, is an intellectual challenge, as I am learning about how the legal process works. I also always enjoy working with bright lawyers.

Some of my earlier government work is now subject to academic analysis, and I have enjoyed reading what is being said. The evaluations are mixed, as is to be expected given the range of academic opinions, but overall it seems that the changes I made have been sustainable and have changed the dynamics towards greater emphasis on social integration and cohesion. In addition, an initiative that my team and I started well over a year ago is now public and getting reasonably good press; my former team has carried that one well. I am not nostalgic for the work environment, but this is a nice reaffirmation that the work I did matters.

My progress on David Landes' book has been slow and steady, but I am enjoying the world view that Landes describes. Movie-wise, my son has been in town again, so we watched a classic old war movie, *The Guns of Navarone*, starring Gregory Peck, David Niven and Anthony Quinn. It is still very watchable after all these years. We also saw Coppola's *The Conversation*, a psychological thriller about a paranoid wiretapper (Gene Hackman) who eventually goes crazy when he is put under surveillance. A good character study, if a bit slow.

Apart from that, I have been getting more e-mails from friends and colleagues recently, which is most appreciated. The 'Contact me' button is proving popular!

Otherwise, I have been continuing my regular routine of walking, eating, and building up strength. Two more weeks to the three-month mark!

WEEK 11 – STILL ON TRACK

October 30, 2011

I had a good clinic visit with the clinical doctor, who was very happy to see that I was 'thriving' – in a medical jargon sense. My appetite is back, I have gained some weight, and my energy is reasonably high. It was fun to hear her quickly review my file from the past month and cover all the ways I in which I have improved – it made me feel even better!

We covered a few points:

- My liver enzymes were up slightly, but nothing to worry about (another GvHD symptom).

- As noted last week, my inter globulin is a bit low (3.9 rather than 4!) so I will start getting IVIG supplements shortly. These treatments may go on for some time, depending on how quickly my overall immunity improves.

- My iron level is too high – 1400, where 600 is normal. This is a consequence of all the transfusions I have had. They will, in essence, 'bleed' me to get this down, but the clinical doctor assured me that they no longer use leeches!

- Everyone in the family and who sees me regularly needs to get flu shots to minimize the risk to me. Surprisingly, I too can get the flu shot in December, as it will provide me with some protection in subsequent months (right now it would not work on me given that I remain on the immunosuppressant, Tacrolimus).

- Finally, compared to my auto SCT, the protocol on re-vaccination has changed, and the process now starts at six months post-transplant rather than one year after, as was the case before. We had a wonderful discussion about 'levels of evidence;' while this change has not been substantiated by a fully randomized trial (that would be unethical!), there is a body of evidence supporting it and the risks involved in administering the vaccines later could be significant.

We also had an interesting discussion about what tests and scans might be necessary. She mentioned that they may consider a CT scan but then, thinking it through, said that a scan would be more appropriate if there was no evidence of GvHD. Since there is evidence that I have GvHD, the scan is optional.

I asked whether a scan would make any difference in terms of treatment decisions. She replied that they have basically given me 'everything they have got' (Total Body Irradiation, very strong chemo) so further treatment options are limited and it is unlikely that a scan would reveal any other possibilities. Since a CT scan would have no treatment implications, I indicated that I prefer not to have a scan at this time. For now, I will focus on the recovery track, and leave the scan to next year when it may be necessary for to compare with your original baseline.

She understood completely – no real advantage now, just increased anxiety – and then amusingly enough ran through all the doctors, noting that 3 out of 4 at least would agree that there is no need for a scan! I made the right call – reading all the articles on unnecessary screening and implications, and understanding my own psychological and emotional need to avoid additional unnecessary worry made all the difference. Of course, if the situation changes (e.g., recurrence of vision problems), it changes, and the relevant scans and tests can be done. But less is more!

We also discussed diet now that I am eating normally. She recommended that I stick with Boost for a few more weeks until I gain another kilo or two (although how I feel is more important than the number), and continue to drink the salty broth for the sake of my kidneys (helps increase the flow) – although she also noted that I can lighten up on salt otherwise (my blood pressure had gone up!).

She then gave me the obligatory reminder that while I am doing 'perfectly,' the relationship with my donor is a lifetime one and I will continue to be monitored closely, given the potential bumps in the road. Still, it was a good, warm and generous discussion overall.

Last weekend, my son and I looked through some of our old family photos and material (he is interested in history) and he prompted me to put all the various bits of information and photos into one integrated document. I now have a project for the next three to four months. I am developing a renewed appreciation for the work of historians as I try to piece together sometimes conflicting information. As with all such projects, there is a management and workflow challenge involved. I have to review the materials and verify them; scan, edit and organize photos; and find some people who can fill in the gaps. Some sides are more thoroughly documented (e.g., my Canadian and British sides), whereas others encountered the disruptions of the Russian and Iranian Revolutions.

While the software (Family Tree Maker) and web sources (Ancestry.ca or Ancestry.com) available make this kind of work a lot easier than it was in the past, there is enough detective work involved to keep me more than engaged – in fact, the project has become all-consuming (and is slowing down my other reading).

I risked my first 'crowd' scene this week to watch my mother-in-law become a Canadian citizen, something that I did not want to miss (I have always liked these ceremonies, and it was nice to attend as a private person rather than as a public servant). Being around so many people felt odd, and half-way through the ceremony I wondered whether I would pay the price by catching something, but so far, so good. I will still be avoiding large groups of people for the next little while, however; this was an exceptional occasion.

This week, we watched *Waste Land*, a fascinating documentary about the efforts of Brazilian photographer Vik Muniz. Muniz films Jardim Gramacho in the favelas (shanty towns) of Rio, and the *catadores* (recycling pickers) that work there, and how Muniz uses his art to change the perspectives and lives of the catadores. Their humanity is inspiring, as is watching their transformation to greater dignity and in some cases, new lives, as is the often funny repartee between Vik Muniz and his 'subjects.'

Another great film that we saw, though quite different, was *No One Knows About Persian Cats*, about the indie music scene in Tehran. It was filmed just before the 2009 Iranian presidential elections and subsequent repression. An incredibly bouncy, energetic and fun film, and the 'music videos' contained within were a searing critique of the kind of life that Iranian youth face. Another film well worth seeing, and it exposes a part of Iranian society that most of us are not familiar with.

One of the fun things about being in the 'recovery' phase is the sense of discovery about what one can and cannot do. As always, the brain assumes and the body corrects. My latest discovery took place when I automatically tried to go up a short flight of stairs two steps at a time, only to find half-way up that those particular muscles were out of commission. I made it to the top but learned my lesson. Now I am trying to get that ability back by gradually training myself at home (the first third of the staircase is doable, the second third I need to work at, and by the third I am dragging – but persevering!).

I expect much of the same in the week ahead in terms of building up my strength. This 'new normal' is nice and allows me to enjoy life without too many constraints. It appears that my countdown was not accurate – one week and six days to the three-month mark, rather than just one week. In any case, I am on the home stretch to this particular milestone, and am relatively relaxed and confident that I will make it!

WEEK 12 – TRANSITIONING TO THE NEXT STAGE

November 6, 2011

I had a good but at the same time frustrating clinic visit this week.

On the good side, the staff remain very happy with my progress post-transplant in terms of how I look and feel and my appetite, activity level, blood counts etc. These could not be better from their perspective, and I am clearly transitioning to the post-three-month stage in their view.

On the frustrating side, the difference of opinion on both minor and major issues between the clinical doctor I saw last week and the senior hematologist this week was striking. Three points where there were differences, from the hematologist's perspective:

- The taking of IVIG (immunoglobulin) to boost my immunity. He said that there is no need for it, and IVIG is not normally given to transplant patients unless there are issues with infection. One less thing to worry about.

- 'Bleeding' me to reduce my iron content. The senior hematologist said that this will not be required until the new year, when my haemoglobin count will be even higher (it is essentially donating blood, and as he put it, if I did so now I would need more than juice and cookies to get up!).

- More significantly, the question of whether or not I should have a CT scan. His answer was categorical: we need to know if there is any disease remaining, which *would* have implications for treatment. In essence, should the scan be negative, we will continue on the same course; if positive, they will take me off the immunosuppressant (Tacrolimus) to ginger a greater reaction, and use immunotherapy more actively. As he put it, while there are few 'arrows remaining in the quiver,' there is a window in the next few months to 'steer' the treatment if needed (better to be 'steered' than to drive myself into the ditch!). This was a sobering reminder that no matter how well I feel now, my life remains on a 'knife's edge' given all the factors that need to be balanced.

There is, of course, a hierarchy of opinions, and the senior hematologist trumps the clinical doctor. Moreover, he is the main hematologist who walked me through the decision-making process, and I have a lot of trust and confidence in him. We then turned to a more philosophical discussion about the difference between medical imperatives (need to know and react) and personal values (do I really want to know, or just live). He knows me well enough to tell me I tend to the pragmatic side, and that since that there is a treatment implication, I should go for the scan. It is hard to disagree – I have come so far down this road that it would be silly not to give it my best shot. Hopefully my Christmas present will be a negative scan, and all this worry will be for naught.

The hematologist also, as he has done in the past, crystallized where I am in the process, noting that there are four indicators as to the success of the transplant process:

1. My blood marrow is working (blood counts are good);

2. My donor likes me (appropriate level of GvHD);

3. No infections; and,

4. No recurrence of my illness (mantle cell lymphoma)

For the first three months, the focus is on the transplant process and the first three factors; in these respects, I am doing well. I am now transitioning to the stage where I have to worry about the fourth factor, hence the scan. This means major progress, though it is scary in many respects – no champagne just yet!

I appreciated my hematologist's explanations and approach. However, the contrast between his opinion and that of the clinical doctor means that they need to get their act together better and be more consistent. I have to remember to keep on probing, asking, and challenging to ensure that I understand the implications of treatments, and that the medical team understands I am using the notes on my iPad to work with them to ensure that I get the best care possible. Remember, never assume, and always repeat questions!

My most popular posts for October:

1. Cancer Terminology and Language – CBC.ca | White Coat, Black Art

2. Organizing And Administering Our Own Care

3. Why Supplement Studies Haven't Panned Out – Health Blog – WSJ

4. Alternative medicine: The illusion of control : Respectful Insolence

5. Hospital social media marketing

My family tree work remains all-consuming and has crowded out my reading time. I find that I need to balance the 'brain' work (historical research, reviewing documents) with the 'brain-dead' work (scanning documents and photos, labelling them). I feel my chemo brain after about an hour of the former, another reminder of what my body has gone through and the nature of the recovery process. Still, it is important for me to have a focus.

We have been blessed with wonderful fall weather which has been great for walking. I am also making progress at climbing two stairs at a time (still hard but not as difficult), am starting to do some basic yoga stretches again, and am working on my arms with weights. I am gaining weight to the extent that I can cut back on my supplements (one Boost rather than two per day), and my hair is starting to grow back!

The rebuilding process takes time, cannot be rushed, and is accompanied by lots of rebuilding behind the scenes after the assault of radiation and chemo – but I am getting there.

We watched a few hard films this weekend. The first was *Sophie Scholl: The Final Days*, based on the true story of German students (the White Rose group) who circulated anti-Nazi pamphlets in Munich in 1942 and were executed or otherwise punished for their actions. It was almost more of a documentary than a historical drama, understated in tone; some of the scenes between the interrogator and Sophie were particularly gripping. It was of interest as a historical film, but not great as a film in itself (no *Downfall*). Whenever I hear about someone who was able to be so steadfast and courageous under such circumstances (one of the 'crazy ones,' in the words of the more banal Apple pop ad), apart from feeling admiration, I always wonder what I would do if faced with similar moral choices.

We also saw *Yol*, a Turkish film set in the 1960s. It chronicles the experiences of prisoners who are on leave for a week, from both a personal level (family and family 'honour' challenges) and on a societal level (overall military presence and oppression). Five prisoners, five different stories, all with their own individual tragedies. Their stories are well, if sparingly, told, and give an insight into the diversity of Turkish society, history and culture.

My formal three-month anniversary is in six days, so to avoid any 'jinx,' I will wait until next week before breaking out the balloons. A more significant milestone is our son turning 20 this week, which we will celebrate during his next visit. These are the milestones that I live for.

In the meantime, there will hopefully be more of the same, and we will see if I get another interpretation or surprise at the clinic next week.

WEEK 13 – MADE IT! 100 DAYS

November 13, 2011

I made it to the three-month mark! While I am far from through with the marathon, the highest risk period is over and I have recovered well from the transplant with manageable GvHD effects. We celebrated by going out to one of our favourite restaurants, which has tables spaced far enough apart that we need not worry about germs. Celebrating each step is part of the process.

This makes me think back to the 'awful' Princess Margaret Hospital consultation on June 20th, when I was presented with a 20 percent mortality rate in the first three months after transplant, and an additional 30-40 percent mortality rate over the next two years since the transplant. The doctors here, while equally clear on the risks, had put them in the more positive context of my general health and previous experience with the auto SCT – and warned me not to get too caught up in the averages, noting that the risks continue to decrease as time passes.

Getting past this big milestone is the first step in my recovery, for which I am truly grateful. Perhaps foolishly, I am less worried about the remaining 30-40 percent risk now that I have made it this far.

The bigger question, as the senior hematologist mentioned last week, is that while we know that the transplant is working, we do not know whether it has enough 'edge' to help fight my disease (i.e., if the transplant is successful in itself but my new immune system fails to 'take on' my mantle cell lymphoma, the whole process will have been somewhat pointless). This is an unfortunate possibility when you think about it, but given the alternative... I try (pretty successfully) not to dwell on the 'what-ifs!'

While during last week's clinic visit we discussed the theoretical option of 'steering' my immunosuppressant dose downward should the CT scan show something of concern, this week's visit began the process of evaluating whether the transplant has served its purpose.

I graduated from weekly to bi-weekly visits (more free mornings for me) and the hematologist halved my immunosuppressant (Tacrolimus) dose to let GvHD flare up a bit more in advance of the scan. This transition is a welcome step. The next milestones are the CT or MRI scan later this month, and then the eventual cessation of the immunosuppressants. As always, there is adequate discussion with the medical team, but then things move more quickly than one would have expected based upon those discussions.

I was examined by a fellow of the hospital (more experienced than an intern, one step removed from being a full doctor) examine me, rather than the regular staff. He did the thorough pre-CT scan physical check of my lymph nodes and found no problems. This is reassuring, pending the scan.

He and I discussed the likely side effects of halving my Tacro dose (last time my dosage was reduced, there was an immediate but temporary increase in my rash). The possible reactions are nothing new: rash, throat pain, diarrhea. To date, I have not had any dramatic side-effects; they are all minor and under control, and the GvHD has mostly manifested itself as some minor stomach issues – enough to know that something is happening, but not enough to make me worry. I see no reason to revert to the earlier dose.

My bone density test came back normal (one less thing to worry about), my blood counts are strong and my hair is getting close to Peter Mansbridge (the leading news anchor in Canada) length. Ironically, in my effort to go up the stairs two at a time, I pulled a muscle, so I am back to being more careful. Fortunately this has not impeded my regular walking.

Amusingly, my weight is increasing so quickly that I now have to get back to being a normal person and watching what I eat. I have gone back to a more conventional diet and am checking labels for how few calories a food item contains, rather than how many!

As always, I watched the annual Remembrance Day ceremony on television. This year it was particularly meaningful for me since, as I go through the family history, I am seeing the names of those who did not make it, those who were luckier and did, and those who remained on the home front but were also affected. I also discovered that the grandfather of our local bakery's owner was one of the Canadians killed in Hong Kong, another reminder of how much the Second World War affected so many of us.

One of the problems with having more time on my hands is that I have become more curmudgeonly about bad customer-service experiences (a bit silly to post this, but given that we all have similar horror stories it is nice to be in a position where I have the time at least to make the point with companies!). Some companies that I have been frustrated with:

- Sears, for not acknowledging that parts should not fail on a fridge that is less than two years old, and for not meeting its commitment to get back to me within three days. I sent off a letter to the CEO laying out the issues and the hopelessness of the customer-service department.

- Best Buy, for having a Price Watch guarantee that apparently guarantees that they will not match prices. Again, no straight answer from customer service, so I forwarded my e-mail to a senior executive.

- Bell Canada, for having call centre staff who could not understand a simple credit issue and took over 20 minutes to transfer the call to someone who was competent, and who assured me that the check was in the mail. It was, and I received it last week, so this was a failure in communications rather than in the actual meeting of customer needs.

- Lastly, a positive example: Ottawa Hydro, which had been massacring one of our trees to save the hydro lines, quickly agreed to cut the tree down to save them future work and save us the unsightliness of a *Nightmare Before Christmas* tree. No fuss, no muss.

I received a number of great e-mails and calls this week, and am starting to go on walks with friends and colleagues again. Crowds are still to be avoided, but I can lighten up a bit while still being careful.

We watched a charming and tender movie, *Departures*, about a concert pianist who becomes an undertaker in rural Japan. While the premise sounds odd, it is a beautiful and moving movie about reconciliation: reconciliation with one's talents, with one's past, with the important people in one's life. Though it was serious, there were moments of humour and above all, tenderness. Well worth seeing – some reviews criticized it for being too sentimental, but there is power in sentiment!

We also watched *My Tehran for Sale*, part of a 'new wave' of Iranian cinema that goes beyond the regime-approved stories of village life and captures the youth scene in Iran. The protagonist ends up in an Australian immigration detention centre (Woomera), with even less freedom than she in Tehran. It was not as strong as *Persian Cats*, but a moving portrait of how youth continue to push limits, how they try to navigate an increasingly repressive and paranoid regime, and of the fact that becoming a refugee brings its own risks. Unfortunately, life imitates art. You may recall media coverage of actress Marzieh Vafamehr, who was sentenced to prison time and lashes for appearing in the film. According to last reports, the sentence was lifted on appeal.

This coming week will be my first clinic-free, and I intend to enjoy it! I have nothing special planned, just the usual building up of strength through walks and the like, despite the colder weather. Overall, life is good!

Chapter 12

Recovery

Month 3 to 6

I begin to slowly recover. I gradually feel less crummy and am able to exercise more. Everything seems to be going well until I encounter a bump in the road that sets me back and reminds me that I will remain on a knife's edge for some time.

WEEK 14 – FIRST CLINIC-FREE WEEK

November 20, 2011

This was my first week without a clinic visit (apart from the regular changing of my Hickman dressing on Friday).

I get the same mixed feeling during any transition, whether hospital to out-patient, weekly check-ups to bi-weekly; a sense that I am losing a 'security blanket' while gaining freedom. It is a great trade-off, but one that brings with it a small sense of loss.

Since my overviews of clinic visits have provided much of the core narrative of my weekly updates, I expect that my posts about clinic-free weeks will be shorter; this is a good thing and it reflects my ongoing progress.

I am no longer taking nutrition supplements and my weight seems to be stabilizing at my pre-transplant, pre-fattened-up level. All the walking I have been doing has caused some muscle pain (I had to stop taking the stairs two at a time for a while), but find that it dissipates after a few days. So I walk on! I have also been experiencing some numbness and tingling in my toes, which is probably a side effect of one of my many medications – I will ask the clinic staff about that next week. I have had some insomnia as well, but nothing that keeps me from my activities during the day.

Ten days out from the reduction in my dose of immunosuppressant (Tacrolimus), there have been no major problems; just some burbling in my stomach.

A reminder of just how fortunate I am to have a good benefits plan (as well as of how much medication I need): I shifted from 20 percent co-pay to catastrophic drug coverage, where I only pay $1 per prescription (including for my most expensive drug, which costs about $3,400 per month). I appreciate what I have.

I have started taking a vitamin supplement (Orthomol Immun) again, which helped me rebuild my strength last time.

I have been emerging from my hermit life and going for more walks with friends. It is a great way to catch up; we all like walking, and it is safer for me to socialize outside than inside since my immunity is still below normal. I received some great messages of support on achieving the three-month mark. One person, who is particularly active on the Leukemia and Lymphoma Society Community Board (among the better forums), told me that the one-year anniversary will be even more sweet (he is past the five-year mark). There are a number of mini-milestones to go before I get there (scan results, getting off the immunosuppressant, the removal of my Hickman line), but that is the next big one. A bit too early to start a countdown, however.

I continue to have a lot of fun organizing the family tree. While I am still going through the somewhat mechanical process of scanning photos, I have also been coming across a number of old letters from various military campaigns or family events, which provide more flavour to the lives lived. My workflow is becoming more efficient as I discovering the ins and outs of Family Tree Maker and some of the apps that are making the process easier (Image Capture, Preview). On the other hand, due to the number and size of the files involved, our four-year-old iMac is starting to feel slow!

We watched several Italian films this week, starting with the charming *Il Postino*. It tells the story of the friendship between a barely literate Italian fisherman and the famous Chilean poet Pablo Neruda, and how poetry helps the fisherman woo his girl. It was nice to watch a romantic film for a change; the movie is well-acted and filmed, and reaffirms the power of words and relationships.

We also saw Luchino Visconti's *Le Notti Bianche* (White Nights), which was adapted from a short story by Dostoyevsky. It follows a lonely man and newcomer in town, Mario (Marcello Mastroianni), and a woman, Natalia (Maria Schell), who is also lonely as she has always lived in isolation. Her loneliness is intensified because she is in love with a man (Jean Marais) who may or may not ever return to her but who continues to occupy her life. Over a period of four nights, Mario gets to know Natalia, falls in love, and in the end, loses her when the lover she has been waiting for returns as promised, after a year's absence. Well-written, directed and acted.

Next week is a clinic week and while I have the usual small questions to address, the bigger questions will be about understanding better why my Tacrolimus dose had to be lowered before we could proceed with any scans (which was not the original plan), and getting a better handle on potential next steps.

Otherwise, our usual activities will continue; I always find it surreal that while technically I am still weak and vulnerable, on the surface, life seems normal – and it is healthier to enjoy it that way.

WEEK 15 – MOVING DOWN THE PATH OF TRANSITION

November 27, 2011

Overall, I have continued on the track of strong recovery, making slow but steady progress.

Having noticed that my attitude about this second transplant appears different, a friend asked me what has changed this time. The spontaneous answer was not that I have been struck by deeper questions about the 'meaning of life' and my priorities, nor have I have felt an enhanced appreciation for family and friends, as the first stem cell transplant brought out both of these.

Instead, what has changed is my appreciation for the little things. These range from walks together with my wife outside (and with other family and friends), to the pleasure of figuring out the intricacies of my family tree, to savouring and enjoying food; and even to mundane chores like washing dishes and shovelling snow. They all remind me that I am alive and am able to do things. I expect that as I continue my recovery I will return to taking these for granted to some extent, but hopefully not completely.

Another change brought about by this second transplant is that I tend to procrastinate less. I have a more acute sense of time (I am aware that I may have less of it) and feel the need to make the most of it, so things get done more quickly and with less delay (I also use lists to keep myself on track). It is funny that when it comes to the bigger things, I have more patience than I did (the universe will unfold in due course…), whereas I am eager to get small things done to make time for what matters most.

This week was a clinic week, and I am transitioning more quickly than expected to the next stage. I am a bit confused and surprised by the constant changes to the roadmap, but I was always warned that my treatment would be more bespoke than standard, and that it would be adjusted according to my body's response. A recap of my last four clinic visits:

- 25 Oct: We discussed whether a CT scan would be necessary with the clinical doctor and came to the conclusion that no scan would be needed given the lack of implications for treatment.

- 1 Nov: The senior hematologist was adamant about the need for a scan to check my lymphoma, saying that there could be treatment implications – specifically the opportunity to 'steer' my immunosuppressant (Tacrolimus) dose to increase GvHD if necessary, to combat my lymphoma.

- 8 Nov: The Fellow cut my Tacro dose in half; a CT scan was still part of the plan for the near future.

- 22 Nov: This week, another senior hematologists took me off Tacro completely and reduced my Entocort dose (steroid to address digestive issues only), with no scan planned until the six-month mark in the new year.

Since managing my treatment is a group effort, and cases are reviewed weekly or biweekly as needed, I am confident that all of this has been hashed out by the doctors. I did talk to the hematologist about the different things I have been hearing from different doctors, and told her that it is confusing to me. She simply stated that there are differences of opinion, and that there is no single right answer to many of the questions involved. The method of choice is apparently to constantly adjust the approach depending on the patient's situation.

On the question of the CT scan, she again noted the different approaches but, with a smile, said that part of the reason for doing scans is to 'complete the file' for research purposes, rather than patient benefit! Bureaucratic procedures are not unique to bureaucracy, it seems (not to diminish the value of research reasons).

In the end, I am not unhappy with the decision to put off the scan, since I prefer fewer scans to more (I have been exposed to more than enough radiation over the past few years) and my treatment is being 'steered' to increase GvHD, and thus fight my lymphoma, in any case. The present arrangement is sort of like having my cake and eating it too!

I have not experienced any major side effects since going off Tacro (burbling in my stomach seems to be the main way that my donor reminds me of his presence, plus some very minor rash activity). I have reached another milestone more quickly than expected (I thought that this step would take place closer to the five- or six-month mark). However, as the hematologist reminded me, I am not out of the woods yet and GvHD could still become a problem; the one-year mark is still the next real milestone.

I asked what about how going off the immunosuppressant will impact my immunity; the hematologist answered that although it will help, it will still be some time before my immunity returns to normal (no Handel's *Messiah* for me this Christmas). For the moment, however, things are going well, and she is pleased with my progress.

I raised the issue of toe-tingling and numbness, as well as my occasional leg cramps and pain. The first may be leftover from chemo and should dissipate over time. The second is the normal reaction to building up muscle strength and should also go away with time (my tests this week were walking up five flights of stairs to avoid a slow elevator – the first three were easy, but after that there was more huffing and puffing! – and shovelling snow, which was easier than expected)

On the trivial milestone side, my access to the hospital wi-fi expired and I realized that I do not need it anymore given the reduced frequency of my visits!

For Woody Allen fans – we watched *Woody Allen: A Documentary* on **PBS** this week. It was a great and sympathetic portrait of his work over the past 40 years, put together from interviews with him, his close collaborators and his critics, interspersed with some great clips from his films. It was really fun to watch how his films (including the clunkers) have developed over the years. I assume that it will eventually be available on iTunes or similar services. Of course, if you are not a a Woody Allen fan, there are better ways for you to spend those three hours!

An update on my curmudgeonly consumer complaints:

- The Best Buy corporate office got back to me, asked a few questions, and quickly resolved the Price Match issue by giving me the appropriate credit. They are back in my good books, especially since they mentioned that they would provide feedback to their call centres on how to deal with future issues.

- Sears continues to fluff it. Corporate referred my inquiry back to the call-centre staff, who offered me less than 10 percent of the repair cost. I refused the offer and told the agent to escalate the issue to her manager – I did not write to the Corporate Office for my concerns to be dismissed in that way. To be continued; the issue is not just the money but respect for clients, and so far, Sears is failing on both counts.

My son and my brother are here this weekend for a belated birthday celebration. As always, it is a real pleasure to have my son around the house and chat about what we are both up to. He and I, along with his sister, used most of our time for chatting together, rather than for watching movies. A good chance to connect.

I am looking forward to my next clinic-free week. While there are a number of movies that we want to see (at deserted matinées – *Margin Call*, *My Week with Marilyn*; at home – catching up with some of the older movies that may no longer be in theatres), the weather has been so good that we have focussed on walks. I never thought I would hope for a day or so of bad weather!

To my American readers: I hope you had a good Thanksgiving with family and friends.

WEEK 16 – ON TRACK

December 4, 2011

Not too much to report this week. In short, things continue to go well; my energy level is good, the GvHD has not gotten worse (minimal rash and the usual stomach burbling), and I have remained reasonably active.

I have started to supplement my walks with time on our indoor bike to exercise other muscles. No muscle pain yet, but I do feel them working. I am gradually trying to get back to going up the stairs two at a time – but am being a bit more sensible by alternating single and double steps.

I have constructed a fairly consistent routine to keep me busy between meals, tea breaks and naps:

- Morning: prepare and post blog articles, exercise on the bike machine, hour-long walk, work on the family tree

- Afternoon: hour-long walk, work on the family tree

- Evening: short walk, watch the news

As a result, I am physically active for about two to three hours per day, and mentally active, thanks to my blog and the family tree, for about four to five hours most days. This makes for fairly full days, when I think about it.

All the activity is helping me sleep deeper, although my sleep is still interrupted and I still wake up early. As is the case with any routine, things can get in the way – some necessary (medical appointments), some fun (seeing people, watching movies). But keeping busy is part of my coping mechanism as it keeps my mind focussed on doing, not ruminating.

It has been a fun week of work on the family tree. I have been merging facts about people with their photos. The matching takes some detective work, and it is satisfying to seeing the project take shape. I am starting to become familiar enough with some people that I can correct the labels on the photos when the dates or faces don't line up with the other material.

I am finding this process so engaging that I have to remind myself of the other items, both minor and important, on my to-do list (not so much due to procrastination as to distraction; that's why I have lists!).

We have started going out to movie matinées, which are sometimes almost like private screenings given how few people are there. We saw *My Week with Marilyn*, the story of Marilyn Monroe's shoot with Sir Laurence Olivier in England. I loved the first part, especially the interplay between the American star and the English actors and crew – witty and entertaining. The second part, however, which explored the love interest between Marilyn and the gopher (assistant third director) Colin Clark, dragged on. Mixed.

We also saw *The Descendants* and really liked it. It struck a good balance between exploring serious issues (end-of-life decision-making, a father coming to terms with his failings and addressing them, the complex nature of family dynamics) and keeping a light touch when telling stories. There were some Kleenex moments, but the film did not play on the heartstrings excessively, and the movie was-acted (Clooney is very good, and the other actors are all credible in their roles). Well worth seeing.

As a follow-up to the Woody Allen documentary, we rented *A Midsummer Night's Sex Comedy*. We are starting to work through the movies that we have not seen for some time.

It is time for my monthly review of which posts interested you most this November. In terms of Page views, the top five (apart from the Home page) were:

1. Why doesn't America like science?

2. Gloves Are No Guarantee Your Doctor's Hands Are Clean

3. About (Preface)

4. Phys Ed: Staying Strong as We Age

5. Medical Hotspotting: When Treating Patients Like Criminals Makes Sense

This coming week is a clinic week, so I will see if we are staying the course or if there has been another surprising change of approach. I will also have a lung capacity test to see if my breathing is at all impaired (I expect some impairment, but hopefully it is only temporary). It is not the most fun test as you have to keep breathing in and out even when you think you can't.

Other than that, I will continue with my routine.

WEEK 17 – GRADUATION

December 11, 2011

It has been a great week.

On Monday, I took the lung test (pulmonary function) that I mentioned in my last post and the results were virtually the same as they were pre-transplant, well within the normal range.

On Tuesday, I formally graduated to the long-term Blood and Marrow Transplant (BMT) clinic, and found out that I will only be visiting it on a monthly schedule after the holidays. I can stop taking three of my drugs immediately, leaving me to continue only two medications for the rest of the year. My blood counts are strong (evidence that the transplant is working) and my creatinine (kidney stress indicator) is the lowest it has ever been – after both transplants. While the tingling in my toes and feet continues, that is normal and takes a long time to dissipate.

Other things that I discussed with the hematologist included getting the go ahead to get my flu shot, whether it is OK for me to travel on short local trips (Paris will have to wait for the one-year mark!), and the question of my getting new glasses (chemo plays havoc on your eyesight, and I was told to get cheap ones because there may be more changes). My Hickman line will stay in until the six-month mark so its removal, along with the scan, will be the next milestone. The number of vials required for my blood work has dropped from six to two, but it takes one poke regardless so there is no practical difference.

The medical team is really pleased with my progress, and my efforts to be active, protect my kidneys (by staying hydrated), and be healthy in my general lifestyle and nutrition have paid off. Hearing that was really validating. There are many elements of this journey that I cannot control, but it is satisfying to see that what I can control has a real impact. I left the clinic with a bounce in my step and a smile on my face, the same feeling that I had at the same stage in my last transplant, in early 2010.

Of course, I am far from out of the woods, and the elephant in the room remains whether or not my new immune system will keep my lymphoma in check. My slight rash and the stomach burbling are still present, so we know that my donor is doing something. While we still do not know about the lymphoma, we have to take the victories and successes that we have, savour them, and enjoy the moment.

Funnily enough, my flu shot gave me a light flu (in addition to the usual sore arm), which then morphed into a slight cold. This has reduced my energy level somewhat, and I need more sleep (I seem to drift off earlier in the evening and wake up later); both of these are reminders that my immunity is still a work in progress.

We watched *The Kings of Pastry*, a doc about the annual *Meilleurs Ouvriers de France* pastry competition. It was intense watching all the preparation that goes into the competition, but the tension was balanced by the chefs' glorious creations (I think I gained a few ounces just from looking at them). A fun film to watch. We also continued our Woody Allen spree with *Zelig*, one of my favourites, which delivers some interesting messages about identity in a documentary format.

We have been going over university options with our daughter (how quickly this moment comes). Our son is back for the weekend, which always livens up the house, and we are preparing for the holidays. I hope to get over this cold quickly – while it does not prevent me from my regular routine of walks, etc., it is one of those small irritations that I could do without.

Overall, I have made it through the transition to this post-immunosuppressant stage reasonably well, and am now at the point of having longer-term care. It will be interesting to see the impact on my energy level over the next few weeks; it is possible that the meds had a slight stimulant effect and that my new normal will mean less energy – but the transition is still a good one overall.

WEEK 18 – ADJUSTING TO BEING OFF THE MEDS

December 18, 2011

After the euphoria of my 'graduation' last week, the effects of being taken off several meds are starting to be felt.

Some of them must have had a slight stimulant effect, as I have felt more tired than before. Not enough to impede my walks and exercise, or my work on the blog and family tree, but enough that I need to be more disciplined to get through my regular activities. On the other hand, my sleep continues to be deeper and more rarely interrupted, so like all changes, this one is a mix of the good and the less-good.

Since being taken off Entocort, the steroid for my stomach, my appetite has dropped from bigger-than-normal to normal, and I have a slight bad taste in my mouth. Again, nothing major, but something noticeable.

I will mention these developments at the clinic next week and see whether they are normal or whether I should go back on some of the meds for a bit longer. None of these effects will prevent me from enjoying Christmas, but it is nonetheless important that I track and report them.

I still have a slight rash, the severity of which sometimes increases and sometimes decreases, reminding me that my donor is active. It is not itchy and has not generalized, so the rash is another thing to note and watch rather than worry about.

After the regular change of my Hickman dressing on Friday, it flared up, becoming red and painful, on Saturday. Though I did not have a fever (the key indicator of infection), I called the hematologist, who gave me sensible advice: since I do not have a fever, I do not need to visit emergency immediately, but I should call him in the morning and can then be set up at the Medical Day Care Unit. Anything to avoid emergency. Although there was less inflammation and pain by Sunday morning, I made a quick visit to the hematologist, who prescribed some antibiotics as a precautionary measure to ensure that I do not have any problems over the holidays. I received great care with no waiting period.

The after-effects of the flu shot have disappeared, including the cold that I understand other people have experienced after getting the flu shot. One less thing to worry about.

I enjoyed some good visits with friends this week; I am glad that my hermit-like existence is over and that I am able to see people. This week one of our friends came to visit with her year-old baby; playing with her was a wonderful reminder of life, energy and growth.

I got a surprise call from the BBC World Service inviting me to be a participant on their program, World Have Your Say. The episode in question was about the language of cancer, prompted by Christopher Hitchens' death (he refused the war metaphors, preferring coexistence). I enjoyed the discussion and the chance to interact with the other panelists (most shared

Hitchens' view), who represented a good range of opinions on issues of attitude, faith and approaches to cancer (whether it is overall a gift, causing one to see life differently, etc.).

We watched the Polanski (creepy guy but good director) film *Frantic*, a thriller set in Paris about an American whose wife is kidnapped. The authorities do not believe him, and he has to discover the truth himself. The plot was not terribly original, but the film was good in terms of maintaining and developing tension. Thrillers keep me awake better than talk films, a plus given my current fatigue!

That being said, we also watched a number of non-thrillers, and I managed to stay awake during both.

First, an Israeli film, *My Father My Lord*, which depicts an ultra-Orthodox family and how the demands of the father's faith lead him to neglect his connection to his life and family. The story is set against the backdrop of the Abraham and Isaac parable, in which Abraham prepares to sacrifice Isaac but is granted a last-minute reprieve. The film has a less-happy ending. Although the film is critical of ultra-Orthodox life, the characters are depicted with compassion and feeling.

Second, we watched *The Company of Strangers*, a charming film about a group of older women who become stuck in the middle of nowhere when their bus breaks down. It captures the conversations, lives, and personalities of each. Many of the women playing the roles are not actors, and the film has a nice authenticity and fluidity as a result. It also strikes a good balance between the serious and the light as the women deal with their current predicament and reflect back on their lives.

This week, apart from my visit to the clinic, will revolve around final preparations for the holidays. I am looking forward to everyone being together – my brothers will also be joining us. This time, in contrast with our last Thanksgiving, I am feeling more than well enough to enjoy the celebrations, so I shall.

Best wishes to all for the holidays, whichever you are celebrating; enjoy and savour the time with family and friends.

WEEK 19 – MERRY CHRISTMAS

December 25, 2011

First of all, Merry Christmas! There is only a dusting of snow today, but it is still that time of year for a good family gathering and seeing friends. Along with both my children, my brothers are here, and we have been making lots of calls to other friends and family who are scattered around the globe. Technology both disperses us and brings us together.

Health-wise, I continue to adjust to this post-med stage. No major changes; at the clinic this week, the clinical doctor said that the effects I mentioned in my last post (increased fatigue, burbling stomach, reduced appetite, etc.) were a result of GvHD acting up, rather than a reaction to the flu shot or something else.

I was given permission to take Entocort again if it helps me enjoy the holiday meals more (so far I see no need to do so, as I am eating normally and my weight is stable). My slight rash has gone away, so the flare-up was a normal, temporary one caused by a reduction in immunosuppressants. In addition, the antibiotics I was prescribed and my own immune system have dealt with the inflammation around my Hickman line.

However, because of the effects that I have experienced since going off my medications, plus a slight dip in my blood counts (perhaps due to my fighting a virus), the clinical doctor put me back on a two-week clinic recall. In other words, I have been 'de-graduated,' or sent to remedial training – whichever metaphor you prefer – for a little while. Another example of the different approaches taken by different doctors: she told me that they do not normally make medication changes so close to holidays, but that the senior hematologist, who I saw two weeks ago and who made the decision to stop the meds, has a more 'just do it' style. I will find out what he thinks about this if I see him in early January!

I am well enough to restart my normal 'maintenance' routine over the next few months: getting my annual physical, seeing the dentist and getting new glasses. The clinical doctor and I also chatted about scans and she is also is of the opinion that these are more 'academic' than necessary.

I mentioned to her that I am willing to talk to other patients about mantle cell lymphoma and stem cell transplants (I have already done that with one person in "real life" and many online). She told me that they do have an informal 'buddy' system and that she will add my name to the roster. She noted that some people prefer an individual approach over group discussion (as do I), so 'buddies' are offered only if requested by a patient.

I watched some great movies this week, starting with *Mr. Smith Goes to Washington*, a wonderful Frank Capra movie about political corruption, starring James Stewart as the one honest and idealistic politician (required viewing this holiday season for those in Washington, Ottawa and other capitals given the level of political discourse these days).

We also watched *The English Patient*, a good adaptation of Michael Ondaatje's novel. A powerful story and great cast, beautiful camera work, and wonderful editing – the narrative goes back and forth between the present and the past. . Although I have not read it, *The Conversations: Walter Murch and the Art of Editing Film* by Michael Ondaatje is apparently an interesting conversation on the similarities and differences between storytelling in novels and in film.

This week, I also wrote my first guest blog for **MD Anderson's** Cancerwise. From a content and writing perspective, it provided another route for reflection since I had to think more carefully about the target audience (and editor). My next guest blog is slated for mid-January.

I am almost done integrating family facts, documents and photos into my family tree. The next phase will be using various web tools to supplement and confirm the information that I already have; it will be interesting to see what the various genealogy-related websites and archives can tell me.

I am looking forward to a nice Christmas Day and holiday week with the family. I hope all of you enjoy this time of societal slowness (aside from Boxing Day's excessive consumerism) to be with family and friends.

WEEK 20 – HAPPY NEW YEAR

January 1, 2012

While marking dates by the earth's orbit around the sun has a certain artificiality to it and does not always mesh well with the events in our lives, it is still what we use to reflect back and look forward.

2011 was a roller coaster year for me. When it started, I was back to my normal personal and professional life. My relapse in February threw all that into question. The year was marked by stabilization chemo, the difficult discussions and decision about whether or not to go for the allogeneic stem cell transplant, the transplant itself and my slow recovery. Overall, 2011 was defined by a sense of how fragile life is, and that fragility – and the beauty that goes with it – was what pushed me to chance the stem cell transplant rather than give up.

Holidays provided some of the markers for this phase of the journey. We worked with the medical team to schedule trips to Paris and Stratford, and celebrated the various birthdays and anniversaries. My progress was illustrated by the contrast between Thanksgiving, when I felt weak and crummy (watching everyone else eat while I pecked miserably at my alternative food!) and Christmas, when I was active and able to eat along with the family. As I move along the path of recovery, the day-to-day and week-to-week progress is harder to measure. Special occasions make the changes more noticeable.

This was also a year of changes for my blog and my level of engagement. On my blog, I shifted from primarily posting weekly updates to curating news clippings; I also had my first interview and wrote my first **MD Anderson** Cancerwise guest blog. These changes shaped the cancer part of my identity. I became bored with the mechanics of cancer and more interested in how we, as cancer patients or as family and friends thereof, deal with cancer and its impact on our lives. The ongoing dialogue and challenges with my medical team also made me more appreciative of my support system, and helped me understand the limits of what medicine can and cannot do for me.

A number of people who 'made a ding in the universe' passed away in 2011: Vaclav Havel, Steve Jobs, Jack Layton and Christopher Hitchens on the good side; Kim Jong-Il, Osama bin Laden and Muammar Ghaddafi on the bad.

My family-tree project, spawned from a chance discussion with my son, provided me with some focus (and an obsession!). I seem to need an intellectual pursuit to match my other physical retraining, as during my last recovery, when I studied Persian.

In the coming year, I hope for 'boredom' where health is concerned; just a steady improvement in my physical and intellectual strength. The major milestones are clear:

- The six-month anniversary of my transplant, in February, when I will be revaccinated and have my Hickman line removed;

- The twelve-month mark in August, when I will get a sense of whether this gambit has worked to manage my lymphoma; and,

- And along the way, the personal, family milestones of birthdays, graduations and holidays to remind me of the joy of life and my love of my family.

One thing I find interesting is how my perspective changed with my second transplant. After my auto transplant, I had more faith in averages (80 percent of auto-transplant patients make it to the five-year mark). This time round, I realized that averages are meaningless to me as an individual, and see life expectancy as more contingent.

As someone who likes to plan for the future (I am still a bit of a control freak), being uncertain about what I can look forward to and how much time I have left remains a challenge. While I can 'live in the moment,' I also wish I could plan ahead. The fact that I cannot really do so is strange and surreal, and plays out in the following areas:

- Making it to the one-year mark. This I almost take for granted given my progress to date. The extent to which I can do make it to the one-year mark will have an impact on my short-term projects of getting stronger, finishing the family tree, and returning to my normal reading routine.

- Transitioning out of long-term disability, assuming that my recovery continues apace and that my energy level largely returns to normal. I expect that my energy level will be one of the key factors in whether or not I can (or should) return to work in some advisory capacity until my pension kicks in (early 2013).

- Thinking about post-retirement. The easy part is catching up on travel and doing fun stuff; the harder question is where and how I want to make a contribution. I expect that short-term projects would me more prudent than long-term for the first few years.

- Deciding the future of my blog and other writings once I reach my 'new normal' in fall 2012. While my lymphoma journey will always be an important part of my identify, and has made me more reflective and appreciative, I am not sure whether I want to 'make a career' out of it. I expect that these reflections will continue as I approach the one-year mark.

In sum, I have a fair amount of reflection ahead, accompanied by the over-riding goal of getting as strong as possible.

As it did last year, this version of 'Stand by Me' best expresses my thanks to all of you who 'stood by me' over the past year. If you haven't seen it, it is well worth watching as a great example of how music can bring people together. Thank you once again.

WEEK 21 – REDISCOVERING SOME UNUSED MUSCLES

January 8, 2012

This was another good recovery week, and my clinic visit confirmed that I am on track. While I have not quite 're-graduated' to the long-term ('survivor's') clinic, I should be able to do so after one more regular clinic visit, in two weeks.

The hematologist is not worried about the symptoms I am living with: lower energy, burbling stomach and a more moderate appetite. As to the first, he simply noted the need to monitor my energy level (this is always the case with allo stem cell transplants). He added that the issue of my appetite, given that my weight remains stable, is not a major concern.

Since he was the hematologist who most strongly advocated CT scans, we reviewed that question. He is relaxed about the scans for the moment, since my treatment has already been 'steered' by my being taken off immunosuppressants. When I see the head of the clinic again, I will have a discussion on the various and somewhat conflicting messages on the need or not for a scan, and I am curious – though pleased with the result.

I will start to be revaccinated next month and in good news, the hematologist agreed that there is no sense keeping the Hickman line in – but he noted wryly that 'if we have trouble, we either blame the Hickman or blame ourselves for having taken it out too early.' Even so, since I am at the five-month mark and the Hickman has not been used for almost four months, the time has come.

All in all, a good, boring visit!

Movie-wise, we risked going out during the holidays to see *Tintin* (Spielberg fun) and *The Artist* (enjoyable and beautifully filmed nostalgia for the era of silent film). We watched a few videos at home as well: *Midnight in Paris* (pure enjoyment), *Recount* (reliving the 2000 election, with a great depiction of the 'back room boys' – and they were mainly 'boys'), and the 1953 version of *Julius Caesar* with John Geilgud and Marlon Brando.

I have also been reading again, starting with the delightful *The Cat's Table* by Michael Ondaatje. Like all his books, it is beautifully written and features absorbing characters, whose lives are expertly woven together.

I have also started cross-country skiing again. It is funny that every time I restart something, I am a bit fearful, as if I were beginning again from scratch. While I fell or almost fell a lot the first day, I felt much more stable on the second, so the skill does come back. Still, it takes time to get all those muscles working in sync, and needless to say, I felt sore for a few days afterwards.

I have noticed that I need an additional hour of sleep lately, and thought of what the clinic nurse told me a while back: I will know if I have pushed myself too hard if I can't get out of bed the day after. I think that so far, though I have been pushing myself, I have not gone overboard (two hours or more of extra sleep would make me start to worry!).

The house will grow quieter when the holidays end, with my son back at university and my daughter back at school. Weather permitting, I hope to cross-country ski most days, which is a pleasant change from only walking (and is nicer than the indoor bike), but I doubt that I will try skating again this year because of the balance issue.

It looks like I am on the straight stretch of the roller coaster, and I hope to keep it that way.

WEEK 22 – DISCOVERING SOME LIMITS

January 15, 2012

It has been an interesting week. A few little blips have reminded me that I am still in recovery mode, no matter how good the overall trend has been.

I ate something that disagreed with me, and was essentially wiped out for a day by fatigue and a weak stomach. I lost a few kilos as well, which reminded me that I should maintain a bit of a fat reserve for now. In the end, it was only an upset stomach and I did not develop a fever – which could have indicated a grave bowel infection or more serious GvHD (the gut is one of the areas most affected).

Ottawa has received a heavy snowfall over the last few days, a great opportunity to build up my strength through shovelling and cross-country skiing. Since the snow was wet and sticky, I got more of a workout I than expected, and consequently experienced more muscle pain and stiffness than usual. However, I am still passing the 'get out of bed' test, so while I did push myself a bit too much, doing so was not a serious mistake. In any case, I am glad that the real winter weather has finally arrived.

Overall, I continue to do well and keep on track. I do want to ask my medical team whether the blips I experience could reflect some form of chronic GvHD, or whether they will dissipate over time. I expect that the answer will be that only time will tell!

One of the benefits of my having been less mobile at the beginning of the week is that I had more time to read. I started with *The Icarus Syndrome*, Peter Beinart's history of American hubris as exemplified by Wilsonian World War I progressivism, Kennedy and Johnson's toughness on Vietnam and their expansion of containment, and the Bush (43) era of neo-conservatism and dominance. It is fascinating to see how each generation is conditioned by its formative experiences (e.g., those who grew up during periods of difficult wars were more cautious than those who did not). Beinart also sheds light on the typical contrast between members of the military, who know what death is, and some of the policy makers, who do not, as well as on the extent to which dissenting views are unwelcome in large organizations.

It helped me understand the caution in the current time, although some of the current political debates suggest that some have not learned the lessons of over-reach.

I also read *Zahra's Paradise*, a graphic novel about the crackdown that followed the 2009 election in Iran. It was heartbreaking and horrific in many ways. The story follows a mother and her son as they try to track down her son/his brother, who disappeared during the protests. However, it also captures Iranians' humanity and sense of humour: while reading, I was often sad or angry, but there were many instances when I burst out laughing at the jokes or the irreverence of the characters.

We have also started to watch *Downton Abbey*. It is delightful and entertaining fluff; the storyline is fast-paced, and we all have a weakness for stately English homes! Movie-wise, we watched *Margin Call*, a fictionalized but authentic-feeling film about the events of fall 2008 and the collapse of all those clever mortgage instruments that 'bundled' or grouped mortgages – and hid – risk. It features a taut script that captures the milieu, and the necessary ruthlessness that goes with it, well, with good acting.

As for my progress on the family tree, I moved on this week to the stage of web research. I have most of the information that I need already, but I use the internet to confirm and occasionally supplement that information (with places of birth, more complete names, etc.). This is a case of how the web simplifies what would otherwise take much more time and effort.

I am looking forward to the upcoming week since I plan to see a number of friends, cross-country sky on the fresh snow, and have my usual check-in at the clinic.

WEEK 23 – A BUMP IN THE ROAD

January 22, 2012

The best laid plans of mice and men...

I was looking forward to a good, active week, and then I caught a stomach bug that knocked me down for the bulk of the week. I could not eat or keep anything down, had no energy (not even for reading), and was stuck in the house – extremely frustrating.

Fortunately, this was my regular clinic week, so it was no trouble for me to chat with the medical team and get a few tests done (abdomen x-ray, stool sample, blood work). It looks like my upset stomach was caused by a bug, not by more GvHD or a C. dificil infection. While this bug has been making the rounds, it may have taken more out of me because of what my immune system has gone through (it is still in the rebuilding stage).

I needed to have hydration administered, but the clinic provided home care. This makes a big difference when you are feeling crummy. Plus, a happy accident: my Hickman line has yet to be removed, so getting hooked up to hydration was easy.

On top of everything, my birthday was this week, so even the timing of my stomach bug was not ideal (it never is). Family plans for the weekend (our son is home) had to be scaled back. However, I seem to be on the mend, and hope to start eating real food and going on walks again soon.

I have another clinic visit next Tuesday just to check that everything is OK (my graduation keeps being postponed!).

My normal 'glass half full' perspective was challenged this week. Intellectually, I know that this is a marathon and that bumps on the road are normal, but I still expected that by five months post-transplant I would be less vulnerable than I am.

Invariably, though I did not have an issue with 'big, dark thoughts,' the worry that I may have to live with some chronic condition that has a major impact on my quality of life came back. The problem with feeling weak is that I can do nothing but rest, and just as the 'devil finds work for idle hands,' he also makes mischief with idle thoughts!

What happened this week is just part of this stage of post-transplant life, and a reminder to take as full advantage of the good moments when I can, as there will be other bad moments like this.

As a result, the week was not a productive one. I did get some nice books for my birthday, which I will read in the weeks ahead. I also watched a Jackie Chan movie on the 1911 Nationalist Chinese Revolution (aptly titled *1911*), which was patriotic and clearly intended for the mainland market, and followed the ups and downs of the South Carolina primary.

221

I will not make any predictions for next week – I only hope that my recovery continues and that I get back to normal!

WEEK 24 – ON THE MEND

January 29, 2012

In the end, my 'stomach bug' was actually a minor (although it didn't feel that way!) flare-up of GvHD. I was prescribed steroids (Prenisone, which is stronger than the Entocort I was on) and, as promised, felt the effects within 24 hours.

My stomach still burbles, but the cramps and the vomiting are gone. While my appetite has improved and my weight has stabilized, the process of getting back to a normal diet has been slow. Whenever I 'push' myself too hard on the food front, my stomach quickly tells me to back off. I tend to dream about the foods that I will be able to eat shortly, rather than try to eat them now!

Getting through my stomach issues and the associated worries was more taxing than I would have anticipated. I spoke to my clinical doctor about this, and she told me not to worry. She assured me that my reaction is normal and that I will get through this, but – there is always a but in this marathon – she also reminded me that, as a transplant patient, I am bound to hit bumps in the road from time to time.

I went through several tests this week: another abdominal x-ray for a quick check that no issues with my stomach and intestines, and my 'graduation' CT scan to 'close' this part of the file. Given my previous discussions about the CT scan, I challenged the necessity of having it done. I was told that it was recommended because of my stomach problems, and to wrap up this first six-month section of my treatment.

My CT scan came back the next day. The results were perfect: no sign of lymphoma. This is excellent news. That should be my last CT scan for a while. I will now be having annual MRIs. The resolution of MRIs is lower, but there is no ionizing radiation involved – a reasonable trade-off since I have been exposed to so much radiation through scans and treatments. I still need a brain and spinal MRI to check for lymphoma there, but no problem so far.

The results of my blood work were good again. No liver or kidney issues, and my counts are strong.

I will likely be on Prednisone – the steroid I was prescribed – for a number of months. Things will hopefully settle down during that time period. Although I am on a quarter-dose, there are long-term side effects associated with continued use (as is always the case with medications) that I would like to avoid if possible.

I hope that with this bump over, I can finally graduate. Two clinic visits in a week is more than I would like, but when they're needed, they're needed.

I have been reading Niall Ferguson's *The Pity of War*, his history of the reasons behind WWI. It is one of his heavier academic books, in contrast to his breezier, popular surveys of historical periods. I found Ferguson's rejection of some of the more traditional theories convincing (though it should be noted that I am no expert on the War). What I find most interesting is the decision-making process in the various countries involved: the imperfect information, the miscalculations, and the political factors that come into play with any international conflict.

My wife and I, along with a friend, went a concert of classical improvised Iranian music by Hossein Alizadeh and Pejman Hadadi. We have seen them both perform before as part of a larger group (Dastan Ensemble) and they delivered another great evening and concert as a duo.

Although the weather has been really bad this past week (freezing rain, etc.), I have been getting out more and am easing back into my walking routine. After spending 10-or-so days cooped up in the house, it feels so good to be outside.

The week ahead will be another recovery week as I continue to build up my weight and strength. I will not have to visit the clinic unless any issues come up – here's hoping.

WEEK 25 – SLOWLY BOUNCING BACK

February 5, 2012

My recovery has been slower than I expected. The Prednisone 'fixed' my gut issues, but the side effects included heartburn and headaches. These caused me a fair amount of discomfort, but not enough to prevent me from resuming short walks, seeing and talking to some friends, and getting back into my regular program of reading and working on the family tree.

The good news is that by the end of the week, I was able to eat more or less what I wanted (in moderation, of course) and work on regaining some of the weight I lost.

I will discuss with the medical team whether – and when – I can start reducing my dose of Prednisone to see if that relieves the side effects. Ideally, I would like to go back on Entocort (the less powerful steroid that only affects the gut), since it worked well for me in the fall (though I was on the immunosuppressant at the time, too, so my situation is different now).

It is worth raising the question with my doctors. I expect that I will have to stay on Prednisone for another two weeks or so before we can start playing with the dosage or changing my medication again.

My wife and I made it out to see *The Iron Lady* which we found, despite the mixed reviews and the controversy about portraying Thatcher's hallucinations in her old age, to be very sympathetic to her human side. The portrayal of her relationship with Dennis was touching, as was her struggle to make it in a party, and a society, where a privileged background was important. The compromises she made in balancing (or not) her career with her children, and the aftermath of these choices, were also sensitively portrayed. A more interesting and successful portrait than I had expected and as usual, Meryl Streep was superb.

We also watched *In the Heat of the Night*, a Norman Jewison film about 1960s Mississippi and the racial and other tensions between Virgil Tibbs, a black policeman from Philadelphia (played by Sidney Poitier) and Bill Gillespie, the local, and prejudiced police chief in Mississippi (player by Rod Steiger). Still a classic, for the characters, the story, and how it captures that period and place in America – not pretty.

I also finally got around to reading *Steve Jobs*, by Walter Isaacson (my hints about what I would like for my birthday were successful). Many of you have likely read excerpts. The book is an easy read, even if Jobs was frustrating and annoying in many aspects of his professional and personal life (e.g., his poor treatment of some of the early Apple employees). However, his genius at being able to focus and simplify, see 'where the puck is going,' and be at that intersection point, as he puts it, of liberal arts and technology, is amazing (disclosure: apart from an old PC, all our products are Apple now).

The book also made me reflect on leadership in general. In the context of government, a different kind of leader is favoured. 'Insanely great' as a goal largely does not work, as government is intrinsically more consensus-based and cautious, with a focus on stewardship over innovation. Leaders who are strong advocates of change are often weeded out, and the complex dynamic between the political and bureaucratic levels also hampers a single focus on innovation (for American readers, Canadian senior officials are part of the public service, not political appointees – think *Yes Minister*).

I was lucky enough to work for a change-focussed leader, and while that approach is not without its downsides, it was incredibly motivating and we did innovative things. But the innovation was too much for the government – concerns about risk trump all – and a more conventional leader was put in place (and I changed jobs and department as the excitement was gone). Similarly, a dynamic government Minister can change everything, and I have been fortunate to have worked for one of those, too. Even in the relatively protected environment that is the government, I gained some appreciation for how quirks (good and bad) and charisma motivate people.

Lastly, on a more mundane level, here are the January stats for the most popular page views (apart from the Home page).

1. Chefs, Butlers and Marble Baths – Not Your Average Hospital Room

2. A Sharper Mind, Middle Age and Beyond

3. Really? The Claim: Listening to Music Can Relieve Pain

4. Secrets of Cancerhood Blog: Things Not to Say

5. Elderly 'Experts' Share Life Advice in Cornell Project **and** A doctor's letter to a patient with newly diagnosed cancer

The latest Leonard Cohen album, *Old Ideas*, came out this week and I really enjoyed discovering it. *Come Healing* is my favourite track (has some echoes of his *Anthem* that also speaks to me about life and meaning). A sample of the lyrics:

> *O see the darkness yielding*
> *That tore the light apart*
> *Come healing of the reason*
> *Come healing of the heart*
>
> *O troubled dust concealing*
> *An undivided love*
> *The Heart beneath is teaching*
> *To the broken Heart above*
>
> *O let the heavens falter*
> *And let the earth proclaim:*
> *Come healing of the Altar*
> *Come healing of the Name*

O longing of the branches
To lift the little bud
O longing of the arteries
To purify the blood

And let the heavens hear it
The penitential hymn
Come healing of the spirit
Come healing of the limb

I had some good visits and chats with friends this week. It always feels good to get out of isolation!

This should be another recovery week if all goes well. My objective is to gain back some of the weight I lost – I now know that I should always have a bit of a reserve!

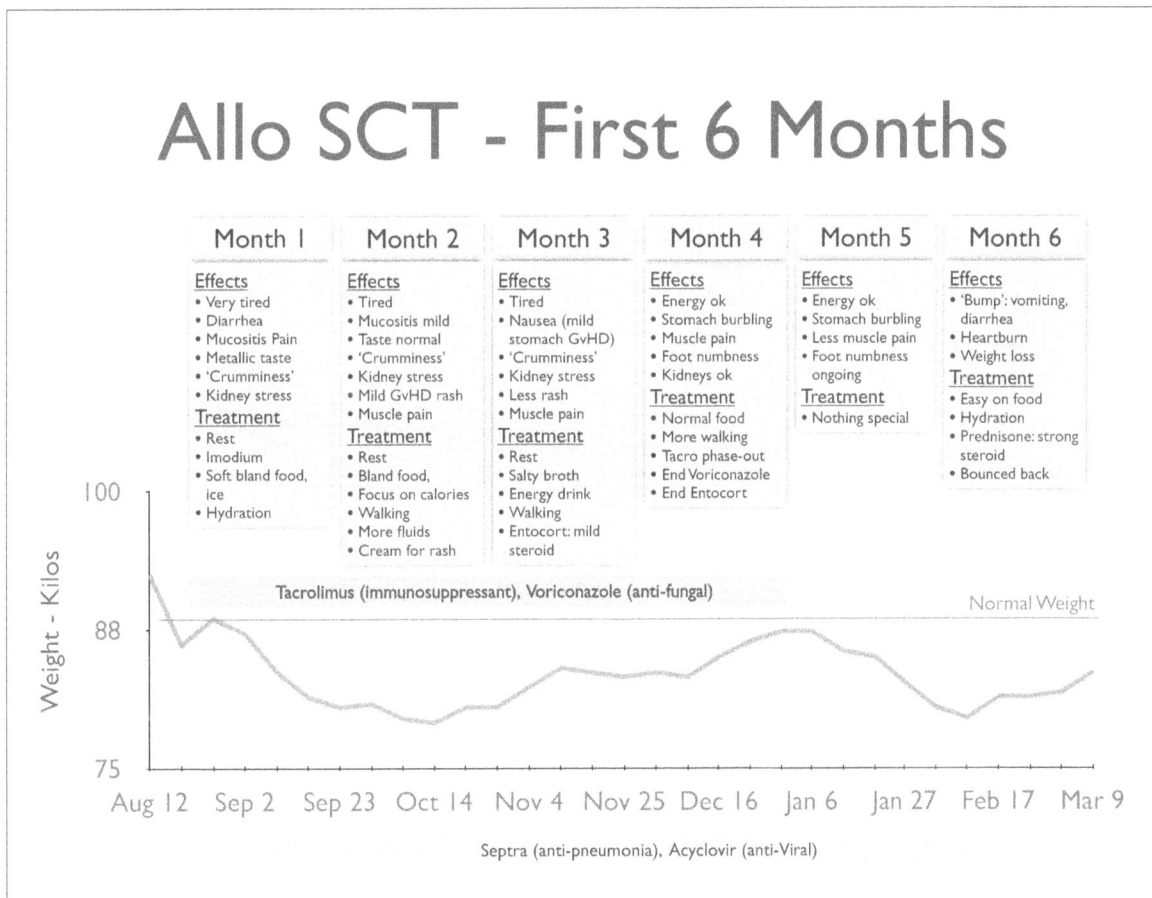

Allo SCT - First 6 Months

	Month 1	Month 2	Month 3	Month 4	Month 5	Month 6
Effects	• Very tired • Diarrhea • Mucositis Pain • Metallic taste • 'Crumminess' • Kidney stress	• Tired • Mucositis mild • Taste normal • 'Crumminess' • Kidney stress • Mild GvHD rash • Muscle pain	• Tired • Nausea (mild stomach GvHD) • 'Crumminess' • Kidney stress • Less rash • Muscle pain	• Energy ok • Stomach burbling • Muscle pain • Foot numbness • Kidneys ok	• Energy ok • Stomach burbling • Less muscle pain • Foot numbness ongoing	• 'Bump': vomiting, diarrhea • Heartburn • Weight loss
Treatment	• Rest • Imodium • Soft bland food, ice • Hydration	• Rest • Bland food, • Focus on calories • Walking • More fluids • Cream for rash	• Rest • Salty broth • Energy drink • Walking • Entocort: mild steroid	• Normal food • More walking • Tacro phase-out • End Voriconazole • End Entocort	• Nothing special	• Easy on food • Hydration • Prednisone: strong steroid • Bounced back

Tacrolimus (immunosuppressant), Voriconazole (anti-fungal)

Normal Weight

Weight - Kilos

100

88

75

Aug 12 Sep 2 Sep 23 Oct 14 Nov 4 Nov 25 Dec 16 Jan 6 Jan 27 Feb 17 Mar 9

Septra (anti-pneumonia), Acyclovir (anti-Viral)

Chapter 13

Getting On

Month 6 to 9

I pull out of the 'bump in the road' and continue on with a largely uneventful recovery. I build up my strength, my immune system is strong enough for me to go out and be with people, and life becomes more enjoyable.

WEEK 26 – 6 MONTHS: ALMOST BACK TO 'NORMAL'

February 12, 2012

My stem cell transplant was exactly six months ago, so I have another anniversary to mark. While this one is not as significant as the three-month mark from a medical perspective (since risk declines with time), it is still worth reflecting on and appreciating.

This week has been good. I have been eating normally and going for walks; my energy level is back up; and the side effects of my medication are diminishing, if not completely gone. Everyone in the family has benefitted from my renewed appetite and interest in food – I am cooking more of our meals!

While I have luckily avoided major mood swings (a side effect), my family makes sure to remind me that I am more irritable than usual! I am trying to be more self-aware and keep the grumpiness, which is not helpful for any of us, in check.

I also had a good clinic visit, and met with the senior hematologist this time rather than the clinical doctor. Some interesting points:

- It is not completely clear that my stomach upset was the result of GvHD, although the symptoms were consistent with that possibility;

- I should not worry about my weight – as long as I drinking and eat normally, it will work itself out (lately I have neither lost nor gained any weight);

- I can reduce my Prednisone dose by one tablet every five days – a gradual process, but so far, so good;

- Vaccinations are postponed for now, since Prednisone has an immunosuppressant effect;

- I have formally graduated (at last!) to the long-term clinic, with clinic visits now only every two-weeks. One of the fringe benefits of this is that my blood will no longer be tested regularly, which means no (or at least fewer) pokes; and,

- The hematologist is still keeping the option of a colonoscopy open, should it be necessary to check out possible reasons for my previous digestive problems but I will question that decision in light of my clear CT scan, that I am eating normally again with no stomach problems, and my desire to avoid an unpleasant procedure.

The doctor's ironic comment, always delivered with a smile, is that we do not want a 'perfect' transplant; a certain number of complications indicate that my donor and I are reacting in the way necessary to keep mantle cell lymphoma at bay.

The other big news is that I finally got my Hickman line out. I can now shower without contorting myself to keep it dry, a small but welcome pleasure.

Blood Counts Over the First 6 Months

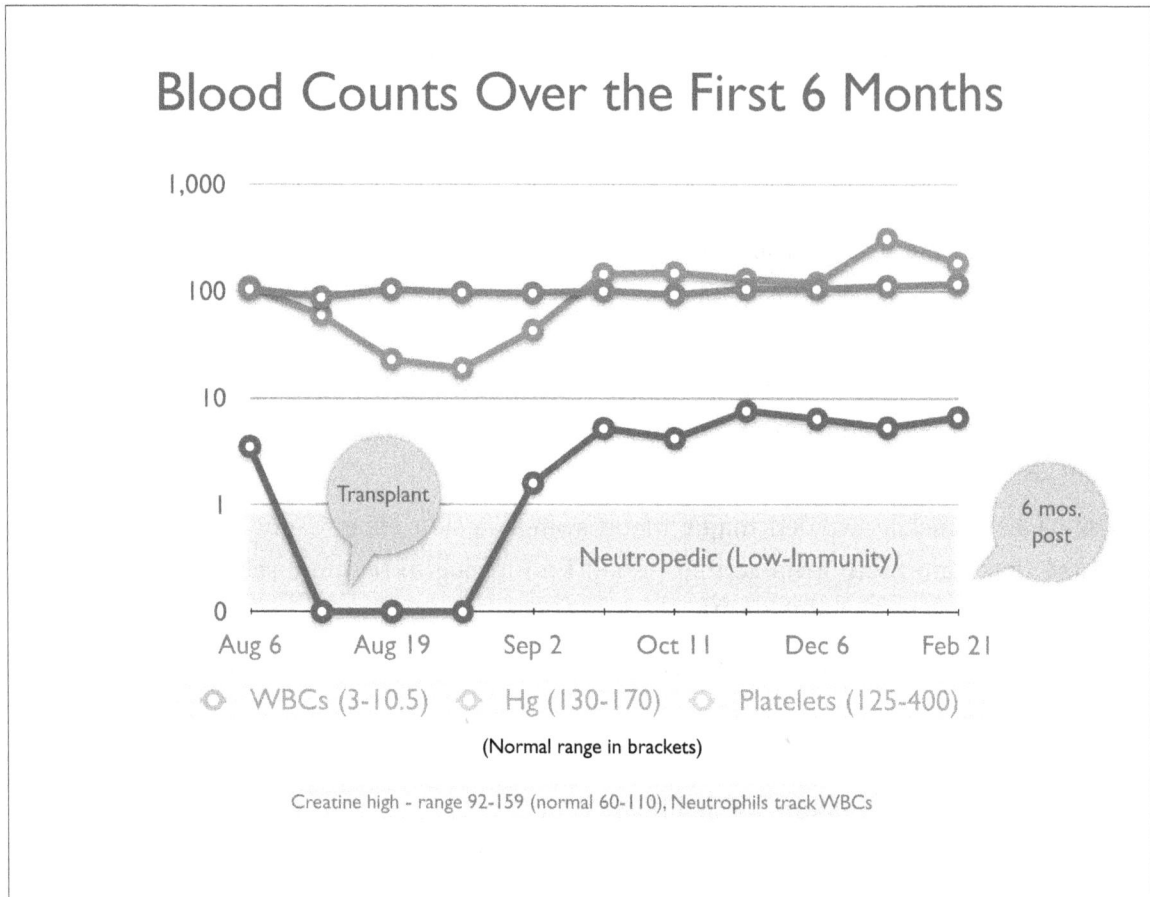

1,000

100

10

1

Transplant

0

Neutropedic (Low-Immunity)

6 mos. post

Aug 6   Aug 19   Sep 2   Oct 11   Dec 6   Feb 21

WBCs (3-10.5)   Hg (130-170)   Platelets (125-400)

(Normal range in brackets)

Creatine high - range 92-159 (normal 60-110), Neutrophils track WBCs

This week has also been good for movies.

We saw Roman Polanski's *Carnage*, adapted from a play, which featured a great cast: Jodie Foster, Kate Winslet, Christoph Waltz and John C. Reilly, who portray two couples trying to resolve a conflict between their sons. The tone of their interactions is initially civilized, but it degenerates progressively as inter- and intra- couple (as well as gender-related) tensions start coming out. Good black humour in parts. For those Crackberry addicts among you, there is a priceless scene that says it all. Although reviews were not great, we really enjoyed it.

We also saw *Tinker Tailor Soldier Spy*, based upon the book by John Le Carré, with a great British cast, and Gary Oldman as Smiley, the main character. It is a bit slow in places, and the editing can be confusing, but it captures so well the atmosphere of the time and place (during the Cold War), and bureaucratic and other games, that it comes all together. A more psychologically- than action-based thriller, and very creepy throughout.

We also rented *Le Bruit des Glaçons (The Clink of Ice)*, a French cancer comedy made directed by Bertrand Blier, and starring Jean Dujardin (of *The Artist* fame). While the premise is engaging – an alcoholic and failed writer (as well as his housekeeper) is visited by cancer in the form of a person – and some of the dialogue has wonderful black humour, it combines excessively silly relationships with a feel-good ending that goes beyond even the Hollywood standard. Now I will have to watch *50/50* to compare the two.

I am reading Daniel Kahneman's *Thinking Fast and Slow*, on the psychology of how we subconsciously make judgements and reach conclusions, which he argues depends on whether we use our automatic 'System 1' (fast) or more considered 'System 2' (slow) kind of thinking. I will have more reflections on Kahneman's book when I finish it next week, but suffice to say that it is an engaging (yet sobering) read.

A number of you were amused by my customer-service complaints (which predate my -induced irritability!). I never heard back from Sears about the fridge, so I wrote them a 'gently scathing' close-off letter that ended with the following paragraph:

> *I recognize that each company has its own service policies and approaches, and equally understand from the business press the challenges facing Sears Canada. I am, however, disappointed in the lack of substantive response from Sears and can only conclude that I am not valued as a customer. As a result, we will not be making any future purchases from Sears and have been sharing our story with family, friends and others.*

This upcoming week will see the further tapering-off of my Prednisone dose, and seeing how that goes; my sixth-month follow-up with the radiation oncologist, which I expect will be uneventful (part of routine procedure); and getting on with the regular 'maintenance' by getting my eyes checked (my prescription may have changed, due to a combination of normal aging processes and chemo).

WEEK 27 – 'NORMAL' AND 'THINKING, FAST AND SLOW'

February 19, 2012

A normal week, at last. There were no major issues; I am eating and drinking well, I went for lots of walks, can take normal showers post-Hickman line and have been able to move on with my projects. Even my weight has started to pick up and the process of tapering down my Prednisone dose has gone well.

I had my six-month recall visit with the radiation oncologist responsible for my Total Body Irradiation (TBI) treatment. It was more a formality than anything. His main area of concern was shortness of breath, since the main short-term risk of TBI is to the lungs, which are more sensitive to radiation than the rest of the body (though they are shielded during TBI to reduce exposure).

The results of my Pulmonary Function Test, as well as my experience with walking and other exercise, show that there are no issues with my lungs. The radiation oncologist noted that my strength should continue to build up over time. The only other thing that he flagged was to watch my thyroid, since thyroids, too, are potentially sensitive to TBI. There are no major precautions for me to take, apart from minimizing sun exposure through sunscreen and clothing (and he said that everyone should do this anyway). Best of all, he told me that I don't need to see him again!

I have finished the necessary but somewhat dry web search for the family tree. It took less time than expected, and I am now on to a more enjoyable step: renewing or making contact with some of the branches of the family to check my work, and more importantly – and interestingly – capture some of the family stories behind the dull stuff. Much more creative and satisfying.

We saw one of the Oscar nominees for best foreign picture, the Iranian film *A Separation* by Asghar Farhadi. Wonderful storytelling, good acting, and great depiction of family and class tensions. It was relatively edgy for an Iranian film made in Iran; while the film is not political, the undercurrents are (there is a great scene where the mother blurts out that she is moving abroad with her daughter to save her from living in 'these conditions,' before quickly retracting her statement). It will be interesting to see the response should it win; I expect mixed feelings from the Iranian government, as they try to stoke up yet manage tension with the 'Great Satan' (the United States in the language of the Iranian regime). Should it lose, it would play more into the narrative of Iranians as victims. Most Iranians would, of course, be proud to see it win. For those interested, I recommend an interesting short film by another Iranian director, Jafar Panahi, a sweet story with similar undertones, The Accordion.

We finally got around to seeing *50/50*, the 'cancer comedy' about a 27-year-old man, Adam, and his diagnosis with cancer. It was written by Will Reiser, and inspired by his own experience with the illness. While there were some funny moments (more light humour than dark), the tone was more serious and less funny than I expected. Overall, I think the film is a credible depiction of someone younger going through their journey, though I did have some quibbles on the details that were included to strengthen the story (e.g., the warm, comic-relief scenes with Adam and older cancer patients having chemo together – the protocols and timing would never work out to have a 'chemo' club and the chairs, at least in my hospital, are too far apart to chat). The most unrealistic part was the young, inexperienced therapist who becomes the (Hollywood) love interest. It is not believable that someone so inexperienced would be assigned to such a patient, let alone that they would fall in love, and I found that aspect of the story more irritating than anything else. The 'happy ending' is getting through the treatment and on with your life; there is no need for an artificial and forced add-on.

I finished *Thinking, Fast and Slow*, by Daniel Kahneman. There is much to recommend in this book. It is especially worth reading for the increased self-awareness it engenders, be it on a personal or professional level, of how one makes decisions or come to conclusions, and of how the automatic 'System 1' dominates the more deliberative 'System 2.'

As part of leadership training, I had been exposed to something similar before, but Kahneman takes it to another level, offering both a thorough explanation of how our thinking works and some practical steps to avoid blind spots. Interestingly, he acknowledges that as individuals, we are notoriously ill-equipped to self-police (he says that this is true even of himself, though he is super aware); however, institutions are better equipped to inoculate themselves (especially when they have to work with other institutions), at least partially, against some of the main patterns:

• tendency to jump to conclusions (System 1);

• exaggerated faith in small sample sizes, which are less reliable or representative than large sample sizes (e.g., we are disproportionately interested in exceptions);

• anchoring effect, where we gravitate to a specific number (e.g., house listing price) rather than a more independent evaluation;

• dramatic, personal or publicized events affect us more than probabilities based on large sample sizes, and tend to be overestimated (e.g., risk of cancer, plane crashes);

• we often forget that most exceptions regress to the mean – so if someone is having a winning streak, it is likely to end;

• expert intuition seems more reliable when concrete (e.g., from firefighters, medical professionals) than when abstract (e.g., from social scientists, financial analysts); and,

• prospect theory, or the fact that we are inclined to take a sure gain but gamble to avoid the risk of a loss (loss aversion).

Kahneman notes that behavioural economics has corrected the classical economic view of people as 'rational' agents given these and other patterns. While the following may be a caricature of how we behave, *Thinking, Fast and Slow* provoked me to reflect on the contrast between political and bureaucratic decision-making. The political variety draws heavily on anecdotes, stories and what 'people on the ground' are saying, and most impressions are formed under System 1. Bureaucratic decision-making, in contrast, draws more heavily on impersonal, large-scale studies and research, or evidence-based policy, making for a wider base of information (System 2).

Of course, many politicians, in developing their political approach, have taken an intellectual journey that is more reflective and deliberative. And many officials, in selecting and citing large-scale studies, have their own automatic System 1 influencing their procedural and methodological choices (see this clip from Yes, Prime Minister at about the one minute mark for an extreme version of this). This is part of how the two systems work together in all of us.

I had experience with what Kahneman describes when I worked on reshaping policies to address one of the government's priorities. Our evidence base, while solid, clearly reflected the priorities of earlier governments. Faced with the opinions of Ministers and political aides, who said that none of the evidence resonated with what they were hearing in their own interactions with a wide range of Canadians, we had to rethink the previous approach and develop a broader evidence base.

Just as decision-making based *only* on anecdotes can lead to poor outcomes (readers from any country can likely think of a few examples), policy that ignores anecdotes and public opinion in favour of a broad base of evidence runs the risk of missing the granularity of the system and can fail to respond to public concern. A combination of research and anecdotes arguably makes for better policy and programs.

I highly recommend Kahneman's book for decision-makers in particular, although everyone should find it interesting and useful.

I am looking forward to my son being home for reading week this coming week. I have my two-week clinic recall, which should confirm that I can continue to taper off the Prednisone. Hopefully, I will stay the course.

WEEK 28 – STAYING THE COURSE

February 26, 2012

Another good week.

I had my regular bi-weekly clinic visit; no problems. I can continue to taper down my Prednisone dose (reduction to four tablets daily this week, and a further reduction to 3 tablets daily next week). Since my stomach problems seem to have gone away, I will not need a colonoscopy, a procedure that I was dreading somewhat (this reinforces the importance of persistently questioning whether tests and treatments are necessary – had I not said anything, they would have run the test!) This is ironic, really, since a study on the effectiveness of the procedure came out just this week (Report Affirms Lifesaving Role of Colonoscopy); but since my CT scan was clear and the symptoms have gone away, there is no need for the additional worry of an additional test.

The only noticeable side effect that remains is some irritability, usually over small things, which I am still trying to manage (by biting my tongue!).

At the clinic, I also asked whether or not I should take Vitamin D, since I have to avoid the sun with clothing and sunscreen. A good question, according to the hematologist, and she told me that everyone, not just those in my situation, is encouraged to take up to 2,000 IU daily. I have started doing this, and all you readers can consider the advice for yourselves.

Another sign of arriving at the six-month mark and making the expected progress: my long-term disability insurance company wrote to my doctor asking for an update on my condition. I respected the process, not discussing what will be in the medical report prior to it being sent in (will ask next clinic visit) but given earlier discussions with my medical team, this is likely to be a further review around the one-year mark (around August).

I filled out the large-scale, comprehensive Ontario Health Study, which is looking how lifestyle, environment and family history may influence our health. I expect that some interesting data will emerge. If any of you are interested in completing the study (it is a bit clunky, particularly the sign-up procedure), check it out.

For my reading this week, I have been going through an old diary and a travel book from different branches of my family, both dating back to the 1800s (five generations ago). The diary is interesting in that some of the subjects are familiar in contemporary life (extreme weather, raising children, money worries) while others are particular to the period (infant mortality).

The travel book, which is essentially the 1800s version of a blog, reflects the biases of the English of the time with respect to Turkey and the Middle East, and especially Islam, although as an account of travel in the period it has its interesting moments. The ancestor who wrote this book appears to have been a bit of a dilettante, neglecting his family to invent (or so he claims) a steam engine, which in the end was neither built nor worked. The things one discovers.

On to movies: we saw *Pink Ribbons, Inc.*, which was a bit too polemical but raised legitimate issues with corporate sponsorship of breast cancer charities, and suggests that the 'false cheeriness' surrounding the topic of breast cancer can be counterproductive. As one person who was interviewed put it, cancer is not cute and cuddly! Perhaps the most powerful parts of the film were some of the interviews with Stage 4 breast cancer patients, and how they reacted to some of the messages.

I find that the film, while respectful of people getting together to raise funds and be part of the cancer community, undervalues the human aspect of people wanting to feel that they are doing something to help. Also, just as I find it annoying that the Congressional hearings on birth control and related issues only had male witnesses, I was also irritated by the lack of interviews with men featured in *Pink Ribbons, Inc.*, given their perspective as husbands, family members and caregivers.

We watched more TV than movies this week: the season finale of *Downton Abbey*, which was predictable but fun; the *Clinton* documentary on PBS, which brought back memories of those years (while there is no excuse for Clinton's behaviour, there is something particular about sex scandals, and the hypocrisy of Gingrich et al.); and the Republican Primary 'Survivor' debate. To put all that in perspective, we also watched some episodes of *Yes, Prime Minister*.

Overall, a good week; lots of walking and time with my son. My wife went skiing out West with a long-time friend, a necessary break after everything we have gone through.

I do not have any medical appointments next week, which is always a good thing, and will continue to see how the Prednisone phase-down goes. Highlights will be seeing my daughter's school musical, and one of my brothers coming here next weekend to catch up and do his three-month review of how I am doing!

Week 29 – Largely on Course

March 4, 2012

Strangely, my 29th week since the transplant is the same week as the leap year February 29th.

This was a good week overall; I went for lots of walks and worked on my regular projects.

The only thing that I need to raise during my clinic visit next week is that I have been having more stomach sensitivity and related issues. This could have something to do with trying out new foods, but it is more likely due to the phase-down of my Prednisone dose (which is now at three tablets, or 15 mg, per day). Hopefully, these stomach troubles are just part of the adjustment process. While not too serious, they are another irritant that I would rather be without. In addition, a rash on my legs has flared up somewhat, another sign of mild GvHD, and that – hopefully – my donor is fighting my lymphoma.

My guest blogs with Cancerwise (MD Anderson) continue, and I have 'graduated' to being on their blogroll – a promotion. I find it fun to try my hand at a different writing style (shorter, more list-based, focussed on the pragmatic), as it forces me to reflect in a different way and communicate accordingly. If there are topics of interest to any of you, let me know and I will add them to my 'to write' list.

I have also been toying with the idea of whether or not to create a book version of the blog this summer, when I hopefully make it past the one-year mark. To that end, I have been importing the blog content (with the exception of the press clippings), to *iBooks Author*, the new Apple textbook-design software. As is typical for Apple products, it is incredibly easy to use (drag and drop, copy and paste), and the formatting is elegant and effortless.

As I read through the weekly updates, dating back to as early as July 2009, I am struck by how much I have evolved in my willingness to share and be open. The early posts were short and general. As the journey wore on, they became more open and reflective, complemented by short summaries of what I was reading and watching. Since relapse, the depth has increased – that is my perception, at least. There is something powerful about seeing them together, rather than desegregated in the blog. Of course, I am partial!

We watched the Oscars this week, naturally, and were pleased with some of the winners, specifically *A Separation*, Christopher Plummer, and Meryl Streep, who along with all the French winners, gave gracious and thoughtful acceptance speeches.

We saw *Monsieur Lazhar* this week. It is a good, well-crafted film about the integration challenges and worries of a refugee (the teacher, M. Lazhar). It captures the nuance of Quebec society and its debates about 'reasonable accommodation' and interculturalism, and also presents a delicately-framed critique of the education system. The film includes some wonderful vignettes, ranging from the borderline racism of one set of parents towards Monsieur Lazhar ('Vous n'êtes pas d'ici donc peut-être vous ne comprenez pas certaines nuances') to the naiveté of one of his colleagues, who in talking about her travels suggests that exile is just like any other journey (he replies curtly, noting that tourists have travel documents!).

We also watched *Les femmes du 6ème étage (The Women of the Sixth Floor)*, a French comedy about the relationship between a staid, bourgeois *bourcier* (stockbroker) and the Spanish maids who live on the 6th floor. A clichéd story in which the humanity and liveliness of the maids awakens the bourgeois family. Light fluff.

I read *Coeur Ouvert* by Élie Wiesel this week. There is a stark contrast between his first book, *La nuit*, in which he was angry and rebelling against his religion, and *Coeur Ouvert*; in the latter, Wiesel draws heavily on his faith to deal with a high-risk heart operation, and reflects on his life and accomplishments (asking himself whether he has done enough). As expected, the book is reflective and moving, as the following paragraphs illustrate (to my anglophone readers: I do not think the English version is out yet – the book was only published in the latter half of 2011 – and Google translate would butcher his beautiful prose):

> *J'appartiens à une génération qui s'est souvent sentie abandonnée de Dieu et trahie par l'humanité. Et, pourtant, je crois qu'il nous incombe de ne nous séparer ni de l'un ni de l'autre.*

> *Est-ce hier – ou autrefois – que nous avons appris combien l'être humain peut attaindre la perfection dans la cruauté plus que dans la générosité? Que, pour les tueurs et les tortionnaires, il est normal, donc humain, de se montrer inhumain? Dès lors, faudrait-il se détourner de l'humanité?*

> *Je crois que la réponse appartient à chacun de nous. Car il incombe à chacun de choisir entre la violence des adultes et le sourire des enfants, entre la laideur de la haine et le désir de s'y opposer. Entre infliger souffrance et humiliation à son semblable et lui offrir la solidarité et l'espoir qu'il mérite. Peut-être.*

> *Je sais – je parle d'expérience – que, même dans les ténèbres, il est possible de créer la lumière et nourrir des rêves de compassion. Que l'on peut se penser libre et libérateur à l'intérieur des prisons. Que, même en exil, l'amitié existe et peut devenir ancre. Qu'un instant avant de mourir, l'homme est encore immortel.*

> *Voilà: je crois en l'homme malgré les hommes. Je crois dans le langage bien qu'il ait été meurtri, déformé et perverti par les ennemis de l'humanité. Et je continue à m'accrocher aux mots parce qu'il nous appartient de les transformer en instruments de compréhension plutôt que de mépris. À nous de choisir si nous souhaitons nous servir d'eux afin de maudire ou de guérir, pour blesser ou consoler.*

> *Juif, je crois en la venue du Messie. Mais cela ne signifie pas que le monde deviendra juif; je pense qu'il deviendra tout simplement plus accueillant, plus humain. Et ce parce que j'appartiens à une génération ayant appris que, quelle que soit la question, l'indifférence et la résignation ne constituent pas la réponse.*

I have enjoyed spending time with my brother from California this weekend. We mainly go for walks together, but it has been nice to be able to see him every three months or so, rather than only once per year.

Lastly, my monthly top posts list for February. In addition to the Home Page and Weekly Updates, more people have been looking at some of my reflection pieces – Dualities, Lessons, Faith – than in recent months. I imagine that this uptick is from people who are new to my blog. The top five apart from these are:

1. Top five regrets of the dying

2. Bill Moyers Talks With Poet Christian Wiman About Living With Cancer And Finding Faith (VIDEO)

3. Susan G. Komen Foundation – Losing its Way?

4. A doctor's letter to a patient with newly diagnosed cancer

5. The Well Quiz: How Adventurous Are You?

Hopefully, the minor troubles (stomach and rash) that I am experiencing will clear up over the next week, but I will ask at the clinic about whether I can continue to phase-out the Prednisone or need to put the process on 'pause' to help my body and donor continue to adjust to each other.

WEEK 30 – SO FAR, SO GOOD

March 11, 2012

This week was surprisingly good. The stomach burbles disappeared almost completely, even as I notched down my Prednisone dose from three tablets per day to two (10 mg). Conveniently, this improvement took place a day or so before my clinic visit on Monday.

I had a good discussion with the clinical doctor about the following points:

- The process of getting off Prednisone will be slightly slower now – I will take two tablets a day for two weeks, rather than one.

- The slight flare-up of the rash on my legs is minor, not an issue, and can be managed with use of hydrocortisone cream as needed.

- The numbness in my feet is due to numbness in my proprioceptors, the sensors that work with my brain and muscles to ensure balance and coordination. Again, this is a normal side effect, and one that may go slowly away – or not. It is manageable. While I have to be a bit more cautious and watch my balance, the numbness has no major impact on what I can and cannot do (biking, for example, will not be an issue).

- I reminded the doctor that my donor had possibly been exposed to Hepatitis C and asked when I should be tested. Apparently, this information was not in the normal follow-up file (reminder to all – one has to track these things oneself!), but she ordered the test as part of my regular blood work that day. Hopefully the result will be negative.

- I asked about which sunscreen to use, and the doctor replied that any sunscreen that provides UVA/UVB protection and has an SPF of 30 is fine.

- My doctor's office will follow up on scheduling the MRI for my brain and spinal cord. I was warned that the previous damage to my leptomeninges may not be reversible – but I will be happy with it not getting worse.

- I can get re-vaccinated now that my dose of Prednisone is low. I started the process on Friday, and apart from two sore arms, I have had no adverse reactions.

- No issues with local travel as long as I take normal precautions.

I also asked about the letter to my long-term disability insurance provider. She said their overall approach is to give their patients time to recover. Her letter described my condition in such a way as to keep the long-term disability insurance coverage until I had more time to recover before having to go back to work. I expect that there will be another review in about four to six months. While I have been feeling good lately (touch wood!), I am aware of the limits on my strength and endurance, and being able to balance physical and intellectual rebuilding without the pressures of work makes all the difference.

Movie-wise, we watched *Moneyball*, the story of how quantitative statistical analysis trumped scouting in baseball and allowed the Oakland Athletics to build a winning team far more cheaply than would otherwise have been possible (it was cited by Daniel Kahneman as an example where the traditional use of scouts, who assess possible players on their build and appearance – representativeness, i.e., they look the part – was replaced by selecting players that other teams overlooked, based on the statistics of their past performance).

We also watched *Game Change*, an HBO film about the 2008 election and the McCain-Palin campaign. It features a good, tight script, and good performances from Julianne Moore (Palin), Woody Harrelson (Schmidt, the campaign manager) and Ed Harris (McCain). I sometimes have to wonder how the strategists, in their rush for a game changer, could omit basic policy questions in the short vetting process. Another case of fast thinking gone wrong.

The film, as some reviewers have noticed, may be overly sympathetic to Palin on the personal level, given that she was thrust into a situation that she was not prepared for without the self-awareness to know it. The ongoing effect of 'pride in ignorance' has, of course, played itself out this primary season, and we are all poorer for the resulting 'dumbing-down' of political discourse. Still, whatever your politics, *Game Change* is a gripping political film.

I have also been listening to the new Springsteen album, *Wrecking Ball*. The contrast between his angry lyrics and warm music is striking; unless one listens to the lyrics, the anger does not come through.

Here is a sample of the lyrics, from *Shackled and Drawn* (some of which applies to aspects of living with cancer):

> *Gray morning light spits through the shade*
> *Another day older, closer to the grave*
> *Closer to the grave and come the dawn*
> *I woke this morning shackled and drawn*
>
> *Shackled and drawn, shackled and drawn*
> *Pick up the rock, son, carry it on*
> *I'm trudging through the dark in a world gone wrong*
> *I woke up this morning shackled and drawn*

I was busy with other projects and also walked a fair amount this week, so I did not have time to do any reading this week. I have started experimenting with Pinterest, but have yet to figure out how best to use it.

Next week, I will be making my first trip since my transplant: a short one to Toronto, to see our son and some friends. It will be nice to have a change of scene.

WEEK 31 – A BREAK

March 19, 2012

I had a nice break in Toronto this week. We did some university tours for our daughter, and spent time with our son, one of my brothers, and some old family friends.

It felt strange to be in a big city again. The crowds, and my apprehension about these given my immunity concerns, made me cut some visits short (e.g., seeing an exhibit on the Maya during March break was probably not a good idea, so I walked through more quickly that I would have normally). One look at the crowds on the subway (metro) made me realize that it would be better to walk!

As a result, I have been walking more than usual and feeling my leg muscles more. A good opportunity for conditioning.

The other thing is that the background noise of the city made my hearing loss (which has been going on for some time) more noticeable, so I tried to take quieter streets when possible. The aging process at work!

I had fun trying new restaurants and food, but I experienced more stomach burbling (mostly while walking, interestingly), which affected my plans a little bit.

My son and daughter, along with my brother and I, saw *High Life*, a cleverly-written play by Lee MacDowell about an attempted heist by four down-on-their-luck drug addicts. It featured some incredibly sharp and funny dialogue, and the characters were believable and well-acted. I stayed engaged and awake throughout, which speaks to the quality of the play – my energy level is weakest in the evening!

Overall, the trip was a good test, in a way, of how I am doing some seven months out from the transplant. Though I am obviously not in the same shape that I was pre-transplant, I am well and strong enough (assuming I have not picked up any infections) to be out and about in and enjoy the world. This is reassuring and encouraging. I also overcame what was almost a fear of climbing out of the shell of my Ottawa routine. It can be hard to strike that fine psychological balance between prudence and paranoia!

Next week is a clinic week, a check-in more than a check-up. I expect to get the go ahead for the final phase-out of Prednisone. Taking one less medication and having fewer side effects will be a welcome change.

To my Iranian readers: an early Eid-e-Mobarak for the Persian New Year this week.

WEEK 32 – REBIRTH AND RENEWAL

March 25, 2012

Spring: rebirth, renewal, regeneration.

These themes are particularly poignant for me. At this time last year, I was confronted with the relapse of my lymphoma, which brought with it the prospect of uncertain and risky treatment, and the reality that my hopes for normal life were dashed yet again.

At the clinic this week, I met with the same senior hematologist who gave me the bad news last year; this time, however, the story was different:

- no signs of lymphoma;
- blood marrow is working well and blood counts are strong;
- no significant ; and,
- looking and feeling well.

While the more conclusive assessment will take place at the one-year mark, my progress is good and 'directionally correct.' Some other bits of good news included:

- no need to worry about Hepatitis C from my donor – the test came back negative;
- the MRI on May 4th will tell us whether there is any lymphoma-related activity in my brain and spinal cord;
- I have progressed from a two-week to two-month recall – another graduation, as it were, and more free Monday afternoons to look forward to; and,
- no issues with biking, yard work or vacuuming, so I can enjoy this spring and summer while being more useful around the house.

I will continue to lower my Prednisone dose, still at a gradual rate: alternating between two tablets (10 mg) and one tablet (5 mg) every other day until my appointment in May.

I came out of the clinic feeling a mixture of giddy euphoria ('this may really work') and more sober realism ('I have been here before'). I have felt a strange mix of emotions all week, especially given the wonderful – and unseasonal – warm spring weather we have been having lately. Flitting between the two extremes is normal after what I have experienced, and it is so much better than last year's bleakness. Of course, I still feel the same awe and wonder about getting this second chance at life.

I showed the senior hematologist some of the graphics and tables that I have been preparing for my book. We had a fun discussion. He started off by saying that I am obviously feeling well if I am able to start producing things like this, and then started a deeper discussion based in part on his experience in teaching.

He is not a great fan of Powerpoint ('deadly,' he called it), noting that its main weakness is that it presents information in a linear fashion, when the reality that he and his colleagues face is more complex. He challenged me to try Prezi, which can capture this complexity more effectively. He suggested that I try thinking in 'parallel' rather than serially, and use my creative side more.

Since my natural disposition is towards more linear, analytic thinking, this is quite a challenge, and I will need a few months to do my 'homework'. My recent post on medical history (Visualize This: An e-Patient's Medical Life History) provides some additional inspiration.

It was impressive to see another side of my hematologist, particularly the teaching side, which he is passionate about. He shared some great asides about the penchant on the part of some students for looking up everything and correcting their professors – even the minor details (e.g, he will say that my white blood cell count is 8.6, and someone will look it up and say, 'no, it is 8.5').

I look forward to showing him my homework on my iPad (he was adamant that it should be on the iPad) in a few months.

With the arrival of warmer weather, I have started biking again. It feels wonderful to be outside, enjoying the sense of freedom that only biking provides – and that it has provided me ever since my childhood. When I bike now, however, as part of the balance between the prudent and paranoid, I am equipped with SPF clothing that covers up as much of my skin as possible. Not as bad as biking in a biohazard suit, but the combination of an SPF cap and a helmet is far from elegant.

Some of you may recall that before my transplant, I kept track of my biking times. My first times this week were horrible, but they started to come down after a few days. I am still about 10-15 percent slower than before, a measure of how much the treatment has taken out of me.

I am not trying to compete with Lance Armstrong (I find some of his tweets about 80 km bike rides less inspiring than irritating, but then again, I expect that some people find my little victories equally irritating!), but with myself. It gives me a better sense of the before and after, and what will be my new normal.

I have been reading Neil Bissoondath's critique *Selling Illusions: The Cult of Multiculturalism in Canada*. He perceptively notes some of the absurdities of extreme multiculturalism; the complexity of culture, identity and ethnicity; and the problems that narrow identities can pose for creativity when taken to the extreme. One of the better quotes on the complexity of ethnicity and its relation to individuals:

> *My point is simple, but it is one usually ignored by multiculturalism and its purveyors – for to recognize the complexity of ethnicity, to acknowledge the wild variance within ethnic groups, would be to render itself and its aims absurd. The individuals who form a group, the "ethnics" who create a community, are frequently people of vastly varying composition. Shared ethnicity does not entail unanimity of vision. If the individual is not to be betrayed, a larger humanity must prevail over the narrowness of ethnicity.*

To preserve, enhance and promote the "multicultural heritage" of Canada, multiculturalism must work against forces more insistent than any government policy. If a larger humanity does not at first prevail, time and circumstance will inevitably ensure that it does.

He may overstate the effects of time and circumstance in today's age of cheap travel, free communications and increased targeted ethnic market segmentation (e.g., banks, broadcasters). He does not acknowledge that Canadian multiculturalism has always had a strong integrative intent (dating from Book IV of the Bi and Bi Commission) in contrast with Europe, where immigration policies (guest workers), lack of immigration culture and identity, and greater traditional identification of ethnicity with nationality, led to a vision of communities living side-by-side, not blending together. Bissoondath also overstates the difference between the US and Canada, where the 'melting pot' and 'cultural mosaic' labels are overstated.

If any public policy runs the risk of extremism, I think that the Canadian tendency, which leans toward over-accommodation, is better than the European one, which leans toward intolerance at best, racism and discrimination at worst.

For a more nuanced view, I recommend this Review of Pax Ethnica by Will Kymlicka, which notes that successful multiculturalism is not just tolerance and the absence of violence, but also more positive integration at both the group and individual levels:

At their best, these cases go beyond mere tolerance or bare co-existence to include positive elements of inter-group solidarity, and this is what makes them harbingers of a better society. The various groups are committed to living together in justice, and to sharing fairly economic opportunities, political representation and cultural recognition.

I received the annual invitation to participate in the Light the Night Walk for blood cancers this week. Although the Leukemia and Lymphoma Society does good work, I did my usual due diligence on the portion of funds that are spent on management and fundraising, as opposed to program spending – 47.5 percent, of which 37 percent is for fundraising. I find it hard to support a charity when one out of every two dollars goes to overhead costs. My hospital has a better ratio (only about one in every five dollars).

The weather is back to seasonal norms, and the brief taste of what is to come remains just that. I have nothing major planned for the week ahead, but I seem to have enough activities and projects to keep me busy and engaged.

WEEK 33 – LIFE CONTINUES

April 1, 2012

Life continues and there no major changes to report – all good.

As expected, Ottawa is back to normal seasonal temperatures, so I have not been cycling (apart from indoors), but am still going on a lot of walks. I treated myself to a good bike tune-up, so I am ready for the warm weather that is yet to come.

My hair was finally long enough – and mad professor enough (think Back to the Future) – to warrant a haircut, and I now have a more 'corporate' look.

I got a great reader comment on my last weekly update:

> *Sounds like you're doing great. I always considered it a good sign when the oncologist started to let down "the wall" and treat me as if I was going to be around for a while! I couldn't blame him for keeping me at arm's length in the beginning, but it sure encouraged me when he started being more personable and less business-like.*

Delightful sense of black humour!

Over the past few weeks, I have ventured out to more group events. Immunity is no longer an issue, but I do become very tired when I have to focus on my hearing in a group or concentrate more when languages other than English are spoken. These social events give me a sense of how I might do in meetings, and clearly I am not ready for them yet. I am better one-on-one or in quiet locations.

I took my hematologist up on his challenge and started using Prezi. It does require a more imaginative way of presenting than the linear Powerpoint/Keynote decks that we are all used to. I have to doodle and sketch out some ideas, rather than working directly on the screen. It pays off, though, and the navigational possibilities – forward, backward, sideways – are better suited to capturing complexity and the somewhat fragmented and iterative structure of my treatment and personal journey.

Interestingly, while my hematologist wanted me to use Prezi for some of my slides about treatment, I am finding it more useful to integrate the personal and the medical. Finding the right balance between the linear and parallel modes of thinking – I need some of both – is proving to be a challenge, but a fair amount of fun, too.

I realized that making good use of Prezi has more in common with filmmaking than with a PowerPoint deck, so I started Michael Ondaatje's *The Conversations: Walter Murch and the Art of Editing Film* (Murch was the editor of *The English Patient*, as well as *Apocalypse Now* and many other films by Coppola and others).

It helps me understand how I might move back and forth between topics while maintaining a coherent storyline, and also happens to be a great read on the creative process. I once did a report that incorporated strong graphics and my boss at the time reminded me, wisely, to be ruthless on the cutting floor. I am not quite there yet – still in the creative phase of getting all the ideas out.

A few sample quotes from Walter Murch to give you a sense of what I am reading:

> Somebody once asked W.H. Auden, "Is it true that you can write only what you know?" And he said, "Yes it is. But you don't know what you know until you write it. Writing is a process of discovery of what you really do know. You can't limit yourself in advance to what you know, because you don't know everything you know.. . . .

> Yes, that's what I call the "Tragedy-of-Job moments" (referring to the cutting out of what initially appear to be key scenes). They are like the good man Job, who does everything – and more – that God requests of him, but God perversely afflicts him and not the bad person who is Job's neighbour. Why me? Job asks. Well, it's because God can see the whole that Job cannot see, and in some mysterious way these afflictions are for the good of the whole, in a way that is invisible to the person.

Lastly, here are my monthly stats on the most popular posts, apart from my weekly updates and views of my Home page:

1. The women behind ideological debates about abortion
2. Why I Won't Get a Colonoscopy | Scientific American Blog
3. A Story About Care – YouTube
4. A doctor's letter to a patient with newly diagnosed cancer
5. Faith

I have some nice get-togethers planned next week to reconnect. I am looking forward to these, as well as to my usual routine and projects.

WEEK 34 – ALL IS WELL

April 8, 2012

Not much new to report – which is good. I have been taking advantage of the walking weather, had some nice get-togethers with friends and colleagues, and filled my days with the usual activities and projects.

As part of the process of turning my blog into a book and preparing my Prezi, I have been working on some graphics to capture the different stages.

These largely reflect 'linear' views to be used in the more 'parallel' Prezi. I enjoy developing the graphics, and experimenting with colour, grouping and 'layering' in Keynote. Without the normal corporate constraints (e.g., templates, culture of bullets), I have the latitude to try a denser approach, encapsulating a lot of information that was presented to me in a more organic and step-by-step process at the time.

For those interested, these are now posted on my blog. Any comments or feedback on how these could be made more comprehensive is appreciated.

I have also been working on a piece that aims to categorize the various terms people with cancer use to describe themselves: warrior, fighter, hero, survivor, student/intern/graduate, and victim.

It has been harder to put together than I expected, as it is these labels are subjective and change throughout the cancer journey – unlike a technical and medical glossary. The process has forced me to do some good thinking, with the help of several friends, and I hope to finalize the piece in the next few weeks. My intent is to create an article that helps the reader reflect on why individuals gravitate to certain terms, and the possible implications of those choices.

Suggestions of any terms I have missed would be appreciated.

I finished *The Conversations: Walter Murch and the Art of Editing Film*. I really enjoyed it, and it makes me want to re-watch most of the movies mentioned and get a hold of some that I haven't seen yet (e.g., *A Touch of Evil*, by Orson Welles, which Murch re-edited according to Welles' original wishes - which were overturned by the studio). Some favourite quotes:

> *I can think of no higher tribute to a film than ... that you sense simultaneously that it's crystalline and organic at the same time. Too crystalline and it's lifeless, too organic and it's spineless...*

> *There's that wonderful line of Rilke's, "The point of life is to fail at greater and greater things." Recognizing that all our achievements are doomed, in one sense – the earth will be consumed by the sun in a billion years or so – but in another sense the purpose of our journey is to go farther each time. ... I think we're always failing, in Rilke's sense – we*

know there's more potential that we haven't realized. But because we're trying, we develop more and more talent, or muscles, or strategies to improve, each time...

When something is successful, everything that went into it, both the good and the bad, tends to get bundled up as the recipe for how to make a success. It becomes very difficult to separate out what was true and what was untrue, what was good and what was bad, what was superficial and what was profound...

The distortions of failure, of course, are the opposite: instead of having everything unjustly accepted, everything is rejected. Or that's the risk, at any rate. Truly great lessons can be learned from work that fails, but failure is stamped on the product and there's a tendency to think everything you did was wrong, and you vow not to go there again. You have to resist this impulse, just as you have to resist the syrupy entanglements of success. These are, almost, religious issues. What the world thinks is a success, what it rewards, has sometimes very little to do with the essential content of the work and how it relates to the author and his own development.

The book was helpful in my attempt to develop some non-linear and more creative ways to tell stories and engage with others, and the reflections within were also good in themselves.

I also have a renewed appreciation for the importance of sound in movies, which was juxtaposed with this short series of quotes on silence, from the book *In Pursuit of Silence*:

The Origin and Cultural Evolution of Silence

When I watched *A Dangerous Method* this week, I found myself focussing on the editing more than usual, as the film itself did not hold my attention (I am curious as to whether the original play, *A Talking Cure*, worked better). I expect that I will never watch movies in quite the same way again.

To those celebrating Easter or Passover, best wishes for this time of reflection and family.

WEEK 35 – 9-MONTH MARK

April 15, 2012

Although the nine-month mark has no specific medical significance, I am so habituated to quarterly reporting that I take this as another milestone! The next big step is the one-year mark, and I am now three-quarters of the way there.

This has been another good week. The weather improved and was able to go for several bike rides. While I would like to claim credit for shaving close to 10 percent from my circuit time, it was more likely the tune-up and higher tire pressure that made the difference.

Part of my return to 'normal' is catching up on the little things. This time, the 'little thing' was my regular dental cleaning. The timing was perfect since I recently read an article on dental x-rays and brain cancer; I politely declined the offer of x-rays, though my reaction was somewhat irrational since I have been exposed to much larger doses of radiation over the past few years.

I had some good visits with friends this week, some of whom have had experiences like mine, some of whom have not. It is always nice to get out of the house and see people again.

I wanted a change in my reading material, so I went back to fiction with Neil Bissoondath's *The Soul of All Great Designs*. A clever concept – the relationship between two people who need to conceal their true identities from each other, the one an interior designer who has to appear gay to attract business, the other an Indo-Canadian whose family expects her to only see or marry another Indo-Canadian. Though the book is beautifully and engagingly written, and the secrecy theme is well-played out, there is something flat about the characters, particularly the interior designer (whose true name we never know). My other complaint is that the ending seemed a bit too neat and contrived (not a spoiler to say that it does not end well).

We went to see the Iranian singer Googoosh in concert last night (she is one of the more famous Iranian pop singers from before the Iranian Revolution). Our son came up to join us for the concert as well, so it was a good family outing. She is in great form, much more energetic than when we last saw her over five years ago. The crowd was alive and enthusiastic, and she clearly enjoyed and fed off that energy. A great evening.

Funnily enough, she always does one song in English (and one in French), and the one she chose to close off the show was 'I Will Survive.' I am not sure whether she chose that song for its 'get on your feet' quality, or whether as a survivor on many levels, it resonated with her. From my perspective, the refrain could easily be applied to an empowering cancer context (just replace anymore with at all, and goodbyes with chemo!):

Go on now go,
Walk out the door,
Just turn around now,
Cause you're not welcome anymore,
Weren't you the one who tried to hurt me with goodbyes
Do you think I'd crumble?
Do you think I'd lay down and die?
Oh no not I

I will survive
Oh as long as I know how to love
I know I'll stay alive
I've got all my life to live
I've got all my love to give
I will survive
I will survive
Hey hey!

WEEK 36 – ANOTHER GOOD WEEK

April 22, 2012

It has been another good week. The weather was good for walking and biking, I did some fun reading, found interesting content for my blog, and saw more people. No complaints.

I have had a busier than usual 'social calendar' this week. I have been visiting with a large number of colleagues, including some that I have not seen for many years. At the personal level, it has been good to reconnect and in many cases, talk about what each others' kids are up to, given that they are of similar ages.

This prompted a number of reflections:

- I realized how much I am 'out of it' when discussion turned to shop talk, corporate culture and peeves. What would once have drawn me in no longer holds any interest. This is in contrast with 2009-2010, after my first round, when I was interested in work and looked forward to getting back to my job. The second time changes everything, and this was a good confirmation that I have truly moved on, with no interest in returning, notwithstanding liking the people and substantive policy issues.

- I thought about the difference between personal and professional relationships. The latter are temporary – you do good things with people in a particular context, and then move on. People are busy in their professional and personal lives, so drifting apart is natural. Hopefully we have good memories, and we can relive them when we meet, but our lives go in different paths.

- While I think I was sensitive when colleagues were going through health challenges, I must have missed being aware of some situations and did not always provide appropriate support. I cannot turn back the clock, but hopefully sharing this can save some of you from making the same mistake.

- We choose the relationships that we wish to deepen and strengthen, and consequently, those which migrate from the professional to the personal. A dinner reunion with colleagues with whom I spent two to three years in an executive training program demonstrated this. Given that they all have busy professional and personal lives, who came and who did not reflected a choice between what was more important: the personal (being there) or the professional (being wedded to one's work).

One of the fun things about being in my position (there have to be some fun aspects!) is that I play a bit of a focus group or mystery shopper role for colleagues who deal with human resource (HR) issues, as I have dealt with HR staff and disability programs from an 'applicant' perspective. I provided my overall positive feedback (HR staff were particularly helpful) and noted my pet peeves: non computer-fileable pdfs (fixed, I subsequently discovered) and duplication of forms between the private insurance companies and the government disability program (Canada

Pension Plan - Disability). This is kind of ironic since, as noted earlier, I myself had been doing analysis on service strategies to reduce duplication and complexity on disability supports.

With encouragement from my colleagues, I decided to provide my feedback more formally, as one way of giving back. While I was tempted to raise my concerns at the political level, I remembered that, as a government official, it was more appropriate to officials, rather than Ministers. I received acknowledgement from the office of client satisfaction within a few hours, and from the chief operating officer the following day. I was pleased with the good service, although the actual resolution of the issues I mentioned will take longer.

I have my regular physical next week (part of my transition to worrying about other health issues!). I was unable to find a good medical history form online, and in my frustration, prepared one myself (blank template here). Major additions to the usual form: objectives (in my case, for example, apart from the obvious 'no relapse,' I included the very practical objective of managing other health issues with minimal interventions and hospital time) and lifestyle (e.g., exercise, diet and monitoring). I will see how my doctor reacts to it and, more importantly, whether there are any other health issues I need to address.

We watched *Hugo*, Martin Scorsese's homage to movie-making. Visually, it is an incredibly beautiful film (some of the shots are breathtaking, as is Scorsese's attempt to capture Paris in the post-WWI period). The story of ingenuity, creativity, depression and almost rebirth is a strong one, but the film, whether through the editing or the script, fails to make it come alive. It drags on in places, and the mix between materials for children and adults is uneven. It is still worth seeing for the visual beauty and the reflections on movie-making, and it passed my 'stay awake' test despite the slow pace of the first half.

I started re-reading *Among the Believers*, V.S. Naipaul's observations about his travels in a number of Muslim countries. I am currently reading the first section, which is about Iran in the early years after the revolution, and it makes for familiar if depressing reading. His depiction of Qom, a medieval centre of theological study, is particularly well done.

I am eagerly waiting for the current streak of rainy weather to end – although it is good for our lawn – so that I can get back to biking.

WEEK 37 – COMPLAINTS ABOUT THE WEATHER

April 29, 2012

Despite my hopes, the weather remains cold and damp; better for walking than biking. It is good that I have arrived to the point of complaining about the weather rather than about side effects or other issues!

I had my regular physical this week. My doctor identified no additional health issues, and she has a very practical attitude towards prescribing tests and discussing what is advisable and what is not necessary. Since she already has my medical history, I did not have the opportunity to test my form, but I am sure that it will prove useful in the future. I had my second round of re-vaccinations, accompanied by the usual sore shoulders and some cold-like symptoms.

After making suggestions on improving the application process for long-term disability support, I received a follow-up call from the group responsible. Bureaucracy is a small place, and sure enough it was a former colleague that called. My issue with the duplicative application procedures for the private insurers and the government program (CPP-D) has been recommended in evaluations and work is underway. Approximately 25 percent of applicants fall into this situation, so it is significant enough to merit attention. I offered to provide any additional feedback as appropriate.

I have been working on a longer reflections piece about 'letting go and acceptance' at multiple levels: professional, personal and medical. While the broad outlines are clear in my mind – I have had more than enough time to reflect – the challenge is expressing my thoughts in a clear, readable fashion, without dumbing it down to an oversimplified list. I am getting there.

We watched several movies this week. First, *Payback*, the documentary version of Margaret Atwood's book of the same name, directed by Jennifer Baichwal. It is a hard book to turn into a film, and my recommendation would be to read the book rather than see the film. However, there are some wonderful sequences, particularly one of tomato harvesting in particular, which captures the pace and intensity of the work, and the end (not really a spoiler) when the interviewees seamlessly read passages from Atwood's book.

I also started watching *Veep*, a satire on American politics, which while it may be overly cynical, rings all too true. The writer, Armando Iannucci of *In the Loop* fame, is incredibly sharp.

The Skin I Live In, the latest film by Pedro Almodovar, has all his trademarks: confused identities, hope, anxiety and betrayal. However, the story about a mad plastic surgeon/scientist and his creation drags on, even by Almodovar standards, and is more off the wall than usual. It is beautifully filmed, and has elements of almost an elegant and sophisticated horror film.

In a much lighter vein, I saw *Music of the Heart*, a feel-good film about a teacher and the violin program she starts in Harlem in the 90s. It was a nice counterpoint to the worrying messages of the other films.

No special plans for the coming week. The weather is supposed to be better, so I will start biking again. I will also get my MRI to see if there has been any change in the previous damage to my central nervous system. My old symptoms of headaches and vision blurring have not returned, so hopefully the MRI will confirm that all is well.

WEEK 38 – UNEVENTFUL = GOOD

May 6, 2012

Another uneventful week, which is good. It was a bit too wet for biking, but I went for some good walks. While I can and do drive, I prefer to walk when I have the choice, and seem to be averaging about 2 hours a day.

I had my MRI, the usual charming jack hammer, and will get the results at my next clinic visit on May 14. It is funny that even though, as I noted earlier, I do not expect any alarming news, lying in the 'tube' for 45 minutes is a sober reminder of what I have been through and does bring back some worries. Hopefully, I will get confirmation at my next clinic visit that my condition remains stable or, even better, that there has been some improvement. We shall see.

I am also looking forward to sharing my Prezi and related slides with my hematologist, to get his feedback and see how else he wants to challenge me. My other 'think pieces' are either done 'What we call ourselves' on cancer terminology, will be posted this week or in good shape, 'Letting go and accepting.' In addition, I now have an ISBN for my forthcoming book and plan to complete it around the time of my one year anniversary this August. Now I just have to do it!

I am still reading *Among the Believers*, and have just finished the section on Pakistan. Reading Naipaul's book 30 years after I first read it, I am disappointed to find that some of the same issues still exist, when so many other parts of the world have shown real progress. One of his milder quotations:

> *The Islamic ideal was the theme of a 1951 book, Pakistan as an Islamic State, which he (Nusrat) had brought as a gift for me. It would help me to understand Pakistan, he said. And the book showed me that thirty years before, the Islamic ideal had been as vague, as much a statement of impracticable intent and muddled history (with interim worldly corruption), as it was now. The Islamic state, I read, was like a high-flying kite, invisible in the mist. 'I cannot see it, but something is tugging.'*

April was a month of high readership on my blog, perhaps because my posting frequency increased slightly. Here are the five most popular posts from April:

1. Life, Interrupted: A Young Cancer Patient Faces Infertility

2. Lessons

3. Is The United States' High Spending For Cancer Care Really Worth It?

4. Healthcare, No, a Universal Cancer Vaccine Was Not Just Developed, and Life and death battle with OHIP

5. Dualities

I will be travelling and largely disconnected from the electronic world next week – good quiet time – so I will not be able to respond to comments or 'Contact Me' messages. I have scheduled a number of articles to post automatically while I am gone; we will see how that works. I will be back to my usual schedule the following week.

Chapter 14

The Home Stretch

Month 9 +

Life is getting better and better. My energy level is relatively high, and I am able to travel. I am coming to terms with my 'new normal,' and realizing that I have been one of the lucky ones.

WEEK 39 – CROSSING THE COUNTRY

May 13, 2012

I took the train across Canada with my son this week. The trip was a marvelous reminder of just how large, rich and varied our country is, and also made for a great Internet-free week to connect and be together. One simply does not get the same appreciation in an airplane.

While some parts of the trip are long (Northern Ontario, the Prairies), one lives the open space, time and distance in a very immediate way. We had some great wildlife sightings (mountain sheep, bears, eagles, beavers, ospreys, elk etc.), another reminder of the richness and diversity of our landscapes.

I also have renewed respect for the generation that surveyed the route and built the railway, without any of our modern tools and technology. I can only imagine how many false turns and detours were taken in the initial surveys to find the best winding route between the lakes of Northern Ontario and through the Rockies, not to mention the risks and challenges of construction.

The train cars themselves are antique, having been built in 1954 with a still contemporary, almost futuristic, stainless steel or aluminum look (most of the passengers appeared to have been 'built' earlier!). The interior seems to have some art-deco influences, as well as reminders of the technology of the day (anyone remember old-style toggle switches?).

I was also reminded of just how dependent our economy is on natural resources. The number of freight trains we passed (or more accurately, passed us, as freight have priority over people), most between 150-200 cars long, was striking; they carried potash, oil, lumber, grains, oilseeds and more. Equally striking was the sheer number of imports from Asia, containers of which were double stacked on the same long trains. A more dramatic way to capture Canadian trading patterns than through dry trade statistics.

Our time off the train in the Rockies, during which we went walking and biking, showed me just how well I am doing – not badly, considering that I had to keep up with my 20-year-old son. There was much more up and down than I am used to, and more uneven terrain, but apart from one steep lookout trail (frequented by mountain goats), I was able to maintain a reasonable pace. I am certainly not at my pre-transplant level, but quite good given all that my body has gone through over the past 10 months.

One of the joys of a lengthy train ride is the reading time. I finished *Among the Believers* (still a good re-read and relevant after all these years) and I went through most of the essays in Christopher Hitchens' *Arguably*. While some of his essays are stronger than others, it is amazing how prolific and consistently good he was. Some of my favourite essays were those on Mark Twain ('American Radical'), animal 'rights' ('Political Animals'), religion and the military ('In Praise of Foxhole Atheists'), replacing the 10 commandments ('The New Commandments'), water boarding ('Believe Me, It's Torture'), Iran ('Long Live Democratic Seismology,' 'The Persian Version'), and Isabel Allende ('Chile Redux'). A great collection to dip in and out of.

This was a wonderful way to spend a week with my son – not from a 'bucket list' perspective (I hate that term) but rather as an opportunity to be together and share.

It was also a good way to wait for my MRI results, which I get tomorrow at the clinic. It is hard to believe that I managed two months between visits, and hopefully everything will continue on track. Less is more in my case.

Week 40 – All Well, Some Cognitive Testing

May 20, 2012

The week started off with a good clinic visit. The new routine seems to be that the nurse, then the hematologist, bound in, take a quick look at me, ask a few questions, and remark that I look well. This is much better than the alternative, and I find it kind of funny that despite all the fancy equipment and tests available, a basic 'look over' says all.

Some specific points:

- My MRI was good and showed no changes. I asked for more detail about whether or not the damage to my leptomeninges had diminished or remained stable, and the hematologist replied that the report simply said that there were no signs of lymphoma. However, he added that the presence or absence of symptoms is a better indicator than an MRI, as the situation can change quickly. In other words, I should not count on the MRI, but getting a clear result is still a good sign.

- A radiologist friend of mine explained the MRI result in more detail. In essence, there has been a slight decrease in the damage to my leptomeninges. He explained that as with any trauma, the healing process is slow; still, it does appear to be taking place. Good news.

- There are no plans to change my Prednisone dose (currently alternating between 5 and 10 g per day), which will provide me with stability over the summer (at least until my SCT 'birthday' in August), seeing as side effects have not been an issue at this low a dose.

- As I noted in a previous entry, the iron level in my liver is higher than normal (reflects my large number of blood transfusions). It is unlikely that they will 'bleed' me to reduce the level, since my overall haemoglobin level is not high enough and there are no major issues with the iron level itself remaining high.

- I asked about sun exposure, noting that I have been careful with SPF clothing and sunscreen, and whether I should err on the side of prudence or paranoia. The hematologist replied that it is 'Never good to be paranoid,' but cautioned that I should be careful.

- I have also been cleared for further travel, and my next clinic appointment is scheduled before a possible trip this summer.

- There was no need for blood work, because I provided the hematologist with my results from the physical I had a month ago.

I showed the hematologist the draft of my Prezi. His interest was in how the technology works, how he could use Prezi to liven up his presentations (the flexible navigation between 'slides' can make presentations more interactive), and how steep the learning curve is (he has a presentation coming up in a few weeks). He noted that my Prezi will likely be of interest to support groups more than to doctors, since some of my slides might be helpful for people who are starting their own 'journey.'

I underwent a cognitive thinking test, part of a study on the medium-term effects of stem-cell transplants (I guess I am at that stage now!). The tasks ranged from simple reflex tests (pressing the space bar when one sees a shape) to more challenging tests that require 'system 2' thinking, to invoke Kahneman's terminology.

Some examples: remembering 15 words or 15 shapes; the Stroop Test (correlating shape and colour); and a sequence-remembering test. I am curious to see my results, which I should get shortly.

In a discussion with the pre-med student conducting the test, I mentioned my own perception, which is that I am not as 'sharp' as before – particularly with respect to short-term memory. She noted that people who have been in jobs that require concentration, analysis and thinking often have this perception, as they notice any difference in their cognitive capacity, even if formal testing shows the change to be very small. We live our own subjective reality. I certainly noticed a difference in my cognitive abilities when I returned to work in 2010 after my first stem-cell transplant, and had to find ways to compensate for it.

While I seem to be able to function quite well now, the test illustrated some of my ongoing vulnerabilities. The intense concentration required to perform the tests left me somewhat exhausted; while I think I did well on the simpler tasks, the more complex tests of working memory were another matter. It is what it is.

One last bit of medical news. I received my file of hospital notes and checklists (yes, they use checklists in cancer care – Atul Gawande would be proud!), a two-inch stack of paper, from my 2009 treatment. There is a lot that I do not need to keep – these are the medical equivalents of log books and notes – but it is somewhat reassuring to see the thoroughness of the methodology and documentation.

We watched *The Weight of the Nation* on HBO this week. The documentary and messages were a bit ponderous and heavy (puns intended), but it is hard to dispute the existence of an obesity epidemic (and this is not just an U.S. issue). The website for the movie has good tools for things that people can do on an individual level.

We also watched *Les neiges du Kilimandjaro* (*The Snows of Kilimanjaro*), a French film about a union leader who, along with other workers, loses his job due to downsizing. He is given money for a wedding anniversary trip to Kilimanjaro, but is robbed by a co-worker. The theft forces him to confront and question some of his past decisions, as well as whether he still has obligations to his co-worker even after the co-worker is charged. The movie was a bit slow, and the end was too 'Hollywood' for my liking.

I have been reading *Disgrace*, by South African writer J.M. Coetzee, the 1999 Booker Prize winner. The main character, a disgraced professor, is thoroughly *antipathique* at first (the book recalls Bissoondath's *The Soul of All Great Designs* in that respect), but starts to become a more sympathetic character during his hearing on harassment charges, as he, while fully admitting his guilt, refuses to play along. Then a different but parallel disgrace happens to his daughter, which weighs down on him, and frames an end to a meaningful life. Bleak, thoughtful, very well written, and keeps one's interest.

I have been taking advantage of the good weather to go biking every day. No real improvement in my time, but I am certainly enjoying myself.

WEEK 41 – NICE AND NORMAL

May 27, 2012

This has just been a nice and normal week: wonderful spring weather, lots of walks and bike rides, and work on my blog and other projects. The only disadvantage of the nice weather is that, in addition to wearing sunscreen and SPF clothing, I need to avoid the peak hours of sun. A small price to pay.

I made it to another milestone. Our daughter turned 18 and has her formal high school graduation next month. To think that at this time last year, I was not sure I would make it (and likely would not, or only barely, have made it had I not opted for the stem cell transplant). From a new-born to a young woman full of promise and potential – my, how the time flies, as the cliché goes. But the time is rich in shared memories lived together.

For those of you who have not seen it, my Cancerwise piece, 'What we call ourselves: Finding the right term for cancer' is on my blog. From the comments on Cancerwise, the most popular term is 'fighter' or its variants. I would have expected this to be more evenly balanced with survivor or other terms. This may reflect that 'fighters' are more disposed to comment than others (MD Anderson Cancer Centre website itself tends to feature the word 'survivor'), or how embedded the fighting metaphor is. I was pleased by the number and tenor of comments that my article generated on the MD Anderson Facebook page (the number of comments was 'huge,' according to my editor at Cancerwise). A fun topic to reflect on and write about.

My wife and I saw the Van Gogh exhibition at the National Gallery. It was a nice, small exhibition, focussing on Van Gogh's love of nature and how his art developed, with complementary displays of photographs and prints that may have influenced him, as well as Japanese prints which definitely did (these were lovely). The exhibit included some wonderful pieces and some great blow-ups of his paintings, which show his technique and brushwork. I am not sure where the exhibition is going after Ottawa, but it is a good one to catch.

I have been reading Gilles Paquet's *Deep Cultural Diversity: A Governance Challenge* (back to non-fiction). At first blush, it paints an overly bleak picture and insufficiently nuanced analysis of highly diverse societies. I will comment a bit more next week when I have finished it – reading this book is part of broadening my perspective and understanding.

Our neighbourhood garage sale took place yesterday (it is a big one and attracts a wide and varied range of people), so we spent a few hours clearing out some of the stuff we have accumulated over the years. The trick is to price things to move, and we shared our spot with friends to generate more traffic and interest. Part of the proceeds go to our local food bank, a reminder of those less fortunate.

The only special event I have planned for next week is a hematology symposium at the Ottawa Hospital, which will give me an opportunity to get an update on developments in treatment for lymphoma and other blood diseases – and see if my hematologist managed to prepare a Prezi (in the end, he did not)!

WEEK 42 – 10 WEEKS TO GO – AND A HEMATOLOGY SYMPOSIUM

June 3, 2012

I have made it to the point where I can start a countdown to the one year mark. Getting there.

As I said I would in my last post, I went to the *Celebrating 60 Years of Hematology in Ottawa* this week. The growth of the Hematology program, while impressive, is a depressing reminder of how much blood cancer rates have increased over the last 60 years.

The presentations provided some good overviews on research and treatment, with a focus on the following points:

- Use of new drugs: e.g., Brentuximab for anaplastic large cell lymphoma (ALCL) and Hodgkin lymphoma (approved in US, approval in Canada pending); trials of Everolimus for breast cancer, gastric cancer, hepatocellular carcinoma and lymphoma; and trials of Bendamustine-R as a lower-side-effect treatment for follicular non-Hodgkin lymphoma (NHL).

- New ways to diagnose, including greater use of PET scans in treatment planning;

- New ways to deliver drugs (e.g., better targeting, see A New Class of Cancer Drugs May Be Less Toxic); and,

- New understanding of cell mechanisms and cancer.

I chatted with one of my hematologists, who mentioned that when he indicated his wish to specialize in blood and marrow transplants some 20 years, his advisers said it was a dead-end. They warned him that leukemia and lymphoma would soon be cured by pills, and there would be nothing left to research. Smiling, and not having lost his enthusiasm, he said, 'we are still learning,' but that he hopes that 10-15 years from now, we could look back at transplants and think of them as a 'barbaric' treatment.

He also recommended the book How Doctors Think, noting, that as outlined in *Thinking, Fast and Slow*, doctors are vulnerable to patterns of thinking, and that mistakes leave such a strong impression that in their commitment not to repeat them, they can sometimes miss important details. Another book for my reading list.

The symposium reminded me of a class reunion, in that I got to see most of the members of my medical team – the doctors, nurses, pharmacists and others who have cared for me during the past few years. A number of them remarked on how gratifying it is to see people like me come back to the hospital for a reason other than treatment, and looking well (this is gratifying on my end, too!). A reminder of how much time has passed: one of the pharmacists who helped me through the transplant process is expecting her first child, due the same date as my transplant in August. From life to life.

I finished reading *Deep Cultural Diversity: A Governance Challenge*. I found it frustrating. Parts approach a rant in substance and tone. Paquet uses phrases like 'fundamentalism of entitlements,' 'idolatry of rights' and 'despotism of political correctness.' He also makes assertions about the Canadian Charter of Rights and Freedoms with minimal discussion of the actual jurisprudence involved, discusses the need for moral codes without much detail on the content of these codes, etc.

Part of his conclusion, however, is nuanced:

> *The more timid and gradualist Canadian way is not necessarily an inferior strategy [compared to Australia], since it fits the Canadian ethos. However, it entails a complex and somewhat erratic process of social learning, where progress comes most of the time by fits and starts, locally, and by trial and error, rather than as a result of broadly debated revolutionary transformation. This often means that social learning is fractured and slower…*

> *However frustrating and ineffective the Canadian way may appear by radical standards, it is not only efficient … but … may even constitute a truly attractive strategy for polyethnic, multicultural, and plural societies in general …*

Or maybe with my chemo brain, I have less ability to appreciate complex academic wording and reasoning!

I watched the schlock that is *X-Men 2* with my daughter. Good escapism, even if the plot, character development and so on are shallow, to put it charitably.

I also watched another light film, by Lebanese director Nadine Labaki (she also directed *Caramel*), which approaches black comedy in parts. *Where Do We Go Now?* is about the quirky efforts by women in an isolated village of Christians and Muslims to keep the peace. The comedy is heavy-handed at times, some of the plot twists and turns defy credibility, and yet the film has a warm humanity and charm that I enjoyed, not to mention a fun kitchen musical number.

The stats on my blog have been good this month. Interestingly, more new people seem to be discovering the blog, given the number of hits on About, Healthcare, Lessons, Faith and Dualities (What we call ourselves hasn't made it yet. Apart from these and the Home page, the top posts of interest were:

1. Progress Report on a Decluttering Project
2. Life, Interrupted by Suleika Jaouad (**individual posts taken together**)
3. Gretchen Reynolds on 'The First 20 Minutes'
4. Jenni Murray: Robin Gibb didn't lose any 'battle'
5. The Bilingual Brain Is Sharper and More Focused, Study Says

Next week will be more of the usual, although I am going to the local Lymphoma Support Group, largely to see if my experience can be helpful to people earlier on in the process.

This day of the Diamond Jubilee is a good opportunity to reflect back on how the world and our society have changed over the past 60 years – largely for the better, I think – and what has remained constant: the importance of family and friends.

Week 43 – My Support Group + Update on Stem Cell Transplants

June 10, 2012

As planned, I went to my local lymphoma support group for the first time this week. The first part, a 'sharing and caring circle,' starts off fairly conventionally: 'my name is _____, and I was diagnosed with _____.'

As always, the richness is in the individual stories – some easier, some harder – and the personalities. I could recognize the former executives in the room by the way they processed information and reacted to it. The group consisted of 20 or so people, most a bit older than me, as I think I was the second youngest in the room (but given the effects of treatment, our physical age may be more than our chronological age).

I had the dubious distinction of being the only to have had both auto and allo stem cell transplants (not a 'prize' one wishes for), but had a good discussion with someone who had to make a similar decision as I did about a year ago, about whether to have an allo SCT (he decided to go ahead, for similar reasons: 'reset' and take the chance on life). There was also a good informal exchange on issues as they came up. The discussion felt less artificial and awkward than I expected, so I will continue to attend once the group starts up again in the fall. One layer of my identity is my lymphoma, and this is a good regular reminder of what to be thankful for, as well an opportunity to help others with their journey.

Update on stem cell transplants

One my hospital's hematologists gave a presentation on current and future stem cell transplant developments to the group (the following may be too much medical info for some). After a brief history, starting with the post-Hiroshima link between radiation and cancers, he noted that early transplant results in the 60s were poor, largely due to lack of knowledge about blood typing, which resulted in bad matches. In the 70s, the major development was the establishment of an international transplant registry, which collected and shared data, providing a knowledge base to inform treatment. There were relatively few transplant centres in the 1980s, but by then studies had shown that the principle of transplanting bone marrow was sound.

Some of the major developments that started to improve success rates were more accurate blood typing (Human leukocyte antigen or HLA) and better antibiotics to manage complications.

The previous distinction between auto SCTs (used when the underlying problem is not bone-marrow related), made viable by the development of drugs such as Neupogen, and allo STCs (used when there is an issue with a patient's bone marrow) still largely applies but, as my case demonstrates, is not iron-clad.

Over the past 30 years, the main barriers to success have not changed:

- Death related to the original disease (i.e., dying from the original cancer, which happens to about 50% of patients);

- Side effects of intensive chemo and radiation, ranging from short to longer-term (causes death in about 20% of patients); and,

- Side effects from the new immune system, including GvHD and infection (the risk is dramatically lower after one year).

However, the improvements that have been made are significant:

- Accurate blood typing thanks to improved technology: a match is really a match;

- Better handling of GvHD because of huge advances in drugs (e.g., immunosuppressants);

- Development of peripheral blood cell collection (transfusion-type process), which makes for a quicker recovery than collection from the bone marrow (quicker recovery means lower risk of infections). The 'price' to pay for use of peripheral blood cell collection (there always is a trade-off) is greater risk of GvHD). In general, for more aggressive cancers, the preference is for quicker recovery and increased new immunity; for less aggressive cancers, bone marrow cells may be used to reduce the risk of GvHD;

- The development of Neupogen, the drug used to stimulate white blood cell production and reduce the duration of low immunity and vulnerability;

- New anti-fungal drugs to reduce risks without 'wrecking' kidneys; and,

- And a few simple changes and developments: use of Zofran for nausea; CMV (Cytomegalovirus) monitoring to prevent pneumonia now replaced by PCR (Polymerase chain reaction) testing; with a shorter time required for Acyclovir (anti-viral drug).

Some other changes that the hematologist highlighted:

- The pendulum keeps swinging between harsh and less harsh conditioning regimes, and is currently swinging back to the full myeloblative regime (harsh) that I had. High radiation, in particular, keeps one's old immune system at bay for about six months, providing enough time for the new system to get strong.

- In general, the tendency is to do transplants sooner rather than later, as the timing affects the success rate. However, complementary treatments and drugs can postpone the need for transplant.

- The former hard rules about age limits for transplants have shifted to looking at individual patient health (physiological age, not chronological – is the patient strong enough?); this is partly due to the an aging population and higher treatment expectations.

- The medical community has a greater understanding of the spectrum and variants of cancers, resulting in more complex treatments.

The overall risk of death from treatment decreased from 40 to 20 percent between 1995-2004, due to better patient selection, better drugs, better supporting care and better managing of complications. The overall survival rates – including non-treatment – have increased from 12 to 15 percent over this period. The progress is incremental, but in the right direction.

Finally, the hematologist mentioned some ongoing challenges and areas for improvement:

- Providing care for 'survivors' as longer-term effects of treatment and transplant emerge;

- Improving cost and other efficiencies in providing care; and,

- Analyzing clinical trials to adjust approach to treatments and transplants.

Beyond all the science – and it is a mix of rocket science, skill and art – I still feel a sense of awe, wonder and gratitude at being able to benefit from these developments, and at being given a second chance and a new life.

We went to a concert by Parissa, the leading Iranian classical singer. A wonderful, powerful voice with real presence, emotion and spirituality. Her site is here for those interested.

We watched the French film *Intouchables* (*The Untouchables*), based on a true story about the relationship between a very rich paraplegic, Philippe, and his caregiver, Driss, who comes from the *banlieu* (different than The Help, a similar dynamic). A comedy, it got panned on this side of the Atlantic for being hopelessly out-of-date and racist in its depiction of white/black relations, but was the top hit in France. I went in with mixed expectations but was pleasantly surprised as I watched the humanity and closeness of the relationship between Philippe and Driss develop and strengthen. There were some funny moments (the opera scene is to die for), and it was very well-acted. Worth seeing.

Otherwise, I continue on the overall recovery track, am active, engaged and generally enjoying life. I had another nice bike ride this morning; the weather was perfect and there was no wind, so my time improved.

Nine weeks to go before my anniversary!

WEEK 44 – A GOOD WEEK

June 17, 2012

This has been a great Father's Day weekend. My daughter had her high school graduation, and my son was home as well, so we were all able to celebrate together. Watching and helping one's kids grow and develop is the best gift a father could get.

While these kinds of occasions always bring out the sentimental side in me, I am more sensitive to them now. Not only are these milestones meaningful in themselves, but so is my being around to witness them. As a result, the emotions that wash over me are all that more intense. She made it, I made it; we all made it together.

I attended a number of fun events this week as well. First, a nice neighbourhood gathering to bid farewell to some long-time residents of our street who are downsizing; then, a new citizen recognition event hosted by our Member of Parliament (who couldn't actually be there due to all-night voting at the House of Commons – his wife hosted). My wife and I saw the Van Gogh exhibit again with my family. There were fewer people there this time, so we were able to appreciate the art even more.

To my surprise, I received a Queen Elizabeth II Diamond Jubilee Medal for my contributions to government service. It was particularly rewarding since I was nominated and selected, along with a number of my colleagues, by my peers. I am well enough to deal with the occasional 'crowd scene,' so I was able to attend the awards ceremony and receive the medal in person. It was good to see and reconnect with my former colleagues and catch up on their news. They were pleased to see me looking relatively well. My standard reply to the question of how I am doing was to answer, with a smile, 'I'm standing and I'm here' – that says it all. Funny how the simple word 'here' can have both factual meaning and existential significance! In sum, the award was one of those smaller things in life that nevertheless make one feel good (and in keeping with the family 'tradition' – my Father received a Silver Jubilee medal for his work in the arts).

I have also been re-discovering my creative side as I continue to work on new material for my lymphoma journey book (enhanced edition). Part of the process is choosing images to break up the major sections, which means looking through old pictures from when I was into photography, selecting and scanning them, and seeing how they fit in with the narrative (I would rather feature beautiful photos than pictures of me in the hospital 'uniform'). The written content is largely ready, apart from a few articles I have to finish for both Cancerwise and the book itself, and, of course, the text will be subject to editing and some 'trusted reader' criticism.

I am working on turning my Prezi into a video, with a narrated script, which is another creative outlet.

There are both risks and benefits involved in the fact that technology – Prezi, iBooks – grants me creative autonomy and allows me to 'do my own thing.' The benefit is that I do not have to worry about reporting relationships and having to conform to the demands of superiors or getting permission to do what I want. The risk is that the final product might be too narcissistic or not critiqued enough to be suitable for public distribution. You can't have everything, and what matters most is that I am having fun.

I finally read the Charles Taylor classic *Multiculturalism and the 'Politics of Recognition'*. Taylor walks the fine line between universalism and relativism, making for a good, nuanced discussion of the issues. A quotation:

> *There must be something midway between the inauthentic and homogenizing demand for recognition of equal worth, on the one hand, and the self-immurement within ethnocentric standards, on the other. There are other cultures, and we have to live together more and more, both on a world scale and commingled in each individual society.*

I have been fighting off a bit of a sore throat this week – this may be a result of too much cycling early in the morning and the 'crowd' events – but am otherwise fine.

Next week I have a clinic visit. I have nothing major to complain about, so I assume that the next appointment will be at my one-year mark in August. Eight weeks to go!

Happy Father's Day to all you fathers out there, and thanks, as always, to the partners who make it all possible.

WEEK 45 – CLINIC VISIT, COGNITIVE TESTING RESULTS

June 24, 2012

Everything was fine at the clinic. This time, I met with the clinical physician, rather than one of the hematologists, which allowed for a more thorough review of the minor issues:

- While my Hep B vaccine is working after two shots, I still need to get a third shot this week as part of the new protocol.

- The slight swelling of my feet is nothing to worry about. It may be caused by the thinning of my blood due to low albumen (the things I learn!), a problem that may diminish over time. Similarly, no concerns about the neuropathy (numbness) in my feet, which may or may not diminish.

- With respect to my sore throat, she provided some antibiotics should it not improve within the next few days (fortunately, it did).

- In response to my question about returning to work after the one-year mark, the clinical physician said that we will review the possibility at that next milestone, once the insurance company formally asks for an update on my condition. She cautioned that I should not just send in the form on my own, but rather request an appointment to discuss it with the medical team, as they treat these reviews seriously for transplant cases.

- I am up to date on most of my tests and scans, but will schedule another in about a month. I told her that I am not worried about my lungs since I have no trouble walking, biking and climbing stairs two at a time.

- In addition, I am still cleared for my upcoming trip, unless my blood work holds any surprises (unlikely).

Finally, when I mentioned that I expect to make it to the one-year mark, the clinical physician was incredibly categoric about there being no doubt of that. While the countdown continues, I can also start looking a bit beyond!

As a result, I had my third series of re-vaccinations and, as usual, the only side effect was a couple of sore shoulders. One more round in a month, and then another in six months or so.

I finally got the results of the cognitive testing I participated in over a month ago. In short, my scores (compared to healthy people of my age group) are as follows:

Test	Score
Verbal Memory	Average
Visual Memory	High Average
Processing Speed	Average
Executive Functioning	Average
Reaction Time	Low Average
Working Memory	Average

Without a 'before' picture, I cannot know what is attributable to the cumulative effects of treatment and what is the same as my 'normal' functioning before treatment. Vanity would have me attribute most of this to treatment!

In all seriousness, however, while my executive position required above-average cognitive thinking, I do not need a test to tell me that I am no longer performing at the same level; even after my first transplant, I had to find ways to compensate for deterioration. Still, in the broader scheme of things, a small price to pay, and I have not noticed any impairment to my deeper and more strategic thinking.

Some of the findings from the Ottawa Hospital data on close to 300 patients:

- About 20 percent report experiencing some cognitive symptoms;

- An individual's perception of their cognitive ability appears to be influenced by their mood, their medications, their treatment, and the lymphoma itself (comment: this means everything and nothing);

- 70 percent reported a decrease in their quality of life, due to factors such as financial stress and pain. The variable that correlated most strongly with a decrease in quality of life appeared to be fatigue; and,

- 12 percent reported an increase in their quality of life, due to factors such as strong family relationships, increased spirituality, change in attitude, and more time to pursue leisure activities.

My sense – and I forget the specific questions on the questionnaire – is that it would not be contradictory for one to report both a decrease and increase in quality of life, as some aspects can worsen while others improve. However, the overall findings correlate with my own experience a fair amount.

I have been having fun reading Bill Maher's *The New New Rules*, a Father's Day gift from my son. I must admit that it plays to my ideological tendencies, and have selected a few quotations to give you the flavour:

New Rule – Killer App: *Since the economy won't come back until we start buying stuff, and the only stuff Americans buy is anything from Apple and guns, Apple has to make a gun. Call it the iKillyou. Although, if you want to get it to NRA members, you probably can't sell it at the genius bar.*

New Rule – False Profit: *Not everything in America has to make a profit. If conservatives get to call universal health care "socialized medicine," I get to call private, for-profit health care "soulless vampire bastards making money off human pain." Now I know what you're thinking: "But Bill, the profit motive is what sustains capitalism." Yes, and our sex drive is what sustains the human species, but we don't try to f*** everything.*

We watched *A Woman, A Gun and a Noodle Shop*. The film is a Chinese remake of the Cohen Brothers' *Blood Simple*, the story of a shop owner's revenge on his wife and her lover. Quite well done, and beautifully filmed – some of the landscape scenes are breathtakingly beautiful.

Due to the heat wave this week and my efforts to get over my sore throat/cold, I refrained from biking, but I did go for some lovely early morning and late evening walks.

We will be travelling over the next few weeks , but I have scheduled a number of posts during that period and will do short weekly updates.

Seven weeks to go!

WEEK 46 – RENAISSANCE

July 1, 2012

I started writing this post on the train between Florence and Milan, watching the Italian countryside, and am finishing it from our apartment overlooking Paris.

My wife and I spent a wonderful few days in Florence, a city that I have not visited for some 35 years (my age is showing). Unlike many places, which have changed for the worse, Florence is timeless, and remains rich in history and unmatched in the beauty and innovation of its art and architecture. While my eyes may not view Florence with the freshness of my first trip to Europe, the city has not lost its capacity to inspire wonder and awe. I am always particularly amazed by how transformative the Renaissance was and the impact it continues to have on the world today. A wonderful, stimulating break, and one that made my wife and I realize just how much stress we have been under in the past year. The change of place helped us unwind and restart.

Fortunately, my body acclimatized well to the new environments (my 'new normal' always causes some worry when I am away). While the plane flights brought my cold back, the dry heat of Florence (33° C) made it go away again. My stomach allowed me to enjoy the food (why does one eat so much better in Europe, even in modest restaurants, than in Canada?). I also took my own real-world : climbing the Duomo (close to 500 steps) and the path to San Miniato al Monte. While there was huffing, puffing and increased heart rate involved, I would give myself a pass (although my lack of confidence in my balance led me to hold on to railings more than usual!). I am not doing too badly, after all.

I read John Coates' *The Hour Between Dog and Wolf*, another in a series of books that I have been reading on behavioral economics. Coates has an interesting perspective, having been both a trader and a researcher. Like much of the other work in this field, (e.g., Kahneman's *Thinking, Fast and Slow*) *The Hour Between Dog and Wolf* largely demolishes the classical economic idea of rational decision-making, as it maps out the links between our conscious and unconscious systems. Quote:

> *Today Platonic dualism [the mind-body divide] … is widely disputed within philosophy and mostly ignored in neuroscience. But there is one unlikely place where a vision of the rational mind as pure as anything contemplated by Plato or Descartes still lingers – and that is in economics.*

> *Many economists … assume our behavior is volitional – in other words, we choose our course of behavior after thinking it through – and guided by a rational mind. According to this school of thought, we are walking computers who can calculate the rewards of each course of action open to us at any given moment, and weigh these rewards by the probability of their occurrence…*

Unearthly ideals, we have learned at great cost, too easily lead to social and political disasters. Equally, otherworldly ideals of economic rationality can too easily lead to the sign of a marketplace fatally prone to financial crises.

His policy recommendations for trading desks largely revolve around increasing diversity (dilute testosterone by including more women and older traders), moving from short- to longer-term compensation, and acknowledging and accounting for the irrationality involved in decision-making. All in all, a good read for those interested in decision-making in any sphere, not only the financial markets.

Here is my usual monthly round-up of blog stats. The top articles of interest, apart from the weekly updates and some of the 'reflection' pages, include:

1. In one man's fight against cancer, safety trumps hope

2. Life, Interrupted by Suleika Jaouad

3. A New Class of Cancer Drugs May be Less Toxic

4. 20 Ways to Relieve Stress

5. Research Shows that the Smarter People Are, the More Susceptible They Are to Cognitive Bias

Happy Canada Day to my Canadian readers.

Six weeks to go!

Week 47 – Paris

July 8, 2012

It has been wonderful to be back in Paris seeing some friends, going for the usual beautiful walks, discovering some new cafes (and rediscovering some old) and enjoying the comfort of familiar surroundings (one of the asides in the Coates book on stress is that a familiar location with people one knows is less stressful than a new location).

We saw some good exhibits at the Parisian museums. At the Beaubourg, we visited a retrospective on the work of German artist Gerhard Richter. He exploits an incredibly wide range of styles, from landscape to portrait to abstract, and his works vary from monochrome to bursting with colour. My favourites were his large abstract pieces, which demonstrate his amazing sense and use of colour.

We saw two very different shows at the Grand Palais. The subject of the first was how our portrayal of animals has changed over time. The second was a a collection of portraits by Helmut Newton, the well-known fashion photographer. Both exhibits were equally interesting in their own ways; I found Newton's portraits particularly impressive.

One of the funny things was that the apartment we stayed in was old and had a very uneven floor, which meant that I really felt the neuropathy in my feet and had to pay attention so as not to lose balance.

Unfortunately, as the week went on, my cough came back. I eventually saw a doctor and now have meds to reduce the cough and the inflammation in my throat. I had a good experience with the French healthcare system: no wait time, a thorough exam, and a charge of only about $30. The cough is nothing serious, but has cramped the last few days of our trip. I should have worn face masks on the various planes and buses, given how much the bacteria circulates. My 'new normal.'

I took advantage of the train ride to Southern France to read Nazanin Afshin-Jan's book, co-written with Susan McClelland, *The Tale of Two Nazanins* (disclosure: I know her professionally). The book is about how Afshin-Jan used her celebrity to save the life of another Nazanin in Iran who, in self-defense, killed a man who attacked her. A combination of class, ethnic, and religious biases meant that the Iranian Nazanin had little chance of acquittal. A sharp contrast to the social milieu of the main family depicted in the Iranian film *A Separation*.

While I understand the literary rationale behind presenting these tales as two parallel stories, highlighting the contrast between the gloss of the Canadian Nazanin and the grittiness of the Iranian Nazanin, the book didn't completely hold together for me until the Canadian side, too, became gritty – when the campaign to free the Iranian Nazanin began. The story of how people were mobilized to help her made the book more compelling.

There were some interesting asides in the book. Afshin-Jan complains about the small number of Iranians who attend her public events during the campaign, without perhaps a full appreciation of the challenges that many Iranians have, given ongoing family and other relationships in Iran (Nazanin's family would appear to have none). Her reaction to criticism that she used the campaign to increase her own profile was perhaps overly defensive – all celebrities do this to some extent, and as long as the cause is sound, there is no shame in such synergy. Her summary of Iranian history skips too quickly from the Arab conquest of Iran in the mid 7th century to the Islamic Revolution of 1979. As a result, she left out key periods like the Safavid Empire (1501-1722), which not only led to an Iranian Renaissance, best exemplified by the art and architecture of Isfahan and the development of Shia Islam, but also spawned a period of relative openness for other religions and groups, many of whom were welcomed for their craftsmanship and talent as artisans.

I was also surprised to find so little discussion, in a book about human rights, of the overall human rights framework in Iran: no mention of the 2009 elections and repressed Green Revolution, and a rather naive suggestion for the creation of a United People of Iran and United People project, which, while useful in highlighting the limits of the UN and international systems, is unlikely to be as effective as individual targeted campaigns can be (as Nazanin showed through her own successful campaign).

Other relatively recent books on Iranian society and the prison and judicial systems there include Marina Nemat's *Prisoner of Tehran*, Maziar Bahari's *Then They Came for Me*, and Haleh Esfandiari's *My Prison My Home*. Each of these provides a deeper understanding of contemporary Iran, and, with the exception of Marina's, have the common thread of outside pressure freeing someone from an Iranian prison (Nazanin's achievement was that she did the same for an unknown).

Despite my cold, I have enjoyed spending the last few days with friends here. Hopefully the flight back to Canada will not be too painful, and I can finally kick this cold and get back to my normal routine.

Five weeks to go!

WEEK 48 – ONE MONTH TO GO

July 15, 2012

This has been a good week back at home.

The flight to Ottawa was better than expected. While my (pink!) face mask attracted some curious looks, particularly from the small children on board, it had the positive side effect of slightly reducing the dryness, and hence my cough. Apart from the normal hassle of air travel these days, no problems.

As a precaution, I did have my family doctor check me out on my return. The diagnosis: just a virus, but she prescribed me some nasal spray and stronger cough syrup, which I was able to stop taking after a few days. Despite the heat, I have started biking again, which is enjoyable as always; however, I always seem to have a bit of a coughing fit afterwards, so the dryness might be bringing out some allergies.

My vacation felt like a normal one, with the pressure to get 'back to work,' as I thought of all the things I need to get done over the next few weeks to keep on track with my book.

That being said, this past week has been productive. I have been reviewing the draft and it is coming together nicely. I am getting through both the bigger – thinking about the conclusion – and smaller – copyright and acknowledgement pages, list of illustrations – tasks involved in finishing it. I am also still fussing over the title. I am not sure whether I should continue with the blog's name, 'My Lymphoma Journey,' or find a more catchy one (without being gimmicky).

On the 'administrative' side, I got my U.S. IRS Employer Identification Number, required to sell the book on Amazon and Apple. There are many little details to attend to. In addition, I have started to think about how I might generate publicity for and market the book, and have had some encouraging discussions on this topic with a few cancer centres. I understand why publishers exist, but it is easier to go the self-publishing route.

I also completed a piece, 'Working with your medical team,' for Cancerwise. I engaged with my medical team before writing it to ensure that I captured their perspective. My discussion with them was good and made the piece stronger. One member made the following comment, which places the respective roles of patient and doctor in context:

> *… I was happy to see your advice about the internet to patients. One of our physicians has a good analogy when dealing with patients who are basing medical decisions on information from the internet or family or friends. When you get on a plane for a trip you don't ever think it is appropriate to go to the cockpit and start questioning the pilot on how he flies the plane. You trust that the pilot and team know what they are doing. …*

None of us feel good when patients succumb to an illness. None of us profit from patients who don't live. I go home every night to my children and hope that I have done the best job I can do to keep my patients healthy and safe.

My wife and I watched the latest Woody Allen film, *To Rome with Love*. While it lacked the unifying theme of nostalgia and the coherence of *Midnight in Paris*, it was still a very enjoyable film. It weaves in out of four largely separate stories, all with some connection to Rome. There were a few parts that I particularly enjoyed: Roberto Benigni's role of an ordinary man (Leopoldo) thrust into celebrity, opera singing in a shower (a fun perversion of the cliché), and the interplay between Alec Baldwin (John) and Jesse Eisenberg (Jack). Baldwin is an older man watching the younger man (Eisenberg) make mistakes, and trying to give him advice. There is the familiar Allen dialogue on intellectual poseurs, but this time through the lens of Eisenberg, who plays the 'younger Woody Allen' type, falling for Ellen Page's character (Monica). Allen's version of a summertime flick!

Apart from catching up with friends next week, I hope that the last traces of this cough and cold will disappear. While there are many worse things than a summer cold, but it just doesn't feel right to have a cold when it's warm!

Four more weeks to go!

WEEK 49 – ANOTHER GOOD WEEK

July 22, 2012

Another good week. My cough is slowly going away, the weather is no longer insufferably hot, and I am back to my regular biking routine, seeing friends, and getting on with my book. Our son is here this weekend, and as always it is nice for everyone to be together.

I have revamped my blog site somewhat, organizing the 'page tabs' at the top to make my various reflection and other pieces more accessible to readers by gathering all of these in one place. I will see from the stats whether this is helpful or not. I never thought that I would need to become a 'webmaster'!

My family and I watched one of our favourite Marx Brothers films, *A Night at the Opera.* Timeless. We introduced our kids to the Marx Brothers when they were small and they still like to watch them with us. The leisurely (overly so) musical pieces are almost a necessary break from the breathtakingly rapid and witty dialogue. I joined my kids in their 'preparations' for *The Dark Knight Rises* by watching the previous two movies with them. Nolan's is a well-done reinvention of the franchise.

I read Salim Mansur's somewhat rambling *Delectable Lie: A Liberal Repudiation of Multiculturalism.* While interesting, the book has a number of weaknesses and misses a number of points:

- His characterization of individual rights brings to mind Margaret Thatcher's comment, 'there is no such thing as society,' in an overly classical-liberal sense. Groups and group identities continue to be part of reality and society.

- In contrast to his view of citizenship as exclusive, globalization means that citizenship is less exclusive and immigration less of a one-way ticket. Whatever our origins, we are more mobile, communications are instantaneous and almost free, and our identities are multi-layered.

- Mansur largely overlooks the fact that group rights are part of the history of Canada and the Constitution (e.g, First Nation treaties, English and French language rights). Many other countries have similar historical 'complexities' that form their reality.

- Canadian multiculturalism is integration- and citizenship-based, and was driven in part by the Ukrainian-Canadian community, which wanted its contribution to nation building in Western Canada – just as British and French immigration built other parts of the country – recognized. Many European countries had more of a guest-worker, 'separate community' model, without an emphasis on integration and citizenship.

- Mansur fixates on Muslim immigration and Muslim Canadians, without adequately comparing and analyzing these factors in relation to past fears of the 'other' (e.g., Irish, Ukrainian, Chinese, Japanese, Jewish, Sikh, etc.).

- Mansur's discussion of religious fundamentalism focusses almost exclusively on Islamist fundamentalism, largely overlooking the fundamentalists of other religions, apart from Sikh Canadians. A deeper, comparative analysis would be helpful; after all, from an individual rights perspective, freedom of religion includes freedom from religion, both between and within communities, and most of the integration issues mentioned for Muslims have parallels in other religious communities.

As with many issues, the question is one of balance. An exclusive focus on individual rights, without taking into account how people see themselves and overall social conditions, is likely to be less effective than one that stresses individual rights but allows for some expression of group rights. Mansur is right, however, to flag the risk of over-emphasizing group rights, which limits the potential for individuals within cultural or religious communities to participate fully in society at large. In addition, Mansur's critique of self-censorship and some of the related 'spinelessness' is on the mark.

Next week I have a regular clinic visit, a (no change expected based on my activity level), and the third injection of my Hep B vaccine. Since the end of the heat wave, it has been easier for me to be active and enjoy the outdoors. I am getting close to the one-year mark, so it will be interesting to see if there are any plans to change my meds or whether, as things are going well, we will stay the course.

I suppose it is a good sign if these weekly updates are becoming more like short book reviews than health updates!

Three weeks to go to my anniversary!

WEEK 50 – CLINIC UPDATE AND THE OLYMPICS

July 29, 2012

This was a good week, since my cough is finally gone.

I had my last clinic visit before my one-year anniversary, and I continue to do well – both in how I feel and in the eyes of my medical team.

We are starting to make some changes related to the upcoming milestone, and the transition is welcome.

Highlights:

- Prednisone (the steroid) will be phased down from alternating between 10 and 5 mg each day to alternating between 10 and 0 mg for one month. This is to 'kick' the adrenal glands into producing cortisol. I may feel crummy for three to four days until my cortisol production ramps up. After one month, the dose will decrease further, alternating between 5 and 0 mg. Of course, should the crumminess continue, they may delay phase down. As of this morning, I have experienced minimal crumminess, so I am lucky once again.

- I will be taken off Septra (which reduces the risk of pneumonia) shortly, either soon after the one-year mark or when stops.

- I will continue to take Acyclovir (which prevents shingles) indefinitely since I have a drug plan. I cannot get a shingles vaccine as it is a live vaccine, which would be too much for my immune system to handle.

- I need to start taking vitamin B12, because the process of rebuilding my bone marrow has depleted my stores. I am only being prescribed vitamins – progress!

- The clinical doctor also reviewed all the tests run on me over the last six months: CT scan, MRI, bone density test. All good. My pulmonary function test (PFT) the day after confirmed what I knew: no issues (given my walking and biking) and even a slight improvement.

- My blood counts from last month were all good and stable. I remain slightly anemic, which is natural post-transplant. My creatinine (kidney stress indicator) level was in the normal range, which is rare and good for me. I will have to see whether any post-Europe bounce was evident in the counts taken this week.

The clinical doctor and I had a good discussion about how I was feeling overall. I said that all things considered, I am feeling very good. I have been able to bike, walk, travel, be intellectually active, and enjoy family milestones like my daughter's graduation (my son's university graduation is the next milestone); I have been too busy to be depressed. She answered that it was very rewarding for her and others in the team to see patients doing as well as I am – a real validation of their work and, of course, my family's support. I noted that we are aware that things can change, and that I tend to think in three- to six-month blocks, so that I have a reasonable planning horizon without jinxing things.

I gave the Blood and Marrow Transplant team at the clinic as well as the team on 5 West (the hematology ward) chocolate from my trip to Europe as a small thank-you. I was amazed at how well this small gesture – though it was truly a heartfelt one on the part of my family and I – was received. I also mentioned my forthcoming book to the clinical doctor as I don't want my medical team to be surprised if my marketing strategy works!

I had another round of 're-vaccinations,' bringing with them sore shoulders and a new reaction: a rash on one shoulder that lasted a few days before going away. No more until next January, and then I will be done.

While my book is being edited, I have been converting my Prezi into a video podcast. While the concept of Prezi is simple, it does not have a straightforward 'save as movie' function, so I have yet another piece of software to learn about (Screenflow). This has given me a renewed appreciation for post-production and the relative effort involved in the creative and fun part on the one hand, and the necessary (but less fun) 'getting it out of the door' part on the other. Hopefully, I will get this task finished next week.

My family and I watched the opening ceremony of the Olympics, of course. While these all too often present a sanitized version of history, the British tradition of storytelling was more refreshing, in terms of not only the quirkiness and wit of the ceremony but also the almost 'subversive' tone, in light of current economic and social orthodoxy. A nostalgic portrayal of the former pastoral life, the grimness and inequities of the Industrial Revolution, the social struggles that followed, the importance of universal healthcare, and a celebration of modern, multicultural Britain (putting Canada to shame, as Vancouver largely missed the opportunity for such a celebration).

It was funny to see that one British MP tweeted 'multicultural leftie crap' (while Downing Street disowned these comments, it should be noted that the British Prime Minister declared last year that 'multiculturalism is dead'). The MP in question, who was already demoted for attending a Nazi-themed stag party, may yet suffer another demotion – but I expect that others may have shared his views, if not publicly. The opening ceremony was not quite Occupy Wall Street (better production values!), but was nonetheless a reminder for viewers worldwide of the importance of equality, the social safety net, and multiculturalism. It was a nice contrast to the absolute 'on message' approach of the Beijing olympics, and highlighted the value of democratic systems and their respect for artistic and institutional independence (Danny Boyle, the producer, confirmed this independence).

The choice of *Hey Jude* to close was interesting. While the song was written to console John Lennon's son during Lennon's divorce, it was also interpreted at the time as a drug song (*The minute you let her under your skin / Then you begin to make it better*) – an unconscious (or perhaps conscious) irony given the Olympic history of performance-enhancing drugs.

David Brooks wrote an interesting piece on the Olympics (here), in which he makes note of the contradictions between cooperative and competitive values (specifically how the opening and closing celebrations represent the former, and the actual events the latter), and how such contradictions are part of human nature and human institutions.

Brooks could have taken this further by examining more social and economic factors. In one sense, the Olympics represent formal equality of opportunity (all athletes are equal with an equal chance to compete), a fundamental liberal concept. However, watching the Parade of Nations, interspersed with all those commercials, one is also struck by the disparities – by country and sport – in the size of teams and the resources available to athletes. Social and economic support makes a difference in getting to the podium. Some professional leagues address this through revenue sharing, which results in improved competitiveness among teams; others, like the Olympics, do not. While we are right to focus on the dedication and commitment of the athletes (and the families and friends who support them), the Olympics do have an aspect that reflects and emphasizes today's increasing inequalities.

Enough editorializing for the week! I will continue to enjoy the summer weather and my usual walking and biking.

Two more weeks to go – almost there, and then on to future milestones.

WEEK 51 – NOT MUCH TO REPORT

August 5, 2012

This was another good week: great weather for biking and walking, and I kept busy and engaged.

The on-off nature of Prednisone (10 mg one day, 0 the next), while it does (mercifully) spare me from feeling crummy, has caused a few minor side effects. My energy level appears to be a bit more variable. Some days I nap, other days I do not; my stomach burbles more than before; my strength seems less consistent, and I have been experiencing a bit more muscle fatigue. My biking time was even slightly higher this week (I don't think I can blame it all on the wind!). This is all part of the adjustment process, and none of the side effects prevent me from doing anything, but they are interesting to experience. I expect that the side effects will diminish once I phase down further to alternating between 5 and 0 mg.

I went to see *Batman: The Dark Knight Rises* with my daughter. It was more conventional than the last one (hard to outdo Heath Ledgers' Joker) and less witty. It featured something of a mish-mash of allusions to Occupy Wall Street and the French Revolution (the people's court), with an overall message on the danger of anarchy (this danger was noted by a number of conservative commentators). There were nonetheless some interesting twists and turns in the plot, and I liked that the ending tied up all the loose ends in a satisfying manner (I would have said credible, but since the whole idea of someone like Batman operating on his own without a large team to support him is not credible...).

On a completely different note, our family watched *Waiting for 'Superman'*, a documentary about education in the U.S. and how, while problems are particularly acute in inner city schools, the U.S. has lost its former competitive advantage in education and has been overshadowed by many other countries. The approach was a bit simplistic – yes, rigidity on the part of teacher unions is a major factor in resistance to change, but the issues also reflect family situations (e.g., parents reading 'Goodnight Moon' and other books to their children to instill a love of reading and books) and broad economic and social conditions (e.g., more affluent families can provide more of the enriched activities than families that are struggling). The documentary is worrying, given the impact that education has had on innovation and mobility. That being said, there were some fairly moving testimonies from families of modest means trying to do their best for their kids and to get them into schools that provide a strong learning environment and focus. As I watched the film with my daughter, who just graduated from high school, it was a good opportunity to discuss her school experience with her (and she recognized how fortunate she has been).

Of course, we have also been catching bits of the Olympics.

I finished reading Guy Vanderhaeghe's *A Good Man* – I needed some fiction for a change, I really enjoyed it. Set in the both the Canadian and American West shortly after the American Civil War and George Custer's defeat, it captures nicely the dynamics across the Canada-U.S. border at a time of 'pacification' of aboriginal populations. The characters are rich and believable, the depiction of the time is engaging (I was not all that familiar with this period), and some of the themes (e.g., aboriginal and 'white' relations) remain pertinent to our time. It is also a bit of a 'page-turner,' as one is so curious to see what happens next. A great read for summer (or any other time).

July was my blog's most popular month ever. The most popular posts (apart from the weekly updates, various reflection pieces and practical tips) were the following:

1. Darcy Doherty and 'Last Chance' treatments (Darcy Doherty: Cancer patient's death strengthens a push for last-chance drugs, Terminally ill patients should have access to last-chance therapies, and In one man's fight against cancer, safety trumps hope)

2. How Stress And Sleep Loss Are Shortening Your Life

3. Life, Interrupted by Suleika Jaouad

4. Is organic food too costly?

5. Patients seek Internet information to start dialogue with physicians and Researchers Find Potential Key to New Treatment for Mantle Cell Lymphoma (MCL)

Hard to believe, but only one week to go to my one year anniversary. Life is sweet.

WEEK 52 – ONE YEAR!

August 12, 2012

A year ago, this possibility felt far, far away, clouded by uncertainty and worry.

Today, looking back over the fears, the ups and downs, and the fundamental question of whether I would make it or not, those times also seem a lifetime away. Part of our survival mechanism as humans is to put bad memories behind us as much as possible.

Revising the edits for my upcoming book reminded me of just how rough the journey has been, but also of the fact that I have been one of the lucky ones: I have experienced no major long-lasting side effects, and no major impairment to my quality of life. The dark days have to be appreciated in that context.

I remain in awe of this second chance that I have been given. The same feeling I had walking out of the hospital one year ago.

Without the stem cell transplant, I would likely not be here today. But I did it, and I am.

I feel a strong sense of gratitude that I am living in a place and a time when such treatment is possible and such a second chance can be given. As I read the horror stories of patients dealing with health insurance in the U.S., I have a renewed appreciation for Canadian medicare and universal coverage. Last, but not least, the support of family and friends has made all the difference.

So where am I, one year out?

- I am doing fine on the four general measures (no signs of lymphoma, blood marrow working with good blood counts, no significant GvHD, and looking and feeling well).

- I have energy levels that allow me to be physically and mentally active, although I need more rest than I did before.

- My emotional state keeps me active and engaged.

- Some neuropathy remains in my feet, which impairs my balance but not my preferred activities of walking and biking.

- I have a reasonably strong immune system that allows me to be with people, in small and larger settings, although with some caution.

All-in-all, life is good, and for that I am truly thankful.

I continue to reflect further on what this all means to me, to my family, and to others as I work on the conclusion to my book. My story, and its meaning for me and and those closest to me, is fairly clear. At the broader level, the meaning is less clear, but does revolve around how we live our lives with others. Some further reflection and hard writing ahead.

Overall, I am more reflective and appreciative, and try to ensure that my day-to-day life reflects this. I always come back to Leonard Cohen, whose words in *Anthem* have helped guide me through this journey:

> *Ring the bells that still can ring*
> *Forget your perfect offering*
> *There is a crack, a crack in everything*
> *That's how the light gets in.*

To celebrate my one-year anniversary, my son came up to visit so that we could all savour the moment – the relief that we all feel, as well as the hope that the worst is behind us – together. We all know what we don't know – what the future will bring – but avoid dwelling on that, and instead live and enjoy the here and now.

In terms of the smaller stuff, last week I was worried that the Prednisone phase down had impacted my energy levels, with my biking times being the measure. This week, I had the best times in over a year. Tangible progress.

My wife and I have again been watching some films with our daughter. First, *The Dead Poet's Society*, which captures the private-school milieu and pressures to conform all too well; and then *The Adventures of Tintin*. Seeing the latter again reminded me of just how visually beautiful it is, and how amazing some scenes are (e.g., the desert into ocean transformation). We also watched *The Ladykillers*, a 1955 film starring a creepy Alec Guinness as the ringleader of a bunch of robbers who pretend to be musicians as they use an old woman's house as their base. It features some great moments and a very young Peter Sellers in a straight role, and was a nice throwback to more intelligent thrillers than the more action-packed ones of today. Lastly, my son and I saw *Waiting for Guffman*, an ensemble piece (the same group that did *Best in Show* and *A Mighty Wind*) and nice offbeat comedy about a small-town theatre production to mark a town's 150th anniversary, and the personalities that come together to put it on.

I do not have much more to say this week, except to thank all of you for your support and encouragement over the past year and longer.

Now I can look forward to my next milestones, which revolve around family events. The next unique ones are a planned trip with my daughter next spring, and my son's university graduation early next summer.

Chapter 15

What We Call Ourselves

We all struggle to find terms that describe our experiences with cancer, whether 'fighter,' 'student,' 'survivor,' 'veteran' or other. Our choice of words depends on where we are on our individual journey. In my case, while I dip into different words when it feels right, I have come to terms with the phrase 'living with cancer.'

Over the past few years, I have reflected on the terms people use to describe their life with cancer. I initially tried to write a glossary of the terms: hero, warrior, fighter, veteran, graduate, survivor, victim or 'living with cancer.'

When I tried the glossary out with a couple of friends (one of whom had been through a comparable experience and one of whom had not), I found that it was not effective. People adopt different terms at different stages in treatment, and a 'journey' approach captures this better than an analytical one.

Rather than use the Kubler-Ross five stages (Denial, Anger, Bargaining, Depression, Acceptance), written for the terminally ill, I started with the framework presented in William Bridges's *Transitions: Making Sense of Life's Changes*, which I found more helpful. Bridges talks about three phases: the ending (or losing and letting go), the neutral zone (an in-between, or ambiguous, phase), and the new beginning (acceptance and embracing). Circumstances change quickly, but transitions take time. Bridges's phases provide a convenient frame for cancer and the move from 'normal' to 'new normal' – a change that we can accept, if not embrace.

Ending, losing and letting go

Our lives fall apart when we are first diagnosed with cancer. Our normal view is shattered, our expectations are crushed, and we have an overwhelming sense of loss. Cancer is not a pink ribbon; slogans like 'cancer sucks' of 'f*** cancer' capture our mood. We tend to be inwardly focussed, coming to terms with our thoughts and feelings.

Victim: We may see ourselves as victims. We have lost our previous healthy life. We are angry ('why me?'). We feel injured, destroyed and even sacrificed, without any reason or cause. Even smokers with lung cancer may say 'Why me?' and 'Why not *x* who smoked more than me?'

Viewing ourselves as victims can be part of our first defense and resistance.

Cancer happened to us — we are powerless. We cede control to medical experts, who do 'things' to us (chemo, radiation, other), and our role is limited to understanding and consenting.

Remaining 'victims' can reduce our responsibility for lifestyle factors (tobacco, diet, exercise) and for how we handle and respond to cancer, its treatment, and the people around us.

The neutral zone

This is the period of realignment and repatterning, and helping ourselves get through our cancer treatment and hopefully recovery.

As we come to terms with our diagnosis and proceed to treatment, war metaphors come into play. We often think, 'I'm going to beat/fight/conquer this' (unless the cancer is terminal). We choose treatments accordingly, agreeing to the most aggressive regime that our bodies can withstand. We learn about our new identity as a patient, and drift away from our previous professional and personal identities.

We also start to form our response to cancer: focussing on what to do, seeking meaning in response to our fear of dying, and thinking about what it all means for our relationships with those closest to us.

Two terms – warrior (or fighter) and hero – best reflect this stage:

Warrior or Fighter (or conqueror, activist): We adopt the 'war against cancer' metaphors. We try to 'will' ourselves through each round of chemo or radiation. We fight the side effects (with help from medications). While we know that cancer is a matter of the body fighting itself, we often consider cancer as somehow external to us, which strengthens the 'battle' metaphor.

We are drawn to the primal nature of the will to survive because of the life and death struggle that we are in.

Fighting empowers us and makes us feel more in control, and we focus on the goal of 'beating this.' We develop a more positive attitude to the 'slings and arrows' of treatment, and try to play a more active role in our recovery (e.g., making an effort to exercise).

Although the treatment and medical team do most of the work, we view them, along with family and friends, as our 'platoon' or 'allies' – supporting us.

Our battle exacts a physical and emotional toll, one that we only become truly aware of during our recovery from treatment.

During this stage, we risk sometimes not knowing when to give up, and when further treatment would not improve our quality of life and longevity.

Hero: As warriors might be, we are admired for our courage in how we deal with cancer, and particularly the character we demonstrate through rough treatment and side effects.

We do not choose cancer, however; it chooses us. We have not voluntarily or professionally thrown ourselves into a dangerous situation (e.g., fire fighters, military), we just find ourselves there. We do, however, choose how we react to our cancer. The term hero reflects the fact that some reactions are more motivating and admirable (for those around us) than others.

As we go transition the neutral zone we are likely starting to identify our future identity.

The new beginning

We stop looking back. We get on with our post-recovery life. We come to terms with what is the same and what has changed. We define our 'new normal.' We keep at the back of our minds the awareness that time is precious and may be limited, and that our cancer could come back.

We use a number of different terms to describe ourselves, reflecting who we are as much as what we have gone through.

Intern, Student and Graduate: As our treatment progresses, so does our personal transition. At a simple level, we move from being interns (diagnosis) to students (treatment) to graduates (recovery and post-recovery). We have learned how to be a patient, we have studied (far too much) information on our cancer and treatment, and at the end of the process, we have picked up a mix of theoretical and 'living through it' knowledge that allows us to graduate (hopefully without ever going back to school!).

This transition also takes place on the emotional level. As interns we may be angry and frustrated, but as graduates we have largely come to terms with what our cancer means for the future. Given the incurable (but not necessarily untreatable) nature of many cancers, our graduation may be more psychological than concrete.

We still need to define what 'graduation' means for each of us; is it truly back to normal, our pre-cancer life, or a 'new normal', with physical and emotional changes that we both are affected by as well as shape ourselves through our attitude.

Survivor: We have undergone difficult and harsh treatment, along with the emotions and life lessons that go with it. We 'made it through' and are back to – hopefully – normal life (prospering) or at least near-normal life (closer to existing). We are recognized by others as survivors, as most people have a sense of the horrors of cancer treatment.

However, we are privileged survivors. We had the care and support of our medical teams, family and friends, unlike survivors of concentration camps and other atrocities.

In response to the widespread use of survivors, some of us use alternates names: 'alivers' or 'thrivers' (which have a more positive and active tone, and some element of 'warriors') or 'diers' (used by some terminally ill people who reject optimistic language).

Veteran: We undergo harsh and unforgiving chemo and radiation treatment, to which the 'war' metaphor applies, for six months to a year or even longer. Relapse can lengthen the ordeal. Recovery takes time, on both physical and emotional levels.

As veterans, we are marked by our experience, given its intensity and the life-altering change in perspective it brings. As when we use the term 'survivor,' in calling ourselves 'veterans' we feel solidarity with others who have had similar experiences, whether with cancer or another disease, and we are recognized in return by others as members of this community.

Our personal 'war against cancer' may or may not be over, depending on whether our cancer is in remission or whether we have suffered ongoing 'collateral damage' in the form of chronic conditions or psychological issues. We either accept this state of being or refuse to do so. Not accepting is akin to remaining a warrior, struggling and fighting.

An ever-changing mix metaphor

As I thought about and worked through these terms, it became more and more clear that there is no one term that works throughout all three phases, from endings through the neutral zone to the new beginning. Each person has to find the terms that best help them at each stage, or use a mixture of terms that continue to resonate.

My preferred term is 'living with cancer,' or, to use Christopher Hitchens' irreverent expression, 'a touch of cancer.' I have largely accepted my 'new beginning' with equanimity.

Other elements remain, however. I started off as a victim, and the warrior or fighter metaphor helped drive, and continues to drive, my recovery, by motivating me to do exercise and other activities. I also consider myself a veteran. I have more knowledge and experience than I desired, and it continues to mark me in many ways.

I feel uncomfortable with the terms hero and survivor, as these may diminish heroes and survivors of more dramatic or worse experiences. However, every now and then, the power of the survivor metaphor hits me, as captured by the song *I will survive*:

> *Go on now go*
> *Walk out the door*
> *Just turn around now*
> *Cause you're not welcome anymore*
> *Weren't you the one who tried to hurt me with goodbyes?*
> *Did you think I'd crumble?*
> *Did you think I'd lay down and die?*
> *Oh no not I*
>
> *I will survive*
> *Oh as long as I know how to love*
> *I know I'll stay alive*
> *I've got all my life to live*
> *I've got all my love to give*
> *I will survive*
> *I will survive*
> *Hey hey!*

Chapter 16

Letting Go and Accepting

We struggle with our choices and options – when to keep fighting, and when to let go – whether in the professional, medical or future realm. We cling to the people who are important to us, and we wonder how we should decide whether or not to accept further treatment, and on what basis.

As I moved from the 'kingdom of the well' to the 'kingdom of the sick' – that 'other place,' to use Susan Sontag's words – I struggled with the issue of when and how I would know when enough was enough, and when I would have to accept my own mortality and the loss of my former life.

This process of letting go and acceptance had a number of different elements to it:

- Professional;

- Treatment options and decisions;

- Thinking about the future;

- What to cling to; and,

- End-of-life questions and overall reflections.

Professional

On the relatively superficial level of professional life, letting go came more or less naturally.

My initial treatment and recovery lasted nine months, but it was clear in my mind that if the treatment worked (four out of five people will be in remission for between three to five years), I would go back to work and my normal life. I had some doubts about how engaged I would be upon my return, and whether I could put up with some of the absurdities of corporate culture. However, these concerns proved to be unfounded, as I quickly found my groove again. Initially, there was no need to let go and accept.

In contrast, my relapse after being back at work for over a year was a real intrusion in my plans. The uncertain odds involved in recovery – first of the salvage chemo (to stabilize me through short-term remission) and second, of the allogeneic stem cell transplant itself (three in five patients die within two years) – changed both the professional and personal dynamics.

It became clear that I would not be able to return to work in a meaningful capacity. I was fortunate to have a good benefits plan with long-term disability insurance, and to be eligible for a pension as of early 2013. Financial concerns were not an issue.

Emotionally, accepting the end of my career took time. My head told me that it was the right thing to do, but my heart missed the people, the issues, and the excitement of working on something. The transition took place on a number of levels:

- First, the 'out of sight, out of mind' phenomenon: my colleagues respected my illness and my need to focus my treatment, but consequently forgot about me and my corporate and historical knowledge and just 'got on with it.' I understood intellectually that this is normal in large organizations, but it was nevertheless humbling since I was accustomed to playing a leadership role.

- Second, the transitory nature of professional relationships became clear. We spend time together working on interesting issues, but then move on to other challenges. Where stronger personal connections have developed, the friendships will continue, but for the most part we move on with our busy lives. I found it striking that despite providing tools to let people know how I was doing and making it clear how and when I welcomed contact, so few people took me up on the offer. It is what it is, and helped me with the process of letting go.

- Third, the odd social occasions with colleagues, and the inevitable shop talk, made it clear to me that I had no interest in returning to work and reinforced how unlikely it was that I would tolerate 'playing the game' again. Several such events took place around the nine-month mark after my allo stem cell transplant helped me finally let go of my professional side without regret. What's gone is gone – move on.

Treatment options and decisions

When it comes to treatment options, the journey is more difficult.

As one would expect, when first diagnosed with (MCL), I spent far too much time searching the web – a depressing activity since MCL is incurable. The comparatively cheery prognosis from my hematologist turned my mood around, and I plunged into the treatment protocol (R Hyper CVAD, auto SCT) with, if not enthusiasm, at least a positive attitude, pushing the dark thoughts of death aside. I assumed that I would have the average three to five years before relapse, a timeframe that, while sobering, I could live with.

My relapse about a year later changed everything.

After the initial shock, anger and depression, one of my first questions to my hematologist was, 'The first time, I spent nine months in treatment and recovery to get about a year. Have I reached the point of diminishing returns?'

As always, the answer was not black and white. The recommended treatment was an allogeneic SCT, but to get there, I needed salvage chemo to place my lymphoma in temporary remission. No longer would I be 'put through' a standard protocol. For the salvage chemo, each round would be subject to evaluation and adjustment as needed – 'bespoke' treatment, to use the fancy term. Fortunately, it worked, and I was able to proceed to the transplant.

The decision process was harder this time and required deeper reflection, given the literally life-or-death stakes. My doctors here in Ottawa were clear that there were no other recommended alternatives. Doctors at Princess Margaret Hospital in Toronto concurred. But these discussions with medical experts highlighted the following:

- Letting go meant that I would likely not survive for more than a year or so. Successive rounds of chemo would become less and less effective.

- Only two out of five patients live for more than two years – although my doctors thought my odds were better, given my general good health, age, and overall positive experience with the auto SCT.

- The choice was almost philosophical: resign oneself to certain death within a year or so, or 'gamble' on the hope that the provided.

- My biggest concern, even more frightening than death, was that I might develop a form of chronic GvHD that would result in a poor quality of life (e.g., respiratory issues that would impede mobility and activities) and make me a burden on my wife and children.

- I also got an overall sense that the choice before me was my last chance at recovery. Choosing to simply live now would come with health complications further down the road, given the harsh nature of treatment () and the cumulative effect of chemo. Of course, without this treatment, I would not get 'further down the road' at all, so while it felt like a trade-off, strictly speaking it was not.

My wish to be here with my wife and our children made the 'gamble' worthwhile, notwithstanding – or perhaps because of – the life and death stakes.

Thinking about the future

Throughout the last year, knowing that there are no more realistic treatment options for me, I have become interested in how people make these kind of choices about treatment. How does one know (not in the medical or clinical sense) when to accept death, and make treatment decisions accordingly? In one sense, I know that one day – hopefully later rather than sooner – I will have to make such a choice.

Studies show that we interpret odds more positively than we should.

> "…the grimmer the prognosis, the more inaccurate and more optimistic the surrogates' responses became. … relatives hearing doctors deliver dire prognoses just didn't accept or believe them. They displayed, in medspeak, "a systematic optimism bias." (Paula Span, New York Times, 8 March 2012)

I displayed an optimism bias in my first round of treatment, but became realistic after relapse.

There are strong testimonies from doctors who have seen the pain and suffering caused by prolonging life unnecessarily:

> *With unrealistic expectations of our ability to prolong life, with death as an unfamiliar and unnatural event, and without a realistic, tactile sense of how much a worn-out elderly patient is suffering, it's easy for patients and families to keep insisting on more tests, more medications, more procedures.*
>
> *Doing something often feels better than doing nothing. Inaction feeds the sense of guilt-ridden ineptness family members already feel as they ask themselves, "Why can't I do more for this person I love so much?" Opting to try all forms of medical treatment and procedures to assuage this guilt is also emotional life insurance: When their loved one does die, family members can tell themselves, "We did everything we could for Mom."*
>
> *In my experience, this is a stronger inclination than the equally valid (and perhaps more honest) admission that "we sure put Dad through the wringer those last few months." At a certain stage of life, aggressive medical treatment can become sanctioned torture. When a case such as this comes along, nurses, physicians and therapists sometimes feel conflicted and immoral. We've committed ourselves to relieving suffering, not causing it. A retired nurse once wrote to me: "I am so glad I don't have to hurt old people any more."* (Craig Bowron, Washington Post, 17 February 2012)

The history of medicine and cancer treatments is replete with examples of excessive medical treatment at the cost of increased suffering to the patient and his or her family. Of course, medical science and knowledge may have progressed as a result, and subsequent patients have benefitted from this.

My assumption is that should I have a further relapse, or serious complications, I will have some time to discuss my wishes with my medical team. In one sense, the process of deciding whether or not to proceed with the was a 'trial run' for the kind of frankness needed, and I was comfortable with how the team responded – they gave my family and I space to reflect and consider. In many ways, it strengthened the relationship and trust we have with each other, and their approach was both direct and supportive. They also 'staged' the discussions appropriately.

The following quotation effectively captures this point in making the choice between further treatment or palliative care:

> *Look at it this way: when a given cancer treatment has a good chance of curing you or of significantly impacting your disease, no responsible oncologist is going to present that option as a "choice". Sure, lots of people get second opinions. Sure, lots of people ask what will happen if they don't go through with the proposed treatment. But doctors only offer you choices when it doesn't actually matter.*
>
> *So when your oncologist says it's "up to you" whether or not to undergo more treatment for cancer, say no. Just go out and do whatever you want for the rest of your life, however*

long or short it may be. Sure, you could be the "one in a million" who responds to the
drugs (bearing in mind that oncologic "responses" are often measured in weeks or
months, generally not in years; we tend to call those "cures"). But the chances of that are
far smaller than you think. Statistically, you're probably better off with hospice. (Lucy
Hornstein, Better Health, 9 November 2011)

The alternative, more combative view, points out the inanity of the phrase 'what does not kill you will make you stronger' in the case of terminally ill patients. In the irreverent, pointed words of Christopher Hitchens:

So far, I have decided to take whatever my disease can throw at me, and to stay
combative even while taking the measure of my inevitable decline. I repeat, this is no
more than what a healthy person has to do in slower motion. It is our common fate.
(Hitchens, Vanity Fair, January 2012)

These readings and reflections have prompted me to take the necessary step of having discussions with my family on my wishes and preparing a 'living directive' that makes this clear. The latter provides them, and medical teams, with as clear an indication of my wishes as possible, in the event that I am not in a position to speak for myself. Most people do not take this step, making it harder on their families and medical teams when the time comes.

What to cling to?

Part of letting go is knowing what it most important, and in a sense knowing what particular aspects of one's life one wants and needs to cling to. Whatever is less important, the secondary, gets pushed into the background. Time becomes more precious and one makes more and more conscious decisions about how to spend one's time.

Of course, energy levels vary, and some time 'wastage' is normal and part of life, but the choice of activities to do and people to see is deliberate. The element of knowing what to cling to has two levels: the personal and the group.

At the personal level, the sense of self becomes more important. One's current identity may be that of living with cancer, but one's previous and broader identity remains. Finding the right balance between these two identities, a balance that may evolve over time, is key. As Mark Dery puts it:

… I've learned one thing at least: the importance of clinging to the rag-
end of your sense of self, however you define it—intellect, sense of humor,
generosity of spirit, a stoicism worthy of Seneca or Mr. Spock, or, in a
writer's case, the mind that makes sense of itself as a reflection in the
mirror of language. (Dery, A Season in Hell, BoingBoing)

Dery also makes an important observation about how much time and effort one should put into being a patient, in the sense of becoming an expert one one's cancer. Most of us start off obsessed with our cancer and research it accordingly. Finding the right balance – between knowing enough to work with your medical team to make informed decisions and trying to 'compete' with their knowledge and experience – becomes important. In Dery's words,

> *Most of all, though, I simply didn't want to allow the disease to metastasize across my*
> *mind, occupying my thoughts as it already had my body.* (*A Season in Hell*,
> BoingBoing)

Setting limits and clinging to your fundamental, pre-cancer identity is part of establishing that balance. Each of us will find a different balance, one that works best for us and those around us.

I personally did become an 'empowered' patient, regularly scanning the internet for articles of interest to me and relevant to my lymphoma. My blog was another way to express my 'cancer identity.' However, as time went on, my interest in cancer- and lymphoma-specific articles and information diminished, and was replaced with a focus on general coping and health issues. I also always maintained, in my book and film choices, what I think was a healthy focus on exploring areas of personal interest. This helped keep me sane, and was, along with keeping active and mobile, fortunately doable during most of my recovery.

Just as we cling to our sense of self, we also cling to our family and those closest to us. Earlier, I mentioned that the key factor in my decision to go ahead with the risky was my wish to be around longer for my family. While I am blessed with good close friends, who have been incredibly supportive and caring, in the end it is my family milestones that are most important to me (although I will be happy to participate in others).

We cling to our family and our family clings to us. Having open discussions with your family, and helping them understand that at some point, both you and they have to let go, is not easy. Preparing an Advanced Medical Directive provides a point of departure for that discussion, but admitting what no one wants to admit is hard. Harold Pollack notes:

> *There are better ways to say: "I love you, and I will miss you" than to beat the heck out*
> *of someone we love through desperation treatments that no longer work.*
>
> *We, the future patients, can help, too. We can reassure the people we will leave behind.*
> *We know that hard decisions will be made in life's endgame we can't completely specify*
> *in advance. We can tell our families: I know that you will do your best. I know that you*
> *love me. It will be sad but okay. Whatever my physical endgame, my life will go on in*
> *you.* (Pollack, The Incidental Economist, February 2012)

End-of-life discussion questions

We are not accustomed to death and are uncomfortable talking about it. Even doctors that have to have these discussions on a regular basis can be uncomfortable with how to initiate the discussion and admit that they can do no more. After all, from a doctor's point of view:

> *We have to acknowledge the impotence of our attempts at some point. "We're not winning. The treatment's not working. She's dying despite our best efforts." People understand if you make it clear that treatment has failed. It's not that we're giving up; it's that we really tried, and we can't save her.* (Interview with Dr. Stephen Workman by Paula Span, New York Times, 14 December 2011)

With medical teams, the best set of questions I have found is (Elaine Waples, KevinMD):

	Question	Purpose
1	Do you understand your prognosis?	Allows the doctor to 'check-in' with the patient and ensure he or she has been clear. A good technique as a patient is to 'replay' what the doctor has said, to ensure that the patient has correctly heard and understood
2	What are your fears about what is to come?	Open-ended question to draw out the concerns and fears of the patient.
3	What are your goals as time runs out?	Another open-ended question to draw-out the patient, but more pointed given the reference to 'as time runs out' and leads into the final question.
4	What trade offs are you willing to make?	With the sharing of fears and goals, channels the patient towards understanding that their will be trade-offs, and his or her input will help the medical team make appropriate recommendations.

Here is a less prescriptive variation with two questions and one point of guidance, for use either by either medical teams or friends and family (Virginia L. Seno, Esse Institute):

1	What is most important to you right now?
2	If there was something you needed done, what would it be?
3	Be quiet and open-minded. Be present. Be available. Be willing to ask and hear and do.

Either set of questions can work well. As a patient, thinking about these earlier rather than later, and discussing them with your family and closest friends, may be helpful in that final stage of letting go and accepting. In my case:

- I have a good understanding of the aggressive nature of my lymphoma and that it is incurable, as well as of the implications and possible complications resulting from my allogeneic stem cell transplant.

- My fears are like most people's: pain and all the personal and family milestones I will miss (e.g., birthdays, holidays, graduations, possible marriages and births).

- My goals are to make the most of the time I have, particularly by spending it with family and friends, but also by sharing my experience to possibly help others.

- I am not prepared to undergo excessively risky treatments should my quality of life be severely impaired, or for a minor increase in longevity. Assessing this in the abstract is easy; making a concrete decision and deciding what 'risky,' 'severely,' or 'minor' mean for me at that time will be harder.

Thoughts and lessons

In the process of looking back, and reflecting on what 'advice' I would give to others before they are themselves confronted by such existential questions, a number of articles have been helpful (e.g., those by Rob A. Ruff, KevinMD). Not surprisingly, the advice ranges from the obvious (spend more time with your family) to the more insightful (start thinking about this possibility early) and reflect/pray/meditate).

The problem with hindsight is that it overlooks the challenges and demands we face as we move through the various stages of our lives. We tend to be building our careers at the same time as our families, which causes work-life balance tensions. Consequently, some looking backward tends towards the naive at best, but with that caveat, I have collected the following thoughts.

But first, an important practical task: prepare an Advanced Medical Directive.

Thought	Elaboration
Reflect upon the contingency of life	As Joni Mitchell says so well: *Don't it always seem to go* *That you don't know what you've got* *Til it's gone* Be more reflective and appreciative, recognizing early on that luck can change and reverse the course of our lives. Take time through prayer, meditation, yoga, walking or whatever gives you the necessary space.
Live more in the moment	For practical reasons, we cannot only live in the moment; we think in the longer term when we have children, buy a house, plan a career, or provide for our retirement. We can nonetheless, however, be more conscious of the moment and make an effort to create more moments.
Focus on people	Life is only as rich as the relationships we have, whether with family, friends or colleagues. Create space and time to strengthen and deepen these, focussing on the most important. Do not forget, with loved ones, (though it can be hard with teenagers) to give those hugs and those words of love: *Please forgive me* *I forgive you* *Thank you* *I love you* Don't focus on 'bucket lists' but rather the people with whom you wish to be with and what you would like to do together.
Explore ideas	I may be biased, but I recommend that you get away from all the distractions of our electronic devices and social networking through the medium of your choice. The religious among us may do so by reading and study Holy books. For the rest of us, there are any number of cultural options to help broaden reflection and understanding.
Be open about trade-offs	We can't have it all. We make work-life trade-offs as we have a family and build our career. We try to live more in the moment while providing for our children's education and our retirement. We try to allocate our time and effort as best we can. We do not have the unique talent and courage of Steve Jobs to "have the courage to follow your heart and intuition" all the way, but we can be more conscious and open about our heart and intuition, as we make trade-offs.

Chapter 17

Living with Cancer

Some final thoughts about what we learn from cancer, what it means to us and others,
and how cancer reminds us of our common humanity.

Life is a journey. Throughout the journey from birth to death, and all the significant milestones along the way, the 'final' destination awaits.

How and when we reach it is, of course, another matter.

For most of us, our reference point is average life expectancy. We conveniently overlook the key word: average. Some of us live less, some live more, some of us have an easier time, some a harder time. We hopefully have more moments of joy than moments of suffering, but both remind us of just how precious life and living are.

Cancer, like a heart attack or other serious illness, is one of those extended moments of suffering that shatters our assumptions about lifespan and marks the beginning of a new journey – living through illness and seeing how it changes our perspective on life.

Our suffering is not to the same degree as that witnessed and experienced by Viktor Frankl in the Nazi concentration camps, but his observations nevertheless apply:

> *If there is a meaning in life at all, then there must be a meaning in suffering. Suffering is*
> *an ineradicable part of life, even as fate and death. Without suffering and death human*
> *life cannot be complete.*

Our individual suffering and cancer journey is reflected in the different ways we refer to this journey and the different words we use to describe ourselves. The journey eventually teaches us how to let go and accept, how to come to terms with our new reality.

My journey is no exception. From the initial shock of diagnosis, to treatment and recovery, the even worse shock of relapse, and yet another cycle of treatment and recovery, my world has turned upside down over the past years. Thinking and writing has helped me through the three phases of transition: ending, neutral zone and new beginnings.

As I journeyed through the transition to new beginnings, I realized that cancer is a sentence, not just a word, to again turn around Robert Buckman's *Cancer Is a Word, Not a Sentence*. Cancer sentences us to a new journey: the lucky ones may be cured, the least lucky will not make it, and for many of us, we will need to 'manage' our cancer as one does a chronic disease, undergoing further treatment as needed.

We are all sentenced, however, to the fear that our cancer will come back.

As time goes on, our memories of the harsh treatment fade, and we either get back to our old lives or discover our new beginning, or 'new normal.' Both are part of the healing process, helping us 'forget' the suffering of the bad days and celebrate being alive with the people and activities we love, which give us meaning and purpose.

Cancer is never a blessing, nor is it a 'learning opportunity' to make us 'better' people. Yet paradoxically, perhaps as a survival mechanism or instinct to seek meaning, many of us take from the experience of cancer a new appreciation for those around us and for what is truly important in our lives. We make it past the sense of loss and accept and are thankful for what we have. Just as our journey has many moments of suffering, there is joy in the moments when we make it to a milestone or create a new family memory.

For me, my transition and journey has two major aspects:

- Coming to terms with my 'new normal' on the physical, emotional and relationship levels, throughout the various stages of treatment and recovery. This has been an ongoing process of discovery and adjustment.

- Reflections on what it all means, if anything; first in terms of myself, my family and those close to me in a personal sense, and second, at the levels of community and society.

As I begin my journey towards my 'new normal,' I am truly one of the lucky ones on all levels:

Physical: I am doing well. I can walk, bike, travel, eat most things, and be engaged and active intellectually. My energy level is lower, my body feels 10 years older, I have to pace myself better, and I have some annoying minor side effects like neuropathy in my feet. Mentally, I am less sharp and quick than before. But I am here, alive and enjoying life.

Emotional: I have made it through the five stages of grieving my previous life (Denial, Anger, Bargaining, Depression, Acceptance). While some regret will always remain, by and large I have moved on and can focus on the here and now. I still have dark thoughts – I have only been treated, not cured – but they are in the background.

I have been able to find a range of activities that provide me with meaning and as much satisfaction, if not more, than my previous professional life – largely because these activities are self-directed, rather than job requirements. I now tend to plan in three- to six-month chunks; any more would appear to be tempting fate.

Relationships: People fill up more space in my life now. This is especially true of my immediate family. We are closer than before in many ways. Part of that closeness is knowing when to put the journey behind us and focus on the moment and simply being. The same holds true for extended family, friends and colleagues, although as is often the case for people living with cancer, some friendships have strengthened while others have withered away. And that's fine.

While cancer hits many of us randomly, in a universe indifferent to our fate, reflecting on and creating meaning, no matter how modest, has been part of my coping mechanism.

As a result, I am more appreciative and reflective when it comes to life, people, and what matters. I take less for granted and, while I cannot completely live in the moment, my focus is more on the here and now than on the future. Life is fragile and contingent, and I have learned to appreciate my 'new normal' – and enjoy it, savour it and above all, live it.

All of those close to me have been similarly affected to some degree, as cancer (or other serious disease) reminds us all of our own mortality and of the fragility of life. Likewise, through some of my exchanges with others through my blog or other online fora, I have found that many others share my experiences and reflections. Mine is an individual experience, but not a unique one.

This brings me to my broadest question: does my experience, and that of so many others, mean anything for society as a whole, or does this collection of individual yet shared experiences, some happier, some sadder, have no broader meaning? Or in other words, what broader meaning do I draw?

At its most basic level, the wider meaning is our common humanity. We all recognize the fragility of life ('there for the grace of God go I') and fear suffering and death.

But what do we do with this shared awareness?

Wherever we live, whether or not we are healthy or fortunate, it comes down to the understanding and compassion that we show towards others.

As I look back on my 'pre-cancer' life, I see that I was far from perfect in this regard, too caught up in my busy professional and personal life – a common affliction. For example:

- My being busy was often an excuse not to help;

- My discomfort with my own mortality made me avoid reaching out many a time;

- My uncertainty about what to say sometimes led me to not call or send an e-mail; and,

- My focus on my own life made me less receptive to support programs and services that help others.

In the end, it has been the support from family, friends, colleagues, blog readers and others that has made all the difference to me, as it has for so many others with cancer. This support provides meaning. Others have also found solace, support and compassion through their faith and faith communities. As Nietzsche said, 'He who has a *why* to live for can bear with almost any *how.*'

Recognizing the importance of this support has led me to get beyond these excuses (though not always perfectly) and make a conscious effort to help others in comparable circumstances.

Just as family and friends suffer when someone close to them gets cancer, society suffers from increased cases of cancer. Fundraising runs and the like tap into this collective feeling – that we need to help people and their families as they live with cancer, supporting them on their way.

As individuals, we all need to find our own way to alleviate suffering, whether this stems from cancer or other serious diseases, or, for that matter, any other issue facing society. While suffering is part of life and part of being human, the same is true of helping others through their difficulties and suffering. Again turning to Frankl:

> … *(self-transcendence) denotes the fact that being human always points, and is directed, to something or someone, other than oneself – be it a meaning to fulfill or another human being to encounter. The more one forgets himself – by giving himself to a cause to serve or another person to love – the more human he is and the more he actualizes himself. What is called self-actualization is not an attainable aim at all, for the simple reason that the more one would strive for it, the more he would miss it. In other words, self-actualization is possible only as a side effect of self-transcendence.*

We all know that the past is past, the now is now, and the future is uncertain. A greater sense of humility in our planning ('The best laid plans of mice and men…') and a greater awareness of the risks we all face can remind us of the need for understanding, compassion and self-transcendence. We can then find our way, our contribution to reducing the suffering of those close to us and of total strangers.

> *O longing of the branches*
> *To lift the little bud*
> *O longing of the arteries*
> *To purify the blood*
>
> *And let the heavens hear it*
> *The penitential hymn*
> *Come healing of the spirit*
> *Come healing of the limb*

Leonard Cohen, *Come Healing*

Annex

READINGS – NON-FICTION

Biography

Afshin-Jam, Nazanin McClelland, Susan	The Tale of Two Nazanins
Esfandiari, Haleh	My Prison My Home
Gilmour, David	The Film Club
Isaacson, Walter	Steve Jobs
Pausch, Randy	The Last Lecture
Wiesel, Elie	Night Coeur Ouvert

Cancer

Frank, Arthur	At the Will of the Body The Wounded Storyteller
Mukherjee, Siddhartha	The Emperor of Maladies: A Biography of Cancer
Sontag, Susan	Illness as Metaphor

Faith

Armstrong, Karen	The Great Transformation: The Beginning of our Religious Traditions The History of God The Spiral Staircase
Eagleton, Terry	Holy Terror

Faith

Lewis, C.S.	Abolition of Man Mere Christianity
Roof, Wade Clark	A Generation of Seekers
Tweed, Thomas	Crossing and Dwelling: A Theory of Religion
Wright, Robert	The Evolution of God

History

Amir & Khalil	Zahra's Paradise
Beinart, Peter	The Icarus Syndrome
Bodanis, David	E=mc2
Cassidy, John	How Markets Fail: The Logic of Economic Calamities
Ebers, Dorothy Harley	Encounters on the Passage: Inuit Meet the Explorers
Ferguson, Niall	Ascent of Money
Ferguson, Niall	The Pity of War
Gotleib, Allan	Washington Diaries
Gwynne, S.C.	Empire of the Summer Moon
Landes, David	The Wealth and Poverty of Nations
MacMillan, Margaret	The Use and Abuse of History
Miller, Aaron David	The Much Too Promised Land
Ralston Saul, John	A Fair Country: Telling Truths About Canada
Snyder, Timothy	Bloodlands: Europe Between Hitler and Stalin

Ideas

Atwood, Margaret	Moral Disorder Payback
Bissoondath, Neil	Selling Illusions: The Cult of Multiculturalism in Canada
Bloom, Allan	The Closing of the American Mind

311

Ideas

Chatwin, Bruce	What am I Doing Here
Eire, Carlos	A Very Brief History of Eternity
Gladwell, Malcolm	The Tipping Point Outliers
Harrison, Lawrence	The Central Liberal Truth
Hitchens, Christopher	Arguably
Maher, Bill	The New New Rules
Mansur, Salim	Delectable Lie: A Liberal Repudiation of Multiculturalism
Ondaatje, Michael	The Conversations: Walter Murch and the Art of Editing Film
Paquet, Gilles	Deep Cultural Diversity: A Governance Challenge
Rubin, Jeff	Why Your World is Going to Get a Lot Smaller
Taylor, Charles	Multiculturalism and the "Politics of Recognition"

Psychology

Coates, John	The Hour Between Dog and Wolf
Frankl, Victor	Man's Search for Meaning
Kahneman, Daniel	Thinking Fast and Slow
Tolle, Eckhart	The New Earth The Evolution of God

Other

Carradine, David	The Kill Bill Diary
Dawkins, Richard	The Greatest Show on Earth
Naipaul, V.S.	Among the Believers

READINGS – FICTION

Atwood, Margaret	The Year of the Flood Oryx and Crake
Bennett, Alan	The Uncommon Reader
Bissoondath, Neil	The Soul of All Great Designs
Boyden, Joseph	The Black Spruce Three Day Road
Coelho, Paulo	The Alchemist
Coetzee, J.M.	Disgrace
Fallis, Terry	The Best Laid Plans
Garcia Marques, Gabriel	Love in the Time of Cholera The General and his Labyrinth
King, Thomas	Green Grass Running Water
McCarthy, Cormac	The Road
McEwan, Ian	Atonement
McGregor, Jon	If Nobody Speaks of Remarkable Things
Nabokov, Vladimir	Invitation to a Beheading
Ondaatje, Michael	The Cat's Table
Ricci, Nino	Origin of Species
Rushdie, Salman	Shalimar the Clown Midnight's Children
Skibsrud, Johanna	The Sentimentalists
Vanderhaeghe, Guy	A Good Man

VIEWINGS

1911

50/50

A Dangerous Method

A Fistful of Dollars

A Matter of Life and Death

A Midsummers' Night Sex Comedy

A Separation

A Night at the Opera

A Single Man

A Woman, A Gun and a Noodle Shop

Adoration

Amélie

An American in Paris

An Education

Another Year

Apollo 13

Avatar

Back to the Future

Batman Begins

Batman: The Dark Knight

Batman: The Dark Knight Rises

Beginners

Biutiful

Black Adder

Black Swan

Blue Valentine

Broken Embraces

Butterfield 8

Carlos

Carnage

Cassandra's Dream

Cat on a Hot Tin Roof

Chinatown

Close Encounters of the Third Kind

Coco avant Chanel

Cool Hand Luke

Crimes and Misdemeanors

Departures

Dial M for Murder

Downton Abbey

Dr Zhivago

El Secreto de Sus Ojos

Entre les murs

Everything You Always Wanted to Know About Sex

Fishing Salmon in the Yemen

Five Easy Pieces

Food, Inc.

Four Lions

Frantic

From Rome with Love

Full Metal Jacket

Game Change

Get Low

Groundhog Day

Hanna

Harry Potter and the Half-Blood Prince

Hereafter

How to Train a Dragon

Hugo

Il Divo

Il Postino

In A Better World

In the Heat of the Night

Incendies

Inglourious Basterds

Inside Job

Invictus

It's a Wonderful LIfe

Judgement at Nuremburg

Julie & Julia

Julius Caesar

Katyn

L'Amour fou

L'Heure d'éte

La jetée

Land without Bread

Lawrence of Arabia

Le bruit des glaçons

Le Notti Bianche

Lemon Tree

Les femmes du 6ième étage

Les Intouchables
Les Invasions Barbares
Les neiges de Kilmanjaro
Limitless
Made in Dagenham
Mao's Last Dancer
Margin Call
Matchpoint
Midnight in Paris
Moneyball
Monsieur Lazhar
Mr. Smith Goes to Washington
Music of the Heart
My Fair Lady
My Father My Lord
My Tehran for Sale
My Week with Marilyn
No One Knows About Persian Cats
Once Upon a Time in America
Once Upon a Time in the West
Paths of Glory
Patton
Payback
Pink Ribbons, Inc.
Potiche
Precious Life
Prêt-à-Porter
Rabbit Hole
Ratatouille
Rear Window
Rebel Without a Cause
Recount
Repulsion
Robin Hood: Men in Tights
Scarface
Singing in the Rain
Social Network
Sophie Scholl: The Final Days
Source Code
Star Trek
Suddenly, Last Summer
Summer Heights High

Sweet Bird of Youth

The Adventures of Tintin

The Artist

The Big Sleep

The Company of Strangers

The Conversation

The Dead Poet's Society

The Descendants

The English Patient

The Fog of War

The Fountain

The Godfather

The Guns of Navarone

The Hurt Locker

The Informant

The Iron Lady

The Kids are All Right

The King's Speech

The Kings of Pastry

The Lady Killers

The Man Who Knew Too Much

The Messenger

The Queen and I

The Skin I Live In

The Station Agent

The Tree of Life

The Wire

Tinker, Tailor, Soldier, Spy

Tristam Shandy

Trois hommes et un couffin

True Grit

Tulpan

Twelve Monkeys

Up

Up in the Air

Valentino: The Last Emperor

Vicky Christina Barcelona

Vision

Waste Land

Whatever Works

When We Leave

Where Do We Go Now?

Where the Wild Things Are
Who's Afraid of Virginia Woolf?
Wild Target
Winter Bone
Winter in Wartime
Woody Allen: A Documentary
X Men 2
Yes Minister
Yes Prime Minister
Yol
Zelig

Acknowledgements

I would like to thank those individuals who helped me, throughout my journey, with my reflections and how best to share them.

To Dennis Fox, Pamela and Guy Levac, and Ian Matheson for their encouragement for the book, their specific suggestions and advice, and for being close and loyal friends supporting me and my family. And Madeleine Levac for her careful and patient editing.

To my blog readers who, either through their comments or the 'stats,' gave me the confidence that this journey had broader interest.

To Cancerwise, in particular Lucy Richardson, who provided me with an additional outlet for reflection and sharing.

To my medical team at the Ottawa Hospital, as well as doctor friends, who were patient with my questions, generous with their answers, and helped me make the necessary decisions and choices.

Lastly, to my family who, although not always comfortable with my degree of sharing, nevertheless humoured me and understood how important this project was for me.

Glossary

A

Acyclovir

Acyclovir is used to decrease pain and speed the healing of sores or blisters in people who have varicella (chickenpox), herpes zoster (shingles; a rash that can occur in people who have had chickenpox in the past), and first-time or repeat outbreaks of genital herpes (a herpes virus infection that causes sores to form around the genitals and rectum from time to time). Acyclovir is also sometimes used to prevent outbreaks of genital herpes in people who are infected with the virus. Acyclovir is in a class of antiviral medications called synthetic nucleoside analogues. It works by stopping the spread of the herpes virus in the body. Acyclovir will not cure genital herpes and may not stop the spread of genital herpes to other people.

Source: MedlinePlus

For transplant patients, it is used to prevent shingles.

Allogeneic stem cell transplant (SCT) or Allo SCT

A procedure in which a person receives stem cells (cells from which all blood cells develop) from a genetically similar, but not identical, donor.

Source: Dana-Farber Cancer Institute

Ara-C

A drug used to treat certain types of leukemia and prevent the spread of leukemia to the meninges (three thin layers of tissue that cover and protect the brain and spinal cord). It is also being studied in the treatment of other types of cancer. Cytarabine blocks tumor growth by stopping DNA synthesis. It is a type of antimetabolite.

Source: Dana-Farber Cancer Institute

ATG (antithymocite globulin)

A protein used to reduce the risk of or to treat graft-versus-host disease.

Source: Dana-Farber Cancer Institute

Ativan

Lorazepam (brand name Ativan) is a drug used for treating anxiety. It is in the benzodiazepine family, the same family that includes diazepam (Valium), alprazolam (Xanax), clonazepam (Klonopin), flurazepam (Dalmane), and others. It is thought that excessive activity of nerves in the brain may cause anxiety and other psychological disorders. Gamma-aminobutyric acid (GABA) is a neurotransmitter, a chemical that nerves in the brain use to send messages to one another. GABA reduces the activity of nerves in the brain. Lorazepam and other benzodiazepines may act by enhancing the effects of GABA in the brain. Because lorazepam is removed from the blood more rapidly than many other benzodiazepines, there is less chance that lorazepam concentrations in blood will reach high levels and become toxic. Lorazepam also has fewer interactions with other medications than most of the other benzodiazepines. The FDA approved lorazepam in March 1999.

Source: MedicineNet.com

Autologous stem cell transplant (SCT) or Auto SCT

A procedure in which blood-forming stem cells (cells from which all blood cells develop) are removed, stored, and later given back to the same person.

Source: Dana-Farber Cancer Institute

B

BEAM Protocol

BEAM is named after the initials of the chemotherapy drugs used, which are:

- carmustine (BiCNU®)

- etoposide

- cytarabine (arabinoside)

- melphalan

Source: Ottawa Hospital

BiCNU

Another term for Carmustine.

Source: MacMillan Cancer UK

Bone Marrow Biopsy

A bone marrow biopsy is the removal of soft tissue, called marrow, from inside bone. Bone marrow is found in the hollow part of most bones. It helps form blood cells.

A bone marrow biopsy may be done in the health care provider's office or in a hospital. The sample may be taken from the pelvic or breast bone. Sometimes, other areas are used.

The health care provider will clean the skin and inject a numbing medicine into the area. Rarely, you may be given medicine to help you relax.

The doctor inserts the biopsy needle into the bone. The center of the needle is removed and the hollowed needle is moved deeper into the bone. This captures a tiny sample, or core, of bone marrow within the needle. The sample and needle are removed. Pressure and a bandage are applied to the biopsy site.

A bone marrow aspirate may also be performed, usually before the biopsy is taken. After the skin is numbed, the needle is inserted into the bone, and a syringe is used to withdraw the liquid bone marrow. If this is done, the needle will be removed and either repositioned, or another needle may be used for the biopsy.

Source: MedlinePlus

Brentuximab

Brentuximab vedotin (INN, codenamed SGN-35 and previously cAC10-vcMMAE) is an antibody-drug conjugate approved to treat anaplastic large cell lymphoma (ALCL) and Hodgkin lymphoma. The U.S. Food and Drug Administration granted the agent an accelerated approval on August 19, 2011 for use against these two diseases. It is marketed as Adcetris.

The compound consists of the chimeric monoclonal antibody brentuximab (which targets the cell-membrane protein CD30) linked to three to five units of the antimitotic agent monomethyl auristatin E (MMAE, reflected by the 'vedotin' in the drug's name). The antibody portion of the drug attaches to CD30 on the surface of malignant cells, delivering MMAE which is responsible for the anti-tumour activity. Hence it is an antibody-drug conjugate.

In a 2010 clinical trial, 34% of patients with refractory Hodgkin Lymphoma achieved complete remission and another 40% had partial remission. Tumor reductions were achieved in 94% of patients. In ALCL, 87% of patients had tumors shrink at least 50% and 97% of patients had some tumors shrinkage.

In August 2011, the U.S. Food and Drug Administration (FDA) approved the use of brentuximab vedotin in relapsed or refractory Hodgkin's lymphoma and relapsed or refractory systemic anaplastic large cell lymphoma.

Source: Wikipedia

C

C. Difficile

C. difficile lostridium difficile (C. difficile) is a bacterium that causes mild to severe diarrhea and intestinal conditions like pseudomembranous colitis (or inflammation of the colon).

When antibiotics destroy a person's good bowel bacteria, C. difficile bacteria can grow. When this occurs, the C. difficile bacteria produce toxins, which can damage the bowel and cause diarrhea. However, some people can have C. difficile bacteria present in their bowel and not show symptoms.

C. difficile is the most frequent cause of infectious diarrhea in Canadian hospitals and long-term care facilities, as well as in other industrialized countries.

Source: Public Health Agency of Canada

Canada Pension Plan – Disability (CPP-D)

Canada Pension Plan (CPP) Disability Benefits provide a monthly taxable benefit to contributors who are disabled and to their dependent children. Most private disability insurance plans in Canada require applicants to also apply to CPP-D, with any CPP-D payments to contributors being deducted from private insurance payments, dependent children payments excepted.

Source: Human Resources and Skills Development Canada and Service Canada

Carmustine

An anticancer drug that belongs to the family of drugs called alkylating agents. Also known as BiCNU.

Source: Dana-Farber Cancer Institute

CMV (Cytomegalovirus)

CMV may cause severe and occasionally life-threatening disease in immunocompromised persons (meaning people with weakened immune systems), such as

- organ and bone marrow transplant recipients,

- cancer patients,

- patients receiving immunosuppressive drugs, and

- HIV-infected patients (see You Can Prevent CMV, A Guide for People with HIV Infection)

A primary (first) CMV infection can cause serious disease in immunocompromised persons. Once a person has had a CMV infection, the virus stays in their body for life. The virus stays dormant (inactive) most of the time, but it can reactivate (become active again) and cause illness. Reactivation of a previous CMV infection is a more common problem for persons with weakened immune systems than primary infection since the majority of people are infected with CMV by the time they are 40 years old.

Immunocompromised patients who are concerned about CMV should consult their physicians about the best ways to avoid problems from CMV infection.

Source: CDC

Colonoscopy

Colonoscopy is the endoscopic examination of the large bowel and the distal part of the small bowel with a CCD camera or a fiber optic camera on a flexible tube passed through the anus. It may provide a visual diagnosis (e.g. ulceration, polyps) and grants the opportunity for biopsy or removal of suspected lesions.

Colonoscopy can remove polyps as small as one millimetre or less. Once polyps are removed, they can be studied with the aid of a microscope to determine if they are precancerous or not.

Source: Wikipedia

Creatinine

A compound that is excreted from the body in urine. Creatinine levels are measured to monitor kidney function and stress.

Source: Dana-Farber Cancer Institute

CT Scan

Computed tomography (CT) is a diagnostic procedure that uses special x-ray equipment to obtain cross-sectional pictures of the body. The CT computer displays these pictures as detailed images of organs, bones, and other tissues. This procedure is also called CT scanning, computerized tomography, or computerized axial tomography (CAT).

Source: National Cancer Institute

Cyclophosphamide

A drug that is used to treat many types of cancer and is being studied in the treatment of other types of cancer. It is also used to treat some types of kidney disease in children. Cyclophosphamide attaches to DNA in cells and may kill cancer cells. It is a type of alkylating agent. Also called CTX and Cytoxan.

Source: Dana-Farber Cancer Institute

Cytarabine

A drug used to treat certain types of leukemia and prevent the spread of leukemia to the meninges (three thin layers of tissue that cover and protect the brain and spinal cord). It is also being studied in the treatment of other types of cancer. Cytarabine blocks tumor growth by stopping DNA synthesis. It is a type of antimetabolite.

Source: Dana-Farber Cancer Institute

D

Dexamethasone

Dexamethasone, a corticosteroid, is similar to a natural hormone produced by your adrenal glands. It often is used to replace this chemical when your body does not make enough of it. It relieves inflammation (swelling, heat, redness, and pain) and is used to treat certain forms of arthritis; skin, blood, kidney, eye, thyroid, and intestinal disorders (e.g., colitis); severe allergies; and asthma. Dexamethasone is also used to treat certain types of cancer.

Source: Medline Plus

Dilaudid

Hydromorphone, a more common synonym for dihydromorphinone, commonly a hydrochloride (brand names Palladone, Dilaudid, and numerous others) is a very potent centrally-acting analgesic drug of the opioid class. It is a derivative of morphine, to be specific, a hydrogenated ketone thereof and, therefore, a semi-synthetic drug. It is, in medical terms, an opioid analgesic and, in legal terms, a narcotic.

Hydromorphone is used in medicine as an alternative to morphine for analgesia, and as a second- or third-line narcotic antitussive (cough suppressant) for cases of dry, painful, paroxysmal coughing resulting from continuing bronchial irritation after influenza and other ailments, inhalation of fungus, and other causes. In general, it is considered the strongest of the antitussive drugs, and was developed shortly after diacetylmorphine (heroin) was removed from clinical use for this purpose in most of the world and banned outright in many countries. The effectiveness of hydrocodone as an antitussive may be partly due to it being partially converted to hydromorphone in the liver.

Source: Wikipedia

Doxorubicin

A drug that is used to treat many types of cancer and is being studied in the treatment of other types of cancer. Doxorubicin comes from the bacterium Streptomyces peucetius . It damages DNA and may kill cancer cells. It is a type of anthracycline antitumor antibiotic. Also called Adriamycin PFS, Adriamycin RDF, doxorubicin hydrochloride, hydroxydaunorubicin, and Rubex.

Source: Dana-Farber Cancer Institute

E

Electroencelphalogram (EEG)

An electroencephalogram (EEG) is a test that measures and records the electrical activity of your brain. Special sensors (electrodes) are attached to your head and hooked by wires to a computer. The computer records your brain's electrical activity on the screen or on paper as wavy lines. Certain conditions, such as seizures, can be seen by the changes in the normal pattern of the brain's electrical activity.

An electroencephalogram (EEG) may be done to:

- Diagnose epilepsy and see what type of seizures are occurring. EEG is the most useful and important test in confirming a diagnosis of epilepsy.

- Check for problems with loss of consciousness or dementia.

- Help find out a person's chance of recovery after a change in consciousness.

- Find out if a person who is in a coma is brain-dead.

- Study sleep disorders, such as narcolepsy.

- Watch brain activity while a person is receiving general anesthesia during brain surgery.

- Help find out if a person has a physical problem (problems in the brain, spinal cord, or nervous system) or a mental health problem.

Source: WebMD

Entocort

Budesonide (brand name Entocort) is a glucocorticoid steroid for the treatment of asthma and non-infectious rhinitis (including hay fever and other allergies), and for treatment and prevention of nasal polyposis. In addition, it is used for Crohn's disease (inflammatory bowel disease). For allo stem cell transplant patients, it is used to calm the digestive tract.

Source: Wikipedia

Etoposide

Etoposide is in a class of drugs known as podophyllotoxin derivatives; it slows or stops the growth of cancer cells in your body. The length of treatment depends on the types of drugs you are taking, how well your body responds to them, and the type of cancer you have. Used as part of the BEAM Protocol

Source: Medline Plus

F

Famvir

Famciclovir (Famvir brand name) is mainly used to treat herpes zoster (shingles; a rash that can occur in people who have had chickenpox in the past), outbreaks of herpes virus cold sores or fever blisters in people, and to treat repeat outbreaks and to prevent further outbreaks of genital herpes (a herpes virus infection that causes sores to form around the genitals and rectum from time to time) in people with a normal immune system.

Famciclovir is also used to treat returning herpes simplex infections of the skin and mucus membranes (mouth, anus) in people with human immunodeficiency virus (HIV) infection as well as in stem cell transplants with low immunity and mucocitis.

Famciclovir is in a class of medications called antivirals. It works by stopping the spread of the herpes virus in the body. However, it may decrease the symptoms of pain, burning, tingling, tenderness, and itching; help sores to heal; and prevent new sores from forming.

Source: Medline Plus

Fluconazole

A drug that treats infections caused by fungi.

Source: Dana-Farber Cancer Institute

G

G-CSf

The scientific term for Neupogen and Neulasta.

Granulocyte colony-stimulating factor (G-CSF or GCSF) is a colony-stimulating factor hormone. G-CSF is also known as colony-stimulating factor 3 (CSF 3).

It is a glycoprotein, growth factor and cytokine produced by a number of different tissues to stimulate the bone marrow to produce granulocytes and stem cells. G-CSF then stimulates the bone marrow to release them into the blood.

G-CSF also stimulates the survival, proliferation, differentiation, and function of neutrophil precursors and mature neutrophils. G-CSF regulates them using Janus kinase (JAK)/signal transducer and activator of transcription (STAT) and Ras /mitogen-activated protein kinase (MAPK) and phosphatidylinositol 3-kinase (PI3K)/protein kinase B (Akt) signal transduction pathway.

Source: Wikipedia Graft-versus-host disease

Graft versus Host Disease (GvHD)

GvHD is a complication that can occur after a stem cell or bone marrow transplant in which the newly transplanted material attacks the transplant recipient's body.

GvHD occurs in a bone marrow or stem cell transplant involving a donor and a recipient. The bone marrow is the soft tissue inside bones that helps form blood cells, including white cells that are responsible for the immune response. Stem cells are normall found inside bone marrow.

Since only identical twins have identical tissue types, a donor's bone marrow is normally a close, but not perfect, match to the recipient's tissues. See: Histocompatibility antigen test

The differences between the donor's cells and recipient's tissues often cause T cells (a type of white blood cells) from the donor to recognize the recipient's body tissues as foreign. When this happens, the newly transplanted cells attack the transplant recipient's body.

Acute GvHD usually happens within the first 3 months after transplant. Chronic GvHD usually starts more than 3 months after transplant, and can last a lifetime.

Rates of GvHD vary from between 30 - 40% among related donors and recipients to 60 - 80% between unrelated donors and recipients. The greater the mismatch between donor and recipient, the greater the risk of GvHD. After a transplant, the recipient usually takes drugs that suppress the immune system, which helps reduce the chances (or severity) of GvHD.

Source: PubMed Health

H

H1N1

'Influenza' A (H1N1) virus is a subtype of influenza A virus and was the most common cause of human influenza (flu) in 2009. Some strains of H1N1 are endemic in humans and cause a small fraction of all influenza-like illness and a small fraction of all seasonal influenza. H1N1 (pronounced "HEE-NEE" by healthcare professionals) strains caused a few percent of all human flu infections in 2004–2005.[1] Other strains of H1N1 are endemic in pigs (swine influenza) and in birds (avian influenza).

In June 2009, the World Health Organization declared the new strain of swine-origin H1N1 as a pandemic. This strain is often called swine flu by the public media. This novel virus spread worldwide and had caused about 17,000 deaths by the start of 2010. On August 10, 2010, the World Health Organization declared the H1N1 influenza pandemic over, saying worldwide flu activity had returned to typical seasonal patterns.[2]

Source: Wikipedia

Hepatitis C

Hepatitis C is a viral disease that leads to swelling (inflammation) of the liver.

Hepatitis C infection is caused by the hepatitis C virus (HCV). People who may be at risk for hepatitis C are those who:

- Have been on long-term kidney dialysis

- Have regular contact with blood at work (for instance, as a health care worker)

- Have unprotected sexual contact with a person who has hepatitis C (this risk is much less common than hepatitis B, but the risk is higher for those who have many sex partners, already have a sexually transmitted disease, or are infected with HIV)

- Inject street drugs or share a needle with someone who has hepatitis C

- Received a blood transfusion before July 1992

- Received a tattoo or acupuncture with contaminated instruments (the risk is very low with licensed, commercial tattoo facilities)

- Received blood, blood products, or solid organs from a donor who has hepatitis C

- Share personal items such as toothbrushes and razors with someone who has hepatitis C (less common)

- Were born to a hepatitis C-infected mother (this occurs in about 1 out of 20 babies born to mothers with HCV, which is much less common than with hepatitis B)

Source: PubMed Health

Hickman line

A Hickman line is an intravenous catheter most often used for the administration of chemotherapy or other medications, as well as for the withdrawal of blood for analysis. Some types of Hickman lines are used mainly for the purpose of apheresis or dialysis. Hickman lines may remain in place for extended periods and are used when long-term intravenous access is needed.

Source: Wikipedia

HLA

The human leukocyte antigen (HLA) system is the name of the major histocompatibility complex (MHC) in humans. The super locus contains a large number of genes related to immune system function in humans. This group of genes resides on chromosome 6, and encodes cell-surface antigen-presenting proteins and has many other functions. The HLA genes are the human versions of the MHC genes that are found in most vertebrates (and thus are the most studied of the MHC genes). The proteins encoded by certain genes are also known as antigens, as a result of their historic discovery as factors in organ transplants. The major HLA antigens are essential elements for immune function. Different classes have different functions:......

HLAs have other roles. They are important in disease defense. They may be the cause of organ transplant rejections. They may protect against or fail to protect (if down regulated by an infection) against cancers. They may mediate autoimmune disease (examples: type I diabetes, coeliac disease). Also, in reproduction, HLA may be related to the individual smell of people and may be involved in mate selection.

Source: Wikipedia

Hydrocortisone

Hydrocortisone is available with or without a prescription. Low-strength preparations (0.5% or 1%) are used without a prescription for the temporary relief of (1) minor skin irritations, itching, and rashes caused by eczema, insect bites, poison ivy, poison oak, poison sumac, soaps, detergents, cosmetics, and jewelry; (2) itchy anal and rectal areas; and (3) itching and irritation of the scalp. It is also used to relieve the discomfort of mouth sores.

Hydrocortisone may be prescribed by your doctor to relieve the itching, redness, dryness, crusting, scaling, inflammation, and discomfort of various skin conditions; the inflammation of ulcerative colitis or proctitis; or the swelling and discomfort of hemorrhoids and other rectal problems.

Source: MedlinePlus

For allo stem cell transplant patients, it is used to treat mild rash resulting from GvHD.

Hyper-CVAD

Hyper-CVAD is named after the initials of the chemotherapy drugs used:

- cyclophosphamide
- vincristine

- doxorubicin, which is also known as Adriamycin®

- dexamethasone, which is a steroid.

Hyper is short for hyperfractionated, which means that more than one treatment (or dose) of the same drug is given in a day.

Hyper-CVAD treatment also includes another two drugs, called methotrexate and cytarabine, that alternate with the above drugs. For this reason, the treatment is sometimes called Hyper-CVAD/MTX-Cytarabine, but this is more commonly abbreviated to Hyper-CVAD.

Source: Macmillan Cancer Support

I

Immunotherapy

Treatment to boost or restore the ability of the immune system to fight cancer, infections, and other diseases. Also used to lessen certain side effects that may be caused by some cancer treatments. Agents used in immunotherapy include monoclonal antibodies, growth factors, and vaccines. These agents may also have a direct antitumor effect. Also called biological response modifier therapy, biological therapy, biotherapy, and BRM therapy.

Source: Dana-Farber Cancer Institute

IVIG or intravenous immunoglobulin

Intravenous immunoglobulin (IVIG) is a blood product administered intravenously. It contains the pooled, polyvalent, IgG (immunoglobulin (antibody) G) extracted from the plasma of over one thousand blood donors. IVIG's effects last between 2 weeks and 3 months. It is mainly used as treatment in three major categories:

- Immune deficiencies such as X-linked agammaglobulinemia, hypogammaglobulinemia (primary immune deficiencies), and acquired compromised immunity conditions (secondary immune deficiencies) featuring low antibody levels.

- Autoimmune diseases e.g. Immune thrombocytopenia ITP and Inflammatory diseases e.g. Kawasaki disease.

- Acute infections.

Source: Wikipedia

L

Lasix

Furosemide (Lasix brand name) is primarily used for the treatment of two conditions: hypertension and edema. It is the first line agent in most people with edema due to congestive heart failure.

- Edema associated with heart failure, hepatic cirrhosis, renal impairment, nephrotic syndrome

- Hypertension

- Adjunct in cerebral/pulmonary edema where rapid diuresis, i.e. lowering body water content by inducing urination, is required (IV injection). Used following some chemotherapy where fluid build-up has been an issue (e.g., following dissolving of tumours)

It is also sometimes used in the management of severe hypercalcemia in combination with adequate rehydration.

Source: Wikipedia

Leptomeninges

The two innermost layers of tissue that cover the brain and spinal cord. The two layers are called the arachnoid mater and pia mater.

Source: MedicineNet.com

Lumbar Puncture

The lumbar puncture, or "LP", is a frequently performed procedure in emergency departments, neurology and radiology clinics and hospital wards. In the emergency department, LP can yield information that can rapidly differentiate benign from emergent conditions.

In general, an LP may be done to:

- analyse the cerebrospinal fluid (CSF)

- measure the CSF pressure

- access the intrathecal space for either drainage of CSF or injection of fluid or to administer medications into the intrathecal space

- to perform myelography

Source: University of Ottawa

M

Mantle Cell Lymphoma (MCL)

An aggressive (fast-growing) type of B-cell non-Hodgkin lymphoma that usually occurs in middle-aged or older adults. It is marked by small- to medium-size cancer cells that may be in the lymph nodes, spleen, bone marrow, blood, and gastrointestinal system.

Source: Dana-Farber Cancer Institute

Melphalan

A drug that is used to treat multiple myeloma and ovarian epithelial cancer and is being studied in the treatment of other types of cancer. It belongs to the family of drugs called alkylating agents. Also called Alkeran.

Used as part of the BEAM protocol.

Source: Dana-Farber Cancer Institute

Methotrexate

A drug used to treat some types of cancer, rheumatoid arthritis, and severe skin conditions, such as psoriasis. Methotrexate stops cells from making DNA and may kill cancer cells. It is a type of antimetabolite. Also called amethopterin, MTX, and Rheumatrex.

Source: Dana-Farber Cancer Institute

MRI

Magnetic resonance imaging (MRI), nuclear magnetic resonance imaging (NMRI), or magnetic resonance tomography (MRT) is a medical imaging technique used in radiology to visualize internal structures of the body in detail. MRI makes use of the property of nuclear magnetic resonance (NMR) to image nuclei of atoms inside the body.

An MRI scanner is a device in which the patient lies within a large, powerful magnet where the magnetic field is used to align the magnetization of some atomic nuclei in the body, and radio frequency fields to systematically alter the alignment of this magnetization. This causes the nuclei to produce a rotating magnetic field detectable by the scanner—and this information is recorded to construct an image of the scanned area of the body. Magnetic field gradients cause nuclei at different locations to rotate at different speeds. By using gradients in different directions 2D images or 3D volumes can be obtained in any arbitrary orientation.

MRI provides good contrast between the different soft tissues of the body, which makes it especially useful in imaging the brain, muscles, the heart, and cancers compared with other medical imaging techniques such as computed tomography (CT) or X-rays. Unlike CT scans or traditional X-rays, MRI does not use ionizing radiation.

Source: Wikipedia

Mucositis

Inflammation and irritation of the mucous membranes.

Source: Dana-Farber Cancer Institute

Myeloblative Treatment

A treatment that uses high doses of chemotherapy and may use radiation therapy to destroy cancer cells, thereby also destroying bone marrow/stem cells, which are then infused (or transplanted) to rebuild blood and the immune system. There are various 'strengths' ranging from full myeloblative treatment (with Total Body Irradiation) to reduced intensity regimes.

Patients who are otherwise healthy and young can undergo treatment that destroys the bone marrow completely, also known as myeloablation. Patients who are older or have other health problems can receive either a reduced-intensity myeloablative treatment or a non-myeloablative treatment. These treatments are less intense and do not destroy the bone marrow completely.

Non-myeloablative transplant: A transplant that uses a lower dose of or reduced-intensity chemotherapy (and no radiation) followed by an infusion of stem cells and lymphocytes.

Source: Dana-Farber Cancer Institute, The MDS Beacon

N

Neulasta

A drug used to increase numbers of white blood cells in patients who are receiving chemotherapy. It is a type of colony-stimulating factor. Also called filgrastim-SD/01 and pegfilgrastim. In contrast to Neupogen, which is delivered in daily doses as required, Neulasta is one dose.

Source: Dana-Farber Cancer Institute

Neupogen

Also known as Neulasta, technical term G-Csf.

Source: Dana-Farber Cancer Institute

Neuropathy

Peripheral neuropathy is damage to nerves of the peripheral nervous system, which may be caused either by diseases of or trauma to the nerve or the side-effects of systemic illness.

The four cardinal patterns of peripheral neuropathy are polyneuropathy, mononeuropathy, mononeuritis multiplex and autonomic neuropathy. The most common form is (symmetrical) peripheral polyneuropathy, which mainly affects the feet and legs. The form of neuropathy may be further broken down by cause, or the size of predominant fiber involvement, i.e., large fiber or small fiber peripheral neuropathy. Frequently the cause of a neuropathy cannot be identified and it is designated as being idiopathic.

Neuropathy may be associated with varying combinations of weakness, autonomic changes, and sensory changes. Loss of muscle bulk or fasciculations, a particular fine twitching of muscle, may be seen. Sensory symptoms encompass loss of sensation and "positive" phenomena including pain. Symptoms depend on the type of nerves affected (motor, sensory, or autonomic) and where the nerves are located in the body. One or more types of nerves may be affected. Common symptoms associated with damage to the motor nerve are muscle weakness, cramps, and spasms. Loss of balance and coordination may also occur. Damage to the sensory nerve can produce tingling, numbness, and a burning pain.

Source: Wikipedia

Neutropedic

A condition (neutropenia) in which there is a lower-than-normal number of neutrophils (a type of white blood cell) and hence low immunity.

Source: Dana-Farber Cancer Institute

Neutrophils

A type of immune cell that is one of the first cell types to travel to the site of an infection. Neutrophils help fight infection by ingesting microorganisms and releasing enzymes that kill the microorganisms. A neutrophil is a type of white blood cell, a type of granulocyte, and a type of phagocyte.

Source: Dana-Farber Cancer Institute

P

Pantoloc

Pantoprazole (Pantoloc brand name) is used for short-term treatment of erosion and ulceration of the esophagus caused by gastroesophageal reflux disease. Initial treatment is generally of eight weeks' duration, after which another eight week course of treatment may be considered if necessary. It can be used as a maintenance therapy for long term use after initial response is obtained.

Source: Wikipedia

PCR (Polymerase Chain Reaction)

The PCR test forms the basis of a number of tests that can answer many different medical questions that help physicians diagnose and treat patients. For example, PCR tests can detect and identify pathogenic organisms in patients, especially those that are difficult to cultivate (for example, HIV and other viruses and certain fungi).

Other doctors order PCR tests to help diagnose genetic diseases, while other doctors use PCR to detect biological relationships such as identifying parents of children. PCR tests are also used to identify and characterize genetic mutations and rearrangements found in certain cancers.

However, PCR tests have been modified and extended into many aspects of scientific investigations including evolutionary biology, genetic fingerprinting, forensic investigations, and many others.

Source: emedicinehealth.com

PET scan

Positron emission tomography (PET) is a test that uses a special type of camera and a tracer (radioactive chemical) to look at organs in the body. The tracer usually is a special form of a substance (such as glucose) that collects in cells that are using a lot of energy, such as cancer cells.

During the test, the tracer liquid is put into a vein (intravenous, or IV) in your arm. The tracer moves through your body, where much of it collects in the specific organ or tissue. The tracer gives off tiny positively charged particles (positrons). The camera records the positrons and turns the recording into pictures on a computer.

PET scan pictures do not show as much detail as computed tomography (CT) scans or magnetic resonance imaging (MRI) because the pictures show only the location of the tracer. The PET picture may be matched with those from a CT scan to get more detailed information about where the tracer is located.

A PET scan is often used to evaluate cancer, check blood flow, or see how organs are working.

Source: WebMD

Prednisone

Prednisone is a glucocorticoid drug that is converted by 11beta-hydroxysteroid dehydrogenase in the liver into the active form, It is used to treat certain inflammatory diseases (such as severe allergic reactions) and (at higher doses) some types of cancer, but has many significant adverse effects. It is usually taken orally but can be delivered by intramuscular injection or intravenous injection.

Prednisone is important in the treatment of acute lymphoblastic leukemia, Non-Hodgkin lymphomas, Hodgkin's lymphoma, multiple myeloma and other hormone-sensitive tumors, in combination with other anticancer drugs.

Source: Wikipedia

Proprioceptors

Proprioception, from Latin proprius, meaning "one's own", "individual" and perception, is the sense of the relative position of neighbouring parts of the body and strength of effort being employed in movement.[1] It is distinguished from exteroception, by which one perceives the outside world, and interoception, by which one perceives pain, hunger, etc., and the movement of internal organs. Proprioceptors are the actual sensors.

Source: Wikipedia

Pulmonary Function Test (PFT)

Pulmonary function tests are a group of tests that measure how well the lungs take in and release air and how well they move gases such as oxygen from the atmosphere into the body's circulation.

How the Test is Performed

Spirometry measures airflow. By measuring how much air you exhale, and how quickly, spirometry can evaluate a broad range of lung diseases. In a spirometry test, while you are sitting, you breathe into a mouthpiece that is connected to an instrument called a spirometer. The spirometer records the amount and the rate of air that you breathe in and out over a period of time.

For some of the test measurements, you can breathe normally and quietly. Other tests require forced inhalation or exhalation after a deep breath. Sometimes you will be asked to inhale the substance or a medicine to see how it changes your test results.

Source: MedlinePlus

R

R-CHOP

A chemotherapy protocol used to treat non-Hodgkin lymphoma. Drugs in the R-CHOP combination:

> R= Rituximab
>
> C= Cyclophosphamide
>
> H= Doxorubicin Hydrochloride (Hydroxydaunomycin)
>
> O= Vincristine Sulfate (Oncovin)
>
> P= Prednisone

Source: National Cancer Institute

Rituximab or Rituxan

A monoclonal antibody used to treat certain types of B-cell non-Hodgkin lymphoma and symptoms of rheumatoid arthritis. Monoclonal antibodies are made in the laboratory and can bind to substances in the body, including cancer cells. Rituximab binds to the protein called CD20, which is found on B-cells, and may kill cancer cells. Also called Rituxan.

Source: Dana-Farber Cancer Institute

S

Septra

This medication is a combination of two antibiotics: sulfamethoxazole and trimethoprim. It is used to treat a wide variety of bacterial infections (such as middle ear, urine, respiratory, and intestinal infections). It is also used to prevent and treat a certain type of pneumonia (pneumocystis-type).

Source: WebMD

T

Tacrolimus (or Tacro)

A drug used to help reduce the risk of rejection by the body of organ and bone marrow transplants.

Also referred to colloquially (among doctors, nurses and patients) as Tacro.

Source: Dana-Farber Cancer Institute

The 'Wall'

Colloquial term used by nurses when low immunity and side effects kick in following a stem cell transplant kick in.

Total Body Irradiation (TBI)

Radiation therapy to the entire body. It is usually followed by bone marrow or peripheral stem cell transplantation.

Source: Dana-Farber Cancer Institute

V

Velcade

A drug used to treat multiple myeloma. It is also used to treat mantle cell lymphoma in patients who have already received at least one other type of treatment and is being studied in the treatment of other types of cancer. Velcade blocks several molecular pathways in a cell and may cause cancer cells to die. It is a type of proteasome inhibitor and a type of dipeptidyl boronic acid. Also called bortezomib and PS-341.

Source: Dana-Farber Cancer Institute

Vincristine

The active ingredient in a drug used to treat acute leukemia. It is used in combination with other drugs to treat Hodgkin disease, non-Hodgkin lymphoma, rhabdomyosarcoma, neuroblastoma, and Wilms tumor. Vincristine is also being studied in the treatment of other types of cancer. It blocks cell growth by stopping cell division. It is a type of vinca alkaloid and a type of antimitotic agent.

Source: Dana-Farber Cancer Institute

Vitamin B12

Vitamin B12 is an essential water-soluble vitamin that is commonly found in a variety of foods, such as fish, shellfish, meat, eggs, and dairy products. Vitamin B12 is frequently used in combination with other B vitamins in a vitamin B complex formulation. Vitamin B12 plays an important role in supplying essential methyl groups for protein and DNA synthesis. Vitamin B12 is bound to the protein in food. Hydrochloric acid in the stomach releases B12 from protein during digestion. Once released, B12 combines with a substance called intrinsic factor (IF) before it is absorbed into the bloodstream.

Used post-allo SCT given stores of B12 have been depleted by the transplant process.

Source: Mayo Clinic

Vitamin D

A nutrient that the body needs in small amounts to function and stay healthy. Vitamin D helps the body use calcium and phosphorus to make strong bones and teeth. It is fat-soluble (can dissolve in fats and oils) and is found in fatty fish, egg yolks, and dairy products. Skin exposed to sunshine can also make vitamin D. Not enough vitamin D can cause a bone disease called rickets. It is being studied in the prevention and treatment of some types of cancer. Also called cholecalciferol.

Source: Dana-Farber Cancer Institute

W

Working Memory

Working memory is the system which actively holds information in the mind to do verbal and nonverbal tasks such as reasoning and comprehension, and to make it available for further information processing. Working memory tasks are those that require the goal-oriented active monitoring or manipulation of information or behaviors in the face of interfering processes and distractions. The cognitive processes involved include the executive and attention control of short-term memory which provide for the interim integration, processing, disposal, and retrieval of information. These processes are sensitive to age; working memory is associated with cognitive development and research shows that its capacity tends to decline with old age. Working memory is a theoretical concept central both to cognitive psychology and neuroscience. In addition, studies done on a neurobiological basis have proven that working memory can be linked to learning and attention.

Source: Wikipedia

Z

Zofran

Zofran (generic name Ondansetron) is used alone or with other medications to prevent nausea and vomiting caused by cancer drug treatment (chemotherapy) and radiation therapy. It is also used to prevent and treat nausea and vomiting after surgery. It works by blocking one of the body's natural substances (serotonin) that causes vomiting.

Source: MedicineNet.com

BIOGRAPHICAL NOTES

Andrew Griffith is a former Canadian government executive for a number of departments with extensive domestic and international experience. His government publications include *From a Trading Nation to a Nation of Traders: Toward a Second Century of Canadian Trade Development* and *Market Access and Environmental Protection: A Negotiator's Point of View*. He has received a number of awards for his government service, most recently the Queen Elizabeth II Diamond Jubilee Medal.

In 2009, he was diagnosed with mantle cell lymphoma and has been in and out of treatment since that time. He lives in Ottawa, Canada, with his wife and two young adult children.

He started his blog My Lymphoma Journey to share his experience and has published in Cancerwise of the MD Anderson Cancer Centre, the Cancer Knowledge Network and KevinMD. He can be followed on Twitter @lymphomajourney.

www.ingramcontent.com/pod-product-compliance
Lightning Source LLC
Chambersburg PA
CBHW080227270326
41926CB00020B/4170